DEPRESSION IN ADOLESCENT GIRLS

Depression in Adolescent Girls

Science and Prevention

Edited by
TIMOTHY J. STRAUMAN
PHILIP R. COSTANZO
JUDY GARBER

THE GUILFORD PRESS
New York   London

Printed in the United States of America

This book is printed on acid-free paper.

Last digit is print number: 9   8   7   6   5   4   3   2   1

Library of Congress Cataloging-in-Publication Data is available from the Publisher.

ISBN 978-1-59385-563-5

About the Editors

Timothy J. Strauman, PhD, is Professor of Psychology and Neuroscience and Professor of Psychiatry and Behavioral Sciences at Duke University. Dr. Strauman is a clinical and social psychologist whose research focuses on translating theories of the social-cognitive processes underlying self-regulation into treatments and preventive interventions for psychological disorders. He is a Fellow of the Beck Institute for Cognitive Therapy and Research, a Van Ameringen Fellow of the Academy of Cognitive Therapy, and a Fellow of the Association for Psychological Science and the Society of Experimental Social Psychology.

Philip R. Costanzo, PhD, is Professor of Psychology and Neuroscience at Duke University, where he is also Associate Director of the Center for Child and Family Policy and Director of the National Institute on Drug Abuse Transdisciplinary Prevention Research Center. Dr. Costanzo is a clinical, social, and developmental psychologist whose research explores parental and peer influences on the social development of children and adolescents.

Judy Garber, PhD, is Professor of Psychology and Human Development at Vanderbilt University. Dr. Garber is a developmental psychopathologist whose research focuses on risks for and prevention of depression in children and adolescents. She has been a William T. Grant Faculty Scholar and has received the Boyd R. McCandless Young Scientist Award from the Division of Developmental Psychology of the American Psychological Association (APA), the David Shakow Young Investigator Award from the Division of Clinical Psychology of the APA, and an Independent Scientist Award from the National Institute of Mental Health.

Contributors

Adrian Angold, MD, Department of Psychiatry and Behavioral Sciences, Duke University Medical School, Durham, North Carolina

Tara M. Chaplin, PhD, Department of Psychiatry, Yale University School of Medicine, New Haven, Connecticut

Anna M. Charbonneau, MA, Department of Clinical Psychology, Seattle Pacific University, Seattle, Washington

Greg Clarke, PhD, Kaiser Permanente Northwest, Center for Health Research Northwest, Portland, Oregon

Bruce E. Compas, PhD, Department of Psychology and Human Development, Vanderbilt University, Nashville, Tennessee

Philip R. Costanzo, PhD, Department of Psychology and Neurosciences, Duke University, Durham, North Carolina

E. Jane Costello, PhD, Department of Psychiatry and Behavioral Sciences, Duke University Medical School, Durham, North Carolina

Lynn DeBar, PhD, Kaiser Permanente Northwest, Center for Health Research Northwest, Portland, Oregon

Lindsay E. Downs, MA, Department of Psychology and Human Development, Vanderbilt University, Nashville, Tennessee

Thalia C. Eley, PhD, Institute of Psychiatry, London, United Kingdom

Rex Forehand, PhD, Department of Psychology, University of Vermont, Burlington, Vermont

E. Michael Foster, PhD, School of Public Health, University of North Carolina at Chapel Hill, Chapel Hill, North Carolina

Judy Garber, PhD, Department of Psychology and Human Development, Vanderbilt University, Nashville, Tennessee

Jane E. Gillham, PhD, Department of Psychology, Swarthmore College, Swarthmore, Pennsylvania

Alice M. Gregory, PhD, Institute of Psychiatry, London, United Kingdom

Brigitt Heier-Leitzell, MS, Center for Health Care and Policy Research, The Pennsylvania State University, University Park, Pennsylvania

Janet Shibley Hyde, PhD, Department of Psychology, University of Wisconsin–Madison, Madison, Wisconsin

Gary Keller, MD, Department of Psychiatry, University of Vermont, Burlington, Vermont

Jennifer Y. F. Lau, PhD, Department of Psychology, Magdalen College, Oxford University, Oxford, United Kingdom

Michelle Little, PhD, Department of Psychology, University of Texas at San Antonio, San Antonio, Texas

Katie McLaughlin, PhD, Department of Health Care Policy, Harvard Medical School, Boston, Massachusetts

Amy H. Mezulis, PhD, Department of Clinical Psychology, Seattle Pacific University, Seattle, Washington

Susan Nolen-Hoeksema, PhD, Department of Psychology, Yale University, New Haven, Connecticut

Alison A. Papadakis, PhD, Department of Psychology, Loyola University Maryland, Baltimore, Maryland

Irwin N. Sandler, PhD, Department of Psychology, Arizona State University, Tempe, Arizona

Erin Schoenfelder, MA, Department of Psychology, Arizona State University, Tempe, Arizona

Jordan Simonson, MA, Department of Clinical Psychology, Seattle Pacific University, Seattle, Washington

Timothy J. Strauman, PhD, Department of Psychology and Neurosciences, Duke University, Durham, North Carolina

Sharlene A. Wolchik, PhD, Department of Psychology, Arizona State University, Tempe, Arizona

Bobbi Jo Yarborough, MA, Kaiser Permanente Northwest, Center for Health Research Northwest, Portland, Oregon

Helena M. S. Zavos, PhD, Institute of Psychiatry, London, United Kingdom

Series Editors' Note

The goal of the *Duke Series in Child Development and Public Policy* is to bring the highest-quality research in the vibrant field of child development to bear on important problems in clinical practice and public policy facing children and families. This volume on *Depression in Adolescent Girls* exemplifies both the innovative research that is being conducted on depression and the impressive ways that this research is being translated to clinical practice and public policy.

The problem of depression in adolescent girls has challenged clinicians and scholars for many years. Many changes occur with the onset of adolescence. Menarche presents both physiological and psychological challenges. Neural developments are rapid, with sudden increases in reward systems and sensation-seeking, which are not countered by self-regulatory control mechanisms until the mid-20s. Most girls make transitions to middle school and then high school, exposing them to new and diverse peer groups, greater independence, and more uncertainty than ever before. The need for peer acceptance and approval is coupled with dramatic influence by peers and the peer group on behavior. Boys, and other girls, are the center of life. At the same time, parental influence wanes but certainly does not dissolve. Academic challenges increase due to changes in the structure of schooling. The task of developing one's identity and future orientation in the midst of these myriad influences looms. Depressive symptoms and depressive disorder rise dramatically, not in all girls, but in a worrisome group.

Understanding the development of depression in adolescent girls is the first task taken up by the authors in this volume. Carefully conducted longitudinal studies, novel procedures for assessing cognitive and behavioral factors, and sophisticated data-analytic methods are used to draw inferences about how depressive symptoms develop during this period. Translating this understanding into preventive interventions and treatments is the second task. Can we identify high-risk groups early enough in development to intervene? Can we alter cognitive styles, improve skills, and change peer-cultural context enough to deflect trajectories of development away from depression? Some of the most exciting work in the field is occurring in prevention science, in which innovative interventions are subjected to rigorous randomized controlled trials to evaluate the efficacy of programs. The third, and least well-developed, task is to translate basic scientific understanding and evidence-based interventions into effective public policy that could have an impact on public health. Can we bring effective prevention programs to scale? Can we restructure the school context to affect girls' development? This volume represents the best in the field and a caption of the state-of-the-science in the developmental psychopathology of adolescent depression in females.

Each volume in the Duke series has grown out of a national conference held at the Center for Child and Family Policy at Duke University. The conference held for this volume was attended by leading scholars and practitioners in the field, both as presenters but also as audience participants. Discussions were lively, indicating the broad interest in this topic. Participants across conferences have included nationally renowned scholars from multiple disciplines, officials in public service who are charged with improving the lives of families and children, and students who are learning how to integrate scholarship with service. We are grateful to those who attended.

Reflecting the goal of intersecting basic behavioral science with public policy, the series itself is a partnership between the Duke University Department of Psychology and Neuroscience and the Duke Center for Child and Family Policy, with Series Editors Martha Putallaz and Kenneth Dodge anchoring these two groups, respectively. Each volume in the series also follows the model of an editorial partnership between scholars at Duke University and leading scholars at other universities. As Series Editors, we owe a great debt to Duke University Professors Tim Strauman and Phil Costanzo and Vanderbilt University Professor Judy Garber, who collaborated to produce this volume.

Like previous volumes, the current volume has benefited from financial support provided by the Duke Provost's Office. We are grateful to Duke Provost Peter Lange, PhD, and Duke Vice Provost Susan Roth, PhD We acknowledge and appreciate the important contributions of conference organizer Erika Layko and Center for Child and Family Policy Associate Director Barbara Pollock.

KENNETH A. DODGE, PhD
MARTHA PUTALLAZ, PhD

Contents

Part III. Prevention Science Perspectives

DEPRESSION IN ADOLESCENT GIRLS

PART I

INTRODUCTION

CHAPTER I

Depression in Adolescent Girls

Challenges for Basic Science and Prevention

Timothy J. Strauman, Philip R. Costanzo, *and* Judy Garber

Depression during adolescence is a significant and growing public health concern. Although prepubertal children show prevalence rates of only 1–2%, the point prevalence of adolescent depression is approximately 8%, with the average episode lasting between 6 and 8 months (Kessler & Wang, 2008). From a clinical perspective, adolescent-onset depression has a chronic, episodic course, marked by frequent recurrences and considerable impairment that account for a substantial proportion of the health care costs incurred by this age group. Moreover, depression in adolescence is associated with many related negative outcomes, including substance abuse, academic problems, cigarette smoking, high-risk sexual behavior, physical health problems, impaired social relationships, and a 30-fold increased risk of suicide (Stolberg, Clark, & Bongar, 2002).

Adolescents who experience mood disorders frequently have recurrences later in adolescence and into adulthood (Lewinsohn, Allen, Seeley, & Gotlib, 1999), with recurrence rates ranging from 45 to 72% over 3–7 years. Because of the high costs associated with depression in adolescence, the last 15 years have seen a growing emphasis on efforts to prevent mood disorders among adolescents. This shift originally was catalyzed by both a mandate issued by the Institute of Medicine (IOM; Muñoz, Mrazek, & Haggerty, 1996) and a natural downward extension of depression treatment research.

Sex differences in rates of depression have been studied from a number of perspectives, but as yet no comprehensive and sufficient explanation exists (Costello & Angold, 2000). The inability of current models of depression to account fully for the greater prevalence of depression in females reflects, in part, the lack of a comprehensive etiological account of the disorder itself. The causes of sex differences in depression, however, are unlikely to overlap completely with the causes of depression per se. Given the public health significance of this sex difference in rates of depression (particularly in adolescence), further investigation of the biological, psychological, and social factors that lead to a greater prevalence of depression among adolescent girls and adult women is warranted. The complexity of this challenge is extensive because of inherent difficulties in establishing risk factors for specific disorders as well as the high degree of comorbidity and shared causal factors for behavioral and emotional problems, particularly in youth.

Studies of adults across a number of countries have established that women suffer approximately one and a half to three times more current and lifetime episodes of unipolar depression than men (Angold et al., 1998). However, this sex difference does not appear until adolescence; unipolar depression onset rates are about equal in boys and girls until puberty, with the emergence of an onset differential for males and females between the ages of 10 and 14. These findings may reflect an increase in girls' rates of depression, a decrease in boys' rates, or both (Angold & Costello, 2001).

Major depressive disorder (MDD) is rare in young children and infrequent during childhood, with rates not reaching those of adulthood until middle adolescence. Estimates of rates of MDD in prepubescent children, obtained through a variety of methods (self-report questionnaire, parent questionnaire, structured interview), range from .03 to 2.5% (Puura et al., 1997). MDD is clearly less common during childhood, but the rates become comparable to adults by middle adolescence. Cohen et al. (1993) observed 1-month prevalence rates of MDD to be *highest* among individuals between 15 and 24 years old compared to all other age groups studied. Thus, many adults with mood disorders likely had their first onset during middle to late adolescence, which appears to be a particularly vulnerable period for first episodes of MDD. The change in rates of depression from childhood to adolescence is striking and raises important scientific and public health questions.

Psychiatric epidemiologists (Kendler, 2006) have suggested that investigators should capitalize on emerging knowledge of developmental and psychopathological variations to pose cross-disciplinary research questions about the processes that determine patterns of prevalence for specific disorders. For example, what are the developmental and/or protective features of childhood that prevent depression from occurring at higher rates during this age period? What happens during the transition into adolescence, as well as across the adolescent period, that increases individuals' risk for depression? What factors combine to account for the change in the sex ratio of depression from childhood to adolescence?

In a now-classic paper, Rutter (1986) proposed several possible mechanisms to explain the rapid rise in rates of depression and the change in the sex ratio from the pre- to postpubertal period, including (1) hormonal changes accompanying puberty, (2) the expression of genetic regulatory processes, (3) alterations in the frequency of environmental stressors, (4) developmentally based changes in the availability of either vulnerability or protective factors such as social support, (5) the possible role of cognitive processes such as learned helplessness and attributional style, and (6) developmental changes in children's experience and expression of emotions. Investigators studying sex differences in rates of depression have tended to focus on a limited number of hypothesized causal factors, often within a single domain (e.g., cognitive processes, social support, morphological changes). The need for a new generation of research, in which the independent and interactive contributions of genetic, biological, psychological, and social factors are modeled in a more comprehensive fashion, is clear (Kessler, Avenevoli, & Merikangas, 2001).

This volume is the result of a conference sponsored by the Center for Child and Family Policy at Duke University, at which basic scientists, who study depression from a number of disciplinary perspectives, and prevention scientists, who study community-based interventions to reduce the incidence of depression, came together to discuss what is known about adolescent depression in girls and what the research agenda should be for the next decade. We are particularly fortunate that the volume is part of the Duke Series in Child Development and Public Policy (Kenneth Dodge and Martha Putallaz, series editors), which is sponsored by The Guilford Press. The intent of the conference, and this edited volume, was to bring together an outstanding and diverse group of scholars working at the cutting edge of theory, research, intervention, and policy to improve our society's ability to prevent girls from becoming depressed during and after the transition to adolescence. It is our hope that the volume will facilitate productive "translational" interactions between basic scientists studying the causes of depression among adolescent girls and prevention/intervention scientists working clinically with adolescent girls. Our goal is not simply to present contributions from a distinguished group of investigators or to systematize existing knowledge pertinent to depression in adolescent girls. Rather, we intend for the volume to significantly advance the nation's research agenda on this important public health challenge.

RESEARCH ON CAUSES OF SEX DIFFERENCES
IN DEPRESSION: A SELECTIVE REVIEW

There is a growing literature examining the emergence of sex differences in depression at adolescence, with hypothesized causes ranging from latent genetic factors (Eaves & Carbonneau, 1998) to societal influences such as poverty (Harris & Marmer, 1996). To date, most studies have focused on a limited number of etiological variables, even though no single explanatory construct likely is sufficient to account for sex differences in depression (Hankin & Abramson, 1999). Furthermore, many of the early studies were not conducted from a developmental perspective. Nevertheless, we highlight here several of the most promising findings used to explain sex differences in depression. Based on this review, we conclude that the time is right for the field to shift research priorities from studies focused on limited sets of etiological factors to a broader, integrative approach in which the independent and interactive contributions of multiple factors can be identified. The purpose of this volume is to facilitate such a shift in priorities.

Biological Factors

Puberty is a robust statistical predictor of sex differences in depression, but the specific mechanisms accounting for this association are unclear. Angold, Costello, and Worthman (1998) reported that Tanner-staged pubertal status was a better predictor of the emergence of the expected sex difference in depression than was age, suggesting that some aspect of puberty itself was important in females' increased risk for depression. Angold, Costello, Erkanli, and Worthman (1999) found an association between rising levels of testosterone and estrogen among girls during mid-to-late puberty and increased rates of depression. These findings are particularly noteworthy because no association was observed between central regulatory neuroendocrine changes (follicle-stimulating hormone and luteinizing hormone levels) and depression rates, or between changes in body morphology and depression. Angold et al. (1999) interpreted these findings as indicating that pubertal increases in testosterone and estrogen levels cause those hormones to surpass a hypothetical threshold at which women are more susceptible to depression, but other exogenous (e.g., life events) and/or endogenous (e.g., cognitive style) factors are required to explain individual episodes of disorder.

Other hormones have been linked to depression in childhood and adolescence. Dahl et al. (2000) reported an association between growth hormone (GH) response to GH-releasing hormone in depressed children and proposed mechanisms by which such abnormalities might be associated with other hormonal factors in the development of MDD. Piccinelli and Wilkinson (2000) reported that gonadal hormone levels were directly associated with negative affect during puberty. Warren and Brooks-Gunn (1989) showed that estradiol levels were associated with depressive symptoms, after controlling for luteinizing hormone and follicle-stimulating hormone, but that the associations were complex, noting the added contribution of stressors and social context to the onset of depression in youth.

Another factor often implicated in the emergence of sex differences in depression is the functioning of the hypothalamus–pituitary–adrenal (HPA) axis. Early life stressors may result in both acute and chronic changes in the activation and regulation of the HPA axis, due to hypersecretion of corticotropin-releasing hormone (CRH). Activation of the HPA axis is a potential mediator of the link between environmental influences on depression onset; the HPA axis tends to be more reactive to stress in females than in males, possibly because of a modulating role of gonadal hormones (Weiss, Longhurst, & Mazure, 1999). In turn, CRH hypersecretion may function as a biological vulnerability to depression in adolescence and adulthood that increases sensitivity and reactivity to interpersonal stressors (Heim & Nemeroff, 2001). Because of the technical and logistical challenges of conducting large-scale prospective assessments of hypothesized biological risk factors for depression in children and adolescents, the role of these factors in causing sex differences in depression (in combination with other exogenous and endogenous factors) remains uncertain. Nonetheless, hormonal processes in early childhood and at puberty appear to be prime candidates for inclusion in a comprehensive developmental model of risk for depression.

Genetic/Familial Factors

Although the importance of both genetic and familial factors in vulnerability to depression per se is well established, recent evidence indicates a possible role of such factors in sex differences in rates of depression. Several studies have found greater heritability for depression in pubertal girls compared with boys. In an influential analysis of data from the Virginia Twin Study, Silberg and colleagues (1999) observed that concordance rates for monozygotic as well as dizygotic twin pairs were higher for pubertal females than for pubertal males, prepubertal males, and prepubertal females. A significant effect for genetic factors was observed for adolescent girls but not for adolescent boys or for preadolescents of either sex. Furthermore, the impact of life events on depression was strongest among adolescent girls, and the long-term stability of depression in adolescent girls was best explained by latent genetic factors. Finally, shared environment was also found to contribute to risk for depression in girls. Other studies (e.g., Thapar & McGuffin, 1994) provide evidence consistent with the intriguing possibility that hormonal and/or environmental changes during puberty may "switch on" latent genetic factors in girls. We view behavior genetics as an essential level of analysis in building a comprehensive model of sex differences in rates of depression.

One of the best predictors of depression during youth is having a depressed mother (Goodman & Gotlib, 1999). Goodyer, Cooper, Vize, and Ashby (1993) showed that both parental psychopathology and recent exposure to negative life events predicted MDD in 11- to 16-year-old girls. Hammen, Shih, and Brennan (2004) noted that whereas any psychopathology in the parents predicts higher rates of depression among offspring, having a mother with a history of MDD is a robust predictor of depression in children and adolescents. Consistent with a model of transmission in which maternal psychological deficits associated with depression lead to increased risk, Garber and Robinson (1997) found that offspring of depressed mothers reported significantly lower self-esteem and a more pronounced depressive attributional style than did children of nondepressed mothers. Hammen and Brennan (2001) similarly reported that depressed adolescents whose mothers had histories of mood disorders displayed significantly more negative interpersonal behaviors and cognitions compared with depressed adolescents with nondepressed mothers. Prospective studies of the origins of sex differences in depression will need to address the likelihood that transmission of depression from mothers to daughters occurs by both genetic and environmental routes of influence.

Stressors

A number of studies have found that adolescent girls both report and experience more negative life events than boys (e.g., Garber, 2007), and that adolescent girls report (and experience) more interpersonal and peer-related negative events than boys (e.g., Rudolph & Hammen, 1999), whereas boys report more negative academic events. Interestingly, Rudolph and Hammen (1999) observed that girls were particularly likely to experience more negative events (especially negative interpersonal events) than boys, beginning at puberty. Possible explanations of this difference include changing role expectations that accompany sexual maturation (including the experience of being perceived in sexualized terms) as well as the impact of sex steroids on acute and chronic negative affect. Sociologists have noted that embedding these developmental challenges in a societal context that emphasizes contradictory aspects of femininity may exacerbate their deleterious effect (Rosenfield, 1999).

Among severe stressors likely to be experienced by children, sexual abuse, though not a specific risk factor for depression, appears to be more strongly associated with later depression among female victims (Weiss et al., 1999). Childhood abuse experiences are hypothesized to operate in concert with individual differences in neurophysiological responses to stress, as well as life stressors and increasing role demands as children grow into adolescents, in producing increased risk for MDD among women, beginning during adolescence (Heim & Nemeroff, 2001). Although little is known at present regarding how common and severe stressors interact with genetic and biological risk factors for depression, such interactions represent a particularly promising focus of research in accounting for sex differences in depression (Rutter, 2002).

Psychosocial Factors

Interest in the interactive influence of psychological and social factors on vulnerability to psychopathology among women has grown substantially in the last two decades. Much of this research has been based on psychological models that focus on cognitive and interpersonal processes as risk factors. Nolen-Hoeksema and Girgus (1994) examined the contribution of maladaptive cognitive styles among women to the emergence of sex differences in depression during adolescence. Girls were more likely than their male counterparts to have a ruminative coping style in response to depressed mood. Nolen-Hoeksema and Girgus proposed that a ruminative style interacts with increasing stressors in early adolescence to produce the differential rates of depression in girls versus boys. Other investigators have identified pubertal bodily changes for girls, increased rates of sexual abuse during adolescence, and increasingly sex-typed expectations from parents and peers as stressors that increase for girls during adolescence (Costanzo, Miller-Johnson, & Wencel, 1995).

Hankin and Abramson (2001) proposed a cognitive vulnerability–transactional stress model of depression to account for sex differences in depression beginning in adolescence. They noted that sex differences in adolescence have been found in a number of causal factors within their model, including baseline levels of negative affect, negative life events, aspects of cognitive vulnerability such as rumination and attributional style, and negative events created through stress generation. Although Hankin and Abramson's model does not identify how biological and genetic factors interact with cognitive vulnerability and stress, it is one of the most comprehensive explanations of sex differences in depression. It also provides guidance regarding the design of prospective research concerning the emergence of sex differences in MDD, and it suggests how relevant levels of analysis can be integrated. In a related program of research, Strauman and colleagues observed how parenting styles and infant temperament predicted individual differences in self-evaluation and emotional vulnerability among grade-school-age children (e.g., Manian, Papadakis, Strauman, &

Essex, 2006). This model, which draws on self-discrepancy theory and its extensions, has been well validated in adults and adolescents and involves a number of developmental postulates relevant to sex differences in depression.

Leadbeater, Kuperminc, Blatt, and Hertzog (1999) proposed a multivariate developmental model to explain the associations among interpersonal depressive vulnerabilities, heightened sensitivities to stressful life events involving others or the self, and the occurrence of internalizing disorders in adolescents. Increases in girls' internalizing symptoms were hypothesized to reflect girls' greater cognitive–interpersonal vulnerabilities; their model appeared to predict internalizing problems in both majority and minority girls. As with Hankin and Abramson's (1999) model, the model by Leadbeater and colleagues does not specify how psychological factors interact with genetic and biological sources of vulnerability; nonetheless, it is particularly useful in explaining similarities as well as differences between boys and girls in vulnerability to internalizing versus externalizing problems.

Cyranowski, Frank, Young, and Shear (2000) presented a theoretical framework to address the dramatic shift in girls' versus boys' rates of depression between the ages of 11 and 13 years. They proposed that social and hormonal mechanisms stimulate affiliative needs in females at puberty, and that heightened affiliative need can interact with adolescent transition difficulties to create a depressogenic diathesis as at-risk females reach puberty. Cyranowski et al. have explicitly incorporated hypotheses concerning interactions among hormonal changes, self-concept, and pressures to conform to gender role expectations within their explanatory framework, and although their hypotheses remain largely untested, the model they proposed has clear heuristic value.

Finally, the influence of environmental variables themselves on intrapersonal and biological risk factors for depression also has been investigated. Eccles and colleagues (e.g., Roeser & Eccles, 2000) have reported that differences in school environments as well as different kinds of school transitions (e.g., from grades K–5 elementary school to 6–8 middle school to 9–12 high school vs. K–8 grade school to 9–12 high school) are associated with lasting differences in vulnerability to both internalizing and externalizing problems. Although the pathways by which the environments in which children and adolescents live influence (and are influenced by) other risk factors for depression have yet to be delineated, the need to view the emergence of sex differences in depression from such a social perspective is clear.

The efforts of the investigators whose work is summarized above provide a solid foundation for determining the causes of sex differences in depression. Nonetheless, a truly integrative developmental model that incorporates the range of risk factors implicated—and explains their independent and interactive effects—has yet to emerge. Moving the field forward will require sustained collaboration among investigators from a range of disciplines, including psychology, psychiatry, behavior genetics, biology, neuroscience, sociology, and anthropology. Such sustained collaboration is required because (1) the most compelling models will be multidisciplinary, and (2) there are likely to be multiple pathways to depression and multiple sources of greater vulnerability in women. This volume is intended to foster such sustained collaborations, with the ultimate goal of developing comprehensive models and translating them into efficacious, cost-effective preventive interventions.

Investigators in the biological, behavioral, and social sciences who have studied the origins of sex differences in depression invariably remark that no one level of analysis will be sufficient to provide a complete understanding of the greater prevalence of depression among women (Bebbington et al., 1998; Rutter, 2002). Furthermore, given recent findings that risk factors at one level of analysis are likely to interact with risk factors at other levels, it is no longer sufficient for investigators to pursue isolated hypotheses. The need for a networked group of investigators to move the field forward is clear. The use of new research technologies, such as functional magnetic resonance imaging, requires specialized expertise and collaboration across disciplines, so that data obtained using those techniques can be maximally useful in answering questions about the nature of psychopathology (Miller & Keller, 2000). In statistical and conceptual terms, multiple levels of coordinated analysis are required to determine how risk factors work together (Kraemer, Stice, Kazdin, Offord, & Kupfer, 2001). Fruitful collaborations among behavioral scientists, epidemiologists, and geneticists suggest new opportunities to ground the study of psychopathology in behavior genetics, and vice versa (Eaves & Carbonneau, 1998). Finally, hybrid areas of research (e.g., biocultural study of normal and abnormal emotions; Worthman, 1999) already have emerged from interdisciplinary collaborations, to the enrichment of contributing disciplines. Our goal for the conference and this volume was to contribute similarly to the enrichment of this vitally important field of research.

OVERVIEW OF THE VOLUME

Adolescence is a challenging period of life under the best of circumstances, but for adolescent girls it carries an increased risk of depression that can lead, in turn, to multiple episodes of illness throughout adulthood.

Basic Science Perspectives

In Chapter 2, E. Jane Costello and Adrian Angold provide a sound and thoughtful introduction to the problem of depression in adolescent girls from a developmental epidemiological perspective. Epidemiology addresses questions about the who, when, and why of disease, with the goal of intervening to prevent its occurrence and reduce its impact. In the case of depression in adolescent girls, the "who" questions address the age and racial/ethnic distribution of cases, their comorbidities, and their level of functional impairment. The "when" questions deal with issues such as age of onset, stage of pubertal maturation, relation to age at onset of comorbid disorders, and questions about changes in prevalence over time—for example, whether there has been a recent increase in the incidence of depression among adolescent girls. Perhaps most importantly, the "why" questions that can be addressed using epidemiological methods include precursors (e.g., genetic vulnerabilities), risk factors, interactions among risk factors, changes in risk over development, and sex differences in risk.

Behavior genetic models and methods are increasingly important in studying the etiology of psychiatric disorders, and Chapter 3, by Helena M. S. Zavos, Alice M. Gregory, Jennifer Y. F. Lau, and Thalia C. Eley, provides a practical introduction to such methods as well as a glimpse at their exciting and productive program of research. Genetic studies are moving beyond simple examination of heritability to consider more complex patterns of risks, such as interactions between genes and the environment. However, few studies have examined more than one level of risk. The series of analyses presented by Zavos and colleagues combines multiple methods and includes assessment of genetic risks, cognitive vulnerability, and environmental stress with regard to the development of depression. Data come from two samples: GENESIS1219 (G1219), an unselected sample of 1,500 adolescent twin and sibling pairs, and the Emotions, Cognitions, Heredity and Outcome study (ECHO), a study of 300 child twin pairs. The cognitive measures included interpretation of ambiguous information, attributional style, and interpersonal cognitions. Measures of stress included social adversity, parental educational level, stressful life events, and parental discipline style. Their analyses revealed associations between threat interpretations, attributional style, interpersonal cognitions, environmental stress, and depression. All measures were genetically influenced, and there were interactions between differing levels of risk. Longitudinal analyses revealed the role of some of the vulnerability factors in the development and change of depressive symptoms over time. Their findings further highlight the importance of incorporating multiple levels of assessment into studies of adolescent depression.

The past several years have seen the emergence of ambitious integrative models of vulnerability to depression that can be applied to the specific question of how sex differences in depression begin to appear during adolescence. In Chapter 4, Amy H. Mezulis, Janet Shibley Hyde, Jordan Simonson, and Anna M. Charbonneau present their ABC model and discuss its implications for the onset of depression per se, as well as for how the profound difference in onset rates emerges around the time of puberty. Their model integrates affective, biological, and cognitive factors into a single framework, which postulates that these vulnerability factors emerge and converge in adolescence to form an overall level of depressogenic vulnerability. In turn, individual differences in such depressogenic vulnerability, in interaction with individual differences in stress, are hypothesized to contribute to the emergence of sex differences in depression.

Although it is relatively rare to find an economic perspective in a book on psychopathology, Chapter 5, by E. Michael Foster, Brigitt Heier, and the Conduct Problems Prevention Research Group, clearly demonstrates the relevance of such a perspective for prevention science. Depression is the most prevalent psychiatric diagnosis in girls; roughly one in five experiences depression during the second decade of life. Whereas the public and social costs of depression among adults have received enormous attention, little is known about these costs in young women. Using data collected as part of the Fast Track project, the chapter by Foster and colleagues examines the societal costs of adolescent depression. These data have some unique strengths, including formal diagnostic assessments rather than the symptom checklists frequently included in epidemiological studies. In addition, the sample is not limited to individuals who have received mental health services; it includes individuals meeting diagnostic criteria but are untreated. Foster and colleagues' analyses reveal that the costs of internalizing disorders and comorbid conditions in young women are substantial. They also examined the role of co-occurring conditions in explaining variation *among* depressed young women.

Cognitive processes and styles have long been thought to contribute to depressive vulnerability, and Chapter 6, by Katie McLaughlin and Susan Nolen-Hoeksema, provides a thorough and provocative examination of how unintended thoughts can be associated with either vulnerability or resilience to depression among adolescent girls. From a statistical perspective, one robust contributor to sex differences in depression is a greater tendency to ruminate in response to distress in women compared to men. Numerous studies of adults and a few studies of adolescents have shown that rumination is a risk factor for depression, and females are more likely than males to ruminate. McLaughlin and Nolen-Hoeksema briefly review these studies and the mechanisms by which rumination appears to exacerbate and prolong depression. They then outline a preventive intervention program designed to reduce maladaptive mood regulation strategies such as rumination and increase more adaptive mood regulation strategies such as problem solving. They discuss how this program could focus specifically on preventing the increase in depression in adolescent girls and how it can be integrated with other programs of research considering etiological influences on adolescent depression.

As noted previously, life events can exert a powerful influence on vulnerability to psychiatric disorders, and the death of a parent is among the most difficult challenges that children and adolescents can face. In Chapter 7, Michelle Little, Irwin N. Sandler, Erin Schoenfelder, and Sharlene A. Wolchik note that bereaved youth are especially vulnerable to depression and are more likely than nonbereaved children to experience high levels of internalizing problems. Furthermore, girls show significantly higher rates of internalizing symptoms after parental death than boys. Understanding the pathways that lead to sex differences in depressive symptoms following parental death has important implications for a broader understanding of sex differences in adaptation to other losses and consequent depression. Little and colleagues describe a theoretical framework of the contextual and psychological processes underlying sex differences in risk for the development of depression after parental death.

In the adult clinical psychology literature, the process of self-regulation—how we use personal goals to evaluate our behavior and social standing and the emotional and motivational consequences of those ongoing evaluations—has been linked to depression and other internalizing disorders. In Chapter 8, Alison A. Papadakis and Timothy J. Strauman provide a conceptual framework for applying theory and research on self-regulation and depression to the particular circumstances of adolescent girls. They offer a series of hypotheses regarding differences between adolescent girls and boys that are relevant for the outcomes of self-regulation, including the tendency for girls to have goals and standards that pull them in different and sometimes mutually exclusive directions (e.g., wanting to be a traditional wife and mother and wanting a successful career at the same time). The authors discuss how such a framework could be translated into therapeutic and preventive interventions targeting teenage girls.

Prevention Science Perspectives

The National Institute of Mental Health has called for translational research linking basic knowledge about vulnerabilities that underlie mood disorders to the development of effective preventive interventions. The chapters in this section review research on risk for depression in children and adolescents to address a series of questions of critical importance to successful preventive intervention. For example, who should be the target of depression prevention programs? Basic epidemiological and clinical research indicates that increased risk for depression is associated with being female, having a depressed parent, subclinical depressive symptoms, and anxiety. Although several existing depression prevention studies have targeted one or more of these risk groups, the efficacy of these various prevention programs for children with different kinds of risk has not yet been investigated (Garber, 2007). Similarly, what should be the content of depression prevention programs? Integrated multilevel models of depression propose that individuals with certain diatheses are at increased risk for developing depression when confronted with stressful life events. Risk factors that contribute to depression include genes, neurobiological dysregulation, personality, negative cognitions, problems in self-regulation and coping, and interpersonal difficulties. These vulnerabilities increase individuals' chances of encountering stress and decrease their ability to deal with the stress once it occurs. Most existing depression prevention programs for youth have used cognitive-behavioral techniques, and have had some success. Other depression prevention strategies have included training in coping, social problem solving, social skills, communication skills, and parenting. The use of emotion regulation techniques in depression prevention programs also should be explored. A comprehensive prevention program is needed that includes multiple intervention components, each of which addresses risk and protective factors across different domains and levels of analysis. Given their potentially different risk profiles, however, should the same interventions be used to prevent depression in females and males?

One way to address this important question is to determine whether some depression prevention programs work better for females than males, and if so, why? Chapter 9, by Judy Garber and Lindsay E. Downs, provides a meta-analysis of over 50 studies aimed at preventing depression in youth and calculates the effect sizes within and across studies as a function of participants' sex. Whereas some depression programs have worked better for girls, others have had greater effects for boys, and still others have found no sex differences in program efficacy. Garber and Downs suggest several possible explanations for these mixed findings, including demographic characteristics (e.g., age), structural features of the intervention (e.g., single-sex vs. mixed-sex groups, duration of the intervention), study design (e.g., sample size, types of control groups), and program content (e.g., cognitive, interpersonal). Overall, despite the fact that the rates of depression are greater in females beginning in adolescence, the effect sizes for depression prevention programs tend to be greater for males.

Chapter 10, by Greg Clarke, Lynn DeBar, and Bobbi Jo Yarborough, takes a particularly interesting approach to prevention of depression in adolescent girls. An increasing body of evidence points to high rates of medical, psychological, and substance abuse conditions associated with, and in many cases preceding, depression in adolescence. To the extent that these comorbid disorders/conditions contribute to an increased risk of secondary mood disorders, depression may be successfully prevented by early treatment or prevention of these primary conditions. Chief among these possibly causal conditions are social phobia, generalized anxiety disorder, subdiagnostic eating disorders, substance abuse or dependence disorders, insomnia and other sleep disturbances, obesity, and physical inactivity. Clarke and colleagues review the literature regarding possible causal relations between these conditions and depression. They also examine the time lines for the relative onset of these primary conditions to best identify periods of greatest increased hazard, in order to establish the windows of opportunity where prevention and/or treatment efforts may be most effective. In addition, Clarke and colleagues review evidence-based interventions that address each of these primary conditions, and they explore how establishing common cause with stakeholders for these other conditions may increase the chances of successful implementation of communitywide depression prevention efforts.

Despite the well-established sex difference in depression, few prevention programs specifically target girls and women. Most depression prevention programs are co-ed group interventions that target risk factors, such as cognitive styles, linked to depression in both girls and boys. Chapter 11, by Jane E. Gillham and Tara M. Chaplin, examines the effectiveness of one co-ed group intervention, the Penn Resiliency Program (PRP), with early-adolescent girls. Their findings suggest that PRP prevents depressive symptoms in both girls and boys, although sex differences in intervention effects have been found in some studies. For example, the initial study of PRP found no preventive effect among girls. However, a more recent evaluation of PRP in a primary care setting found significant preventive effects among girls but not boys. The authors discuss the possible limits of co-ed prevention programs, along with research suggesting that PRP may be more effective for girls when delivered in a girls-only format. Finally, new directions for depression prevention in girls are discussed, including the need for interventions to focus on risk factors (e.g., body image) and contextual factors (e.g., media and cultural messages) that may be particularly relevant to depression in girls.

No discussion of depression in adolescent girls would be complete, either from a basic science or intervention perspective, without a focus on family as a level of analysis. In Chapter 12, Bruce E. Compas, Gary Keller, and Rex Forehand provide a concise and highly translational discussion of how depression runs in families and the implications of family-level processes for preventing depression in children and adolescents. Parental depression poses a significant risk for the development of depression and other internalizing and externalizing disorders in offspring; this chapter presents data on two critical mechanisms of risk in families of depressed parents. In addition, the authors describe the development of, and preliminary findings from, a preventive intervention to address these sources of risk. Specifically, the effects of stressful parent–child interactions in families of depressed parents and the ways adolescents react to, and cope with, this stress are described, and options for translating knowledge regarding those processes into preventive interventions are explored. Compas and colleagues present a new cognitive-behavioral intervention for families and report promising initial data on the effects of this intervention.

CONCLUSION

Each of the expert presentations that emerged from this conference, and the associated chapters that constitute this volume, has been directed at a face of the Rosetta stone of depression in adolescent females. Not only is the emergence of depression in teen girls a vexing problem for researchers and practitioners alike, it also appears to constitute a "gateway" disorder which is a prime associate of, or contributor to, multiple forms of distress for women across the lifespan. The gender disparity in the emergence of depression—and in particular, the appearance and widening of that disparity during adolescence—both constitute prime clues to the contributing factors that foreshadow and perpetuate depression.

If we ask "Why females?" and "Why teens?", we are invariably confronted with the panoply of potential answers that our authors consider. As the narrative above implies, these clues will lead to the confluence of biology, individual differences, culture, cognition, and socialization processes that conjointly alter adaptive demands at the transition to adolescence. Whereas these alterations in requirements for successful adaptation to the social world may well have profound effects on developing girls, knowledge of the developmental dynamics of these multiple factors should help us unravel the mysteries of depression for boys and girls alike.

In addition, although the emergence of puberty might be a reasonable common locus of influence for these various antecedents of depression, from the standpoint of prevention science, one would be wise to postulate that the onset of the biological, social, cognitive, and cultural processes ushering in adolescent depression likely are occurring during childhood—perhaps beginning as early as conception in some instances. The chapters in this volume not only describe our most recent knowledge about the various correlates, mediators, and causes of adolescent depression among girls, but they also suggest those phenomena that warrant careful attention in the early stages of the development of the child. The chapters provide prescient suggestions about premorbid indicators of depression that likely precede both the initial depressive episode as well as the transition to adolescence itself. For example, perhaps the depressive phenotype that becomes evident at puberty has an associated genotype established at conception that induces vulnerability to both the stresses of life in general and the stresses of pubertal change in particular. Similarly, the cognitive biases and hopelessness that intensify during the pubertal transition likely have origins that precede their overt expression. The cultural and social expectations that present girls with contradictory social identity expectations and demands as well as regulatory deficits are likely transmitted during childhood by parenting and other forms of socialization. One might say that adolescent depression is like a developmentally gathering storm that reaches gale force with the transition to adolescence. Indeed, the storm gathers itself from the multiple and interacting building blocks that co-determine vulnerability to depression as development ensues.

It is the hope of the editors of this volume and the conveners of this conference that the contributions of this diverse but complementary group of scholars, who have lent their expertise to the exploration of depression in adolescent girls, will provide multiple rays of light that enhance our understanding of a personally painful and socially costly disorder. We are confident that the chapters to follow will enlighten readers from a range of professions and backgrounds with an understanding of how depression emerges for adolescent girls—and ultimately, how we might prevent its occurrence as well as effectively treat it when it does occur.

REFERENCES

Angold, A., & Costello, E. J. (2001). The epidemiology of depression in children and adolescents. In I. Goodyer (Ed.), *The depressed child and adolescent* (2nd ed., pp. 143–178). Cambridge: Cambridge University Press.

Angold, A., Costello, E. J., Erkanli, A., & Worthman, C. M. (1999). Pubertal changes in hormone levels and depression in girls. *Psychological Medicine*, 29, 1043–1053.

Angold, A., Costello, E. J., & Worthman, C. M. (1998). Puberty and depression: The roles of age, pubertal status, and pubertal timing. *Psychological Medicine*, 98, 51–61.

Bebbington, P. E., Dunn, G., Jenkins, R., Lewis, G., Brugha, T., Farrell, M., et al. (1998). The influence of age and sex on the prevalence of depression conditions: Report from the National Survey of Psychiatric Morbidity. *Psychological Medicine*, 28, 9–19.

Cohen, P., Cohen, J., Kasen, S., Velez, C. M., Hartmark, C., & Johnson, et al. (1993). An epidemiological study of disorders in late childhood and adolescence: I. Age and gender specific prevalence. *Journal of Child Psychology and Psychiatry*, 34, 851–867.

Costanzo, P. R., Miller-Johnson, S., & Wencel, H. (1995). Social development. In J. S. March (Ed.), *Anxiety disorders in children and adolescents* (pp. 82–108). New York: Guilford Press.

Costello, E. J., & Angold, A. (2000). Developmental psychopathology and public health: Past, present, and future. *Development and Psychopathology, 6,* 599–618.

Cyranowski, J. M., Frank, E., Young, E., & Shear, M. K. (2000). Adolescent onset of the gender difference in lifetime rates of major depression. *Archives of General Psychiatry, 57,* 21–27.

Dahl, R. E., Birmaher, B., Williamson, D. E., Dorn, L., Perel, J., Kaufman, J., et al. (2000). Low growth hormone response to growth hormone-releasing hormone in child depression. *Biological Psychiatry, 48,* 981–988.

Eaves, L. J., & Carbonneau, R. (1998). Recovering components of variance from differential ratings of behavior and environment in pairs of relatives. *Developmental Psychology, 34,* 125–129.

Garber, J. (2007). Depression in youth: A developmental psychopathology perspective. In A. Masten (Ed.), *Multilevel dynamics in developmental psychopathology: Pathways to the future* (pp. 181–242). New York: Taylor & Francis/ Erlbaum.

Garber, J., & Robinson, N. S. (1997). Cognitive vulnerability in children at risk for depression. *Cognition and Emotion, 11,* 619–635.

Goodman, S. H., & Gotlib, I. H. (1999). Risk for psychopathology in the children of depressed mothers: A developmental model for understanding mechanisms of transmission. *Psychological Review, 106,* 458–490.

Goodyer, I. M., Cooper, P. J., Vize, C. M., & Ashby, L. (1993). Depression in 11–16-year-old girls: The role of past parental psychopathology and exposure to recent life events. *Journal of Child Psychology and Psychiatry and Allied Disciplines, 34,* 1103–1115.

Hammen, C., & Brennan, P. A. (2001). Depressed adolescents of depressed and nondepressed mothers: Tests of an interpersonal impairment hypothesis. *Journal of Consulting and Clinical Psychology, 69,* 284–294.

Hammen, C., Shih, J., & Brennan, P. A. (2004). Intergenerational transmission of depression: Test of an interpersonal stress model in a community sample. *Journal of Consulting and Clinical Psychology, 72,* 511–522.

Hankin, B. L., & Abramson, L. Y. (1999). Development of gender differences in depression: An elaborated cognitive vulnerability–transactional stress theory. *Psychological Bulletin, 127,* 773–796.

Hankin, B. L., & Abramson, L. Y. (2001). Development of gender differences in depression: An elaborated cognitive vulnerability–transactional stress theory. *Psychological Bulletin, 127,* 773–796.

Harris, K. M., & Marmer, J. K. (1996). Poverty, paternal involvement, and adolescent well-being. *Journal of Family Issues, 17,* 614–640.

Heim, C., & Nemeroff, C. B. (2001). The role of childhood trauma in the neurobiology of mood and anxiety disorders: Preclinical and clinical studies. *Biological Psychiatry, 49,* 1023–1039.

Kendler, K. (2006). Reflections on the relationship between psychiatric genetics and psychiatric nosology. *American Journal of Psychiatry, 163,* 1138–1146.

Kessler, R. C., Avenevoli, S., & Merikangas, K. R. (2001). Mood disorders in children and adolescents: An epidemiologic perspective. *Biological Psychiatry, 49*, 1002–1014.

Kessler, R. C., & Wang, P. S. (2008). The descriptive epidemiology of commonly occurring mental disorders in the United States. *Annual Review of Public Health, 29*, 115–129.

Kraemer, H. C., Stice, E., Kazdin, A., Offord, D., & Kupfer, D. (2001). How do risk factors work together?: Mediators, moderators, and independent, overlapping, and proxy risk factors. *American Journal of Psychiatry, 158*, 848–856.

Leadbeater, B. J., Kuperminc, G. P., Blatt, S. J., & Hertzog, C. (1999). A multivariate model of gender differences in adolescents' internalizing and externalizing problems. *Developmental Psychology, 35*, 1268–1282.

Lewinsohn, P. M., Allen, N. B., Seeley, J. R., & Gotlib, I. H. (1999). First onset versus recurrence of depression: Differential processes of psychosocial risk. *Journal of Abnormal Psychology, 108*, 483–489.

Manian, N., Papadakis, A. A., Strauman, T. J., & Essex, M. J. (2006). The development of children's ideal and ought self-guides: The influence of parenting on individual differences in guide strength. *Journal of Personality, 74*, 1619–1645.

Miller, G. A., & Keller, J. (2000). Psychology and neuroscience: Making peace. *Current Directions in Psychological Science, 9*, 212–215.

Muñoz, R. F., Mrazek, P. J., & Haggerty, R. J. (1996). Institute of Medicine report on prevention of mental disorders: Summary and commentary. *American Psychologist, 51*, 1116–1122.

Nolen-Hoeksema, S., & Girgus, J. S. (1994). The emergence of gender differences in depression during adolescence. *Psychological Bulletin, 115*, 424–443.

Piccinelli, M., & Wilkinson, G. (2000). Gender differences in depression. *British Journal of Psychiatry, 177*, 486–492.

Puura, K., Tamminen, T., Almqvist, F, Kresanov, K., Kumpulainen, K., Moilanen, I., et al. (1997). Should depression in young school-children be diagnosed with different criteria? *European Child and Adolescent Psychiatry, 6*, 12–19.

Roeser, R. W., & Eccles, J. S. (2000). Schooling and mental health. In A. J. Sameroff, M. Lewis, & S. M. Miller (Eds.), *Handbook of developmental psychopathology* (2nd ed., pp. 135–156). New York: Kluwer Academic/Plenum.

Rosenfield, S. (1999). Gender and mental health: Do women have more psychopathology, men more, or both the same (and why)? In A. Horwitz & T. Scheid (Ed.), *Handbook for the study of mental health: Social contexts, theories, and systems* (pp. 348–360). New York: Cambridge University Press.

Rudolph, K. D., & Hammen, C. (1999). Age and gender as determinants of stress exposure, generation, and reactions in youngsters: A transactional perspective. *Child Development, 70*, 660–677.

Rutter, M. (1986). The developmental psychopathology of depression: Issues and perspectives. In M. Rutter, C. E. Izard, & P. B. Read (Eds.), *Depression in young people* (pp. 3–30). New York: Guilford Press.

Rutter, M. (2002). Nature, nurture, and development: From evangelism through science toward policy and practice. *Child Development, 73*, 1–21.

Silberg, J., Pickles, A., Rutter, M., John, H., Simonoff, E., Maes, H., et al. (1999).

The influence of genetic factors and life stress on depression among adolescent girls. *Archives of General Psychiatry, 56,* 225–232.

Stolberg, R. A., Clark, D. C., & Bongar, B. (2002). Epidemiology, assessment, and management of suicide in depressed patients. In I. H. Gotlib & C. L. Hammen (Eds.), *Handbook of depression* (pp. 581–601). New York: Guilford Press.

Thapar, A., & McGuffin, P. (1994). A twin study of depressive symptoms in childhood. *British Journal of Psychiatry, 165,* 259–265.

Warren, M. P., & Brooks-Gunn, J. (1989). Mood and behavior at adolescence: Evidence for hormonal factors. *Journal of Clinical Endocrinology and Metabolism, 69,* 77–83.

Weiss, E. L., Longhurst, J. G., & Mazure, C. M. (1999). Childhood sexual abuse as a risk factor for depression in women: Psychosocial and neurobiological correlates. *American Journal of Psychiatry, 156,* 816–828.

Worthman, C. M. (1999) Emotions: You can feel the difference. In A. L. Hinton (Ed.), *Biocultural approaches to the emotions: Publications of the Society for Psychological Anthropology* (pp. 41–74). New York: Cambridge University Press.

PART II

BASIC SCIENCE
PERSPECTIVES

CHAPTER 2

Contributions from Epidemiology

E. Jane Costello *and* Adrian Angold

In order to marshal the resources needed to prevent a disorder, it is critical to understand the size of the problem and the burden it imposes on public health. This is one of the tasks of epidemiology. Once we have an understanding of the size of the problem, epidemiologists can often use the data collected for that purpose to propose some hypotheses about why the distribution of the disorder in the population takes the pattern that it does; that is, it can go from describing the problem to suggesting and perhaps testing causal hypotheses.

Thus, epidemiology addresses questions about the *who*, *when*, and *why* of a disease. "Who" questions address number individuals with the disorder in the population and their characteristics (age, sex, race/ethnicity, etc.). "When" questions deal with timing of onset, especially in relation to the onset of other disorders, cumulative incidence over time, and cohort effects (e.g., is depression in adolescent girls more prevalent now than it was 30 years ago?). "Why" questions deal with causal factors. Who, when, and why questions intersect when researchers seek to understand why, for example, the prevalence of depression changes over development in different ways in boys and girls.

"WHO" QUESTIONS: PREVALENCE, COMORBIDITY, AND SOCIAL BURDEN

The prevalence of depression in girls is low during childhood, but increases sharply around age 13. Although studies vary widely in their estimates, a meta-analysis of 20 studies that include data for girls born between 1950 and 1990 shows that after controlling for the taxonomy (ICD-9, ICD-10, DSM-III-R, DSM-IV), assessment instrument, and the time frame considered (current, past 3 months, past 6 months, past 12 months), the estimated prevalence for girls ages 13–18 was 5.9% (SE = 0.3%) (Costello et al., 2006). Most of this rate was accounted for by major depression and minor depression (or depression not otherwise specified [NOS] in the DSM-IV). Dysthymia had a median prevalence estimate of 1% in adolescents of both sexes. Bipolar disorder was too rare to be estimated.

Depression is highly comorbid with other psychiatric disorders in every age group. A meta-analysis of comorbidity (Angold, Costello, & Erkanli, 1999a) found that across childhood and adolescence, controlling for comorbidities among other disorders, the odds ratio (ORs) for comorbidity with anxiety disorders was 8.2 (95% confidence interval [CI] 5.8, 12.0), with conduct disorder OR = 6.6 (95% CI = 4.4, 11.0), with ADHD OR = 5.5 (95% CI = 3.5, 8.4), and with substance use disorders (SUDs) OR = 4.0 (95% CI = 2.1, 5.9).

Unfortunately, very few studies have published comorbidity rates for adolescent girls alone, and even fewer have controlled for the disorders comorbid with depression. Data from the Great Smoky Mountains Study (GSMS), a longitudinal study of a community-based sample of 1,420 participants (630 girls), show that depression in adolescent girls was highly comorbid with conduct disorder (OR = 20.0, 95% CI = 4.0, 99.2), oppositional defiant disorder (OR = 7.3, 95% CI = 2.2, 24.8), and above all anxiety (OR 33.8, 95% CI 13.5, 84.4). However, it was not significantly comorbid with SUD after controlling for other comorbidities (OR 1.0, 95% CI 0.2, 6.4). Rates of comorbidity with SUD, after controlling for conduct disorder, vary across studies (Costello, Sung, Worthman, & Angold, 2007a; Pardini, White, & Southamer-Loeber, Roberts, & Xing, 2007; Roberts et al., 2007; Wittchen et al., 2007), and more work is needed on gender differences.

The third "who" question that epidemiology needs to address relates to the question of the public health and social impact of a disorder: How big a burden does it cause, as measured by pain and suffering; the economic costs to the individual, the family, and society; and the opportunity costs in lost educational and work potential? Estimates of the World Health Organization (WHO) of the disease burden are calculated in disability adjusted life years (DALYs), a measure of the years of productive life lost because of the illness (Murray & Lopez, 1996). Data are available in broad age categories only, but among women ages 15–44 in the developed regions of the world, WHO estimates that unipolar depression is responsible for more DALYs than any other disorder, accounting for nearly 20% of all DALYs.

The WHO system of accounting does not take account of comorbidity; a more limited study of treatment costs associated with adolescent depression found that most of the economic costs of treatment for adolescents with depression were spent on youth with comorbid disorders. Using GSMS data, we calculated that the average annual cost per 100,000 young adolescents would be about $2 million for those with pure depression, compared with $18 million for those with comorbid depression (Costello, Copeland, Cowell, & Keeler, 2007). This means that, to the extent that depression increases the risk of other disorders, especially disruptive behavior disorders, it increases the economic burden of mental illness even beyond what it causes in itself.

"WHEN" QUESTIONS: TIMING, DURATION, AND HISTORY

"When" questions deal with such issues as age at onset of the first episode of depression, length of episodes, and intervals between episodes. They also address issues about changes in prevalence over time—for example, whether the "epidemic of depression" that has received much media coverage recently is real or not.

Age at Onset

It is becoming increasingly clear that depression, like many other psychiatric disorders, frequently begins in childhood or adolescence. However, there is a lack of longitudinal studies covering the whole age range that would be necessary to make an accurate estimate of the mean age of onset in the population. Studies covering childhood and adolescence have found mean onset ages around 14 for MDD and minor depression, and about a year earlier for dysthymia (Costello, Erkanli, Federman, & Angold, 1999; Lewinsohn, Duncan, Stanton, & Hautzinger, 1986). By the time the Lewinsohn et al. sample was 24, the median age at onset had risen to 16.9. An analysis of 10 surveys of adults from around the world found a median onset age of 20–25 (Andrade et al., 2003). Clearly, depression is a disorder with pre-adult onset for very many people (Insel & Fenton, 2005).

For the purposes of prevention it is important to know when the first symptoms develop in girls who later develop the full depressive syndrome. In the GSMS the age at onset of the first depressive symptom, in girls who had a depressive episode by age 16, was over 2 years earlier than the onset of the full disorder (11.7 years [SD = 3.7] compared with 14.1 years [SD = 2.2]) (Costello, 2009). This finding suggests that for many girls with adolescent depression the first symptoms occur before puberty.

Effects of Comorbidity on Age at Onset

Another important question from the viewpoint of prevention is whether other psychiatric disorders lead to earlier onset of depression in girls, or vice versa. The evidence from nearly all longitudinal epidemiological studies shows that depression has, on average, a later onset than most psychiatric disorders of childhood and adolescence. The exceptions are SUD, panic disorder, and schizophrenia (Lewinsohn, Clarke, Seeley, & Rhode, 1994; Lewinsohn, Hops, Roberts, Seeley, & Andrews, 1993; Rohde, Lewinsohn, & Seeley, 1991). In general, in the GSMS the age at onset of both first symptom and full diagnosis of depression was earlier in girls with anxiety disorders, conduct disorder, or oppositional defiant disorder than in those with no disorder (Costello, 2009). The difference was about 2 years in the case of conduct or oppositional disorder, and a year in the case of an anxiety disorder. Girls who would later develop an SUD did not have earlier onset of depression than others. There were no girls in the sample who had both ADHD and depression.

Recurrence of Early Depression in Girls

As Lewinsohn (Lewinsohn et al., 1994; Lewinsohn, Rohde, Klein, & Seeley, 1999; Lewinsohn, Rohde, Seeley, Klein, & Gotlib, 2000) and others have pointed out, recurrence is a serious risk in early onset depression. Recurrent cases tended to have an earlier onset of the first episode (Pettit, Lewinsohn, & Joiner, 2006), but this study did not find that the severity of the first episode predicted recurrence. In the GSMS, 29.4% of girls with depression had more than one episode by age 21, and 15.2% had more than two.

Changes in Prevalence Over Time: Is There an Epidemic of Depression?

If one were to judge by nonspecialist media reports, one would conclude that the prevalence of adolescent depression, especially in girls, has increased dramatically in recent years. Certainly, prescriptions of medications for depression, especially selective serotonin reuptake inhibitors (SSRIs), have increased, particularly, in the United States (Zito et al., 2006). Other suggestive evidence is an increase in teen suicides in the United States between 1950 and 1990, a British study showing a nonsignificant increase in "emotional problems" (anxiety and depression) across three birth cohorts assessed between 1974 and 1999 (Collishaw, Maughan, Goodman, & Pickles, 2004), and reports from cross-sectional studies of adults of increasing lifetime rates of depression in younger cohorts (e.g. Kessler, 2003; Klerman

& Weissman, 1989; Leaf, Holzer, Myers, & Tischler, 1984; Wickramaratne, Weissman, Leaf, & Holford, 1989).

We set out to test this conclusion by reviewing all the community-based studies of adolescents that had carried out structured or semistructured psychiatric assessments of depression using one of the accepted taxonomies (ICD or DSM). We found 18 datasets that permitted estimates to be made for adolescent girls (ages 13–18). The earliest cohort had subjects born in 1965, and the most recent had subjects born in 1982. We conducted a meta-analysis of prevalence over time controlling for diagnostic taxonomy (ICD-9, ICD-10, DSM-III, DSM-III-R, DSM-IV), the interview used, the time frame of the interview, the number of informants (parent, child, teacher), and the median age of the subjects in a sample.

The results (Costello, Erkanli, & Angold, 2006) showed absolutely no effect of birth cohort, which would have been a sign of an increase or decrease in prevalence over time. There was a higher prevalence when interviews with a longer time frame (e.g., 6 months) were used rather than interviews with a shorter time frame (e.g., 3 months). This finding indicates that the analysis had adequate power to detect meaningful effects. Our conclusion was that, while there is good reason to be concerned about the rate of depression in children and adolescents, 30 years of research suggests that, for as far back as we have reliable assessments, a similar proportion of children has been depressed, albeit largely unrecognized by clinicians until recently.

"WHY" QUESTIONS: CAUSES AND CORRELATES

Any causal theory of female adolescent depression has to explain (1) why the difference between rates of male and female depression appears only around age 13; (2) why the increase follows the rise in gonadal hormones (Angold, Costello, & Worthman, 1999b); and (3) why the impact of most individual stressors is the same in prepubertal and postpubertal depression.

Epidemiological research has both strengths and weaknesses for causal research. On the one hand, it is rarely possible to use the most rigorous randomized controlled study designs to deal with the risk that other variables confound the risk–outcome pathway. On the other hand, community-based studies often have a level of ecological validity that laboratory studies cannot match, particularly for genetic studies, where clinical samples may suffer from a range of selection biases.

Studies of causes and correlates can focus on factors at many different levels of explanation, from genes to intrauterine development to the family, school, and community. Behavioral epidemiology has used genetically informative samples to show that depression is quite strongly familial in both adolescents and adults (Kendler et al., 1993), and that this familiality is largely genetic. However, it has also become clear that life events of the kind known to increase risk for depression (Brown & Harris, 1978) are also influenced by genetics (Kendler, Hettema, Butera, Gardener, & Prescott, 2003; Kendler & Karkowski-Shuman, 1997; Kendler, Kuhn, & Prescott, 2004). Recently, molecular genetics studies have begun to suggest that a serotonin transporter gene moderates risk of depression in the presence of maltreatment (Kaufman et al., 2004) or life stress (Caspi et al., 2003), although the evidence is far from unanimous.

It is not yet clear whether the incident cases of depression in teenage girls show the same pattern of genetic and environmental risk that childhood- and adult-onset cases do. One exploration of this area focused on the finding that girls weighing 2,500 grams (2.5 lbs.) or less at birth were at very high risk for depression when they reached adolescence (Costello, Worthman, Erkanli, & Angold, 2007b). Among girls of normal birthweight, 8.4% had one or more episodes of DSM-IV depression between the ages of 13 and 16; among low birthweight girls the prevalence was 36.5%. A review of other potential risk factors for depression showed that there was a much stronger effect of other risk factors on low birthweight adolescent girls, whereas in the absence of any other risk factors there were no cases of adolescent depression in either group. A single additional risk factor increased the rate to 30% in low birthweight girls, compared with 5% in normal birthweight girls, and the difference in girls with two adversities was even more marked (84 vs. 20%). This finding suggests that low birthweight increased vulnerability to stressors in girls at a time of developmental change, an example of the "Barker hypothesis" that links intrauterine stress to later stress response (Barker, 2003).

IMPLICATIONS FOR PREVENTION

Prevention researchers identify three strategies for introducing preventive interventions. *Primary* or *universal* prevention programs operate across the whole of society, without attempting to identify high-risk groups. Familiar examples are seat belts to prevent trauma in car accidents, or fluoride in drinking water to prevent dental caries. *Secondary* or *targeted* prevention, as the name suggests, focuses on high-risk groups. Examples are dietary restriction to prevent mental retardation in children with the PKU gene, and folate supplements for pregnant women. *Tertiary* or *indicated* prevention is restricted to those who have the disease or are at very high risk, with the goal of protecting society (if the disease is infectious or dangerous) and preventing recurrence and functional disability.

Adolescent depression can benefit from prevention programs at every level. Primary prevention programs to reduce the risk of perinatal dangers, including low birthweight, could have an impact on depression as well as other conditions. Indicated programs have been successful with high-risk groups such as bereaved children (Sandler et al., 2003) and the children of depressed parents (Beardslee et al., 1992). Tertiary prevention of recurrent episodes is now being tested in adults (Frank et al., 2000).

The evidence from this brief review of the epidemiology of female adolescent depression is that this is a disorder with worryingly high prevalence, many clearly identified risk factors, and several promising preventive approaches. It should be a target for serious public health intervention in the next decade.

ACKNOWLEDGMENTS

The work presented in this chapter was supported in part by grants from the National Institute of Mental Health (Nos. MH06367, MH063970), the National Institute on Drug Abuse (No. DA011301), a NARSAD Distinguished Investigator Award to E. Jane Costello, and the NARSAD Ruane Prize for Child and Adolescent Psychiatry to Adrian Angold and E. Jane Costello.

REFERENCES

Andrade, L., Caraveo-Anduaga, J. J., Berglund, P., Bijl, R. V., De Graaf, R., Vollebergh, W., et al. (2003). The epidemiology of major depressive episodes: Results from the International Consortium of Psychiatric Epidemiology (ICPE) surveys. *International Journal of Methods in Psychiatric Research, 12*, 3–21.

Angold, A., Costello, E. J., & Erkanli, A. (1999a). Comorbidity. *Journal of Child Psychology and Psychiatry, 40*, 57–87.

Angold, A., Costello, E. J., & Worthman, C. M. (1999b). Pubertal changes in hormone levels and depression in girls. *Psychological Medicine, 29*, 1043–1053.

Barker, D. (2003). The developmental origins of adult disease. *European Journal of Epidemiology, 18*, 733–736.

Beardslee, W. R., Hoke, L., Wheelock, I., Rothberg, P. C., van de Velde, P., & Swatling, S. (1992). Initial findings on preventive intervention for families with parental affective disorders. *American Journal of Psychiatry, 149*, 1335–1340.

Brown, G. W., & Harris, T. O. (1978). *The social origins of depression: A study of psychiatric disorder in women.* New York: Free Press.

Caspi, A., Sugden, K., Moffitt, T., Taylor, A., Craig, I., Harrington, H., et al. (2003). Influence of life stress on depression: Moderation by a polymorphism in the 5-HTT gene. *Science, 301*, 386–389.

Collishaw, S., Maughan, B., Goodman, R., & Pickles, A. (2004). Time trends in adolescent mental health. *Journal of Child Psychology and Psychiatry, 45*, 1350–1362.

Costello, E. J. (2009). The nature and extent of the problem. In M. E. O'Connell & K. E. Warner (Eds.), *Preventing mental, emotional, and behavioral disorders among young people: Progress and possibilities* (pp. 35–57). Washington, DC: National Academies Press.

Costello, E. J., Copeland, W., Cowell, A., & Keeler, G. (2007). Service costs of caring for adolescents with mental illness in a rural community, 1993–2000. *Archives of General Psychiatry, 164*, 36–42.

Costello, E. J., Erkanli, A., & Angold, A. (2006). Is there an epidemic of child or adolescent depression? *Journal of Child Psychology and Psychiatry, 47*, 1263–1271.

Costello, E. J., Erkanli, A., Federman, E., & Angold, A. (1999). Development of psychiatric comorbidity with substance abuse in adolescents: Effects of timing and sex. *Journal of Clinical Child Psychology, 28*, 298–311.

Costello, E. J., Sung, M., Worthman, C., & Angold, A. (2007a). Pubertal maturation and the development of alcohol use and abuse. *Drug and Alcohol Dependence, 88*, S50–S59.

Costello, E. J., Worthman, C., Erkanli, A., & Angold, A. (2007b). Prediction from low birthweight to female adolescent depression: A test of competing hypotheses. *Archive of General Psychiatry, 64*, 338–344.

Frank, E., Grochocinski, V. J., Spanier, C. A., Buysse, D. J., Cherry, C. R., Houck, P. R., et al. (2000). Interpersonal psychotherapy and antidepressant medication: Evaluation of a sequential treatment strategy in women with recurrent major depression. *Journal of Clinical Psychiatry, 61*, 51–57.

Insel, T. R., & Fenton, W. S. (2005). Psychiatric epidemiology: It's not just about counting anymore. *Archives of General Psychiatry, 62*, 590–592.

Kaufman, J., Yang, B. Z., Douglas-Palumberi, H., Houshyar, S., Lipschitz, D., Krystal, J. H., et al. (2004). Social supports and serotonin transporter gene moderate depression in maltreated children [see comment]. *Proceedings of the National Academy of Sciences of the United States of America, 101*, 17316–17321.

Kendler, K. S., Hettema, J. M., Butera, F., Gardener, C. O., & Prescott, C. S. (2003). Life event dimensions of loss, humiliation, entrapment, and danger in the prediction of onsets of major depression and generalized anxiety. *Archives of General Psychiatry, 60*, 789–796.

Kendler, K. S., & Karkowski-Shuman, L. (1997). Stressful life events and genetic liability to major depression: Genetic control of exposure to the environment? *Psychological Medicine, 27*, 539–547.

Kendler, K. S., Kuhn, J., & Prescott, C. A. (2004). The interrelationship of neuroticism, sex, and stressful life events in the prediction of episodes of major depression. *American Journal of Psychiatry, 161*, 631–636.

Kendler, K. S., Neale, M., Kessler, R., Heath, A., & Eaves, L. (1993). A longitudinal twin study of 1-year prevalence of major depression in women. *Archive of General Psychiatry, 50*, 843–852.

Kessler, R. C. (2003). Epidemiology of women and depression. *Journal of Affective Disorders, 74*, 5–13.

Klerman, G. L., & Weissman, M. M. (1989). Increasing rates of depression. *Journal of the American Medical Association, 261*, 2229–2235.

Lewinsohn, P. M., Clarke, G. N., Seeley, J. R., & Rohde, P. (1994). Major depression in community adolescents: Age of onset, episode duration, and time to recurrence. *Journal of the American Academy of Child and Adolescent Psychiatry, 33*, 809–818.

Lewinsohn, P. M., Duncan, E. M., Stanton, A. K., & Hautzinger, M. (1986). Age at first onset of nonbipolar depression. *Journal of Abnormal Psychology, 95*, 378–383.

Lewinsohn, P. M., Hops, H., Roberts, R. E., Seeley, J. R., & Andrews, J. A. (1993). Adolescent psychopathology: I. Prevalence and incidence of depression and other DSM-III-R disorders in high school students. *Journal of Abnormal Psychology, 102*, 133–144.

Lewinsohn, P. M., Rohde, P., Klein, D. N., & Seeley, J. R. (1999). Natural course of adolescent major depressive disorder: I Continuity into young adulthood. *Journal of the American Academy of Child and Adolescent Psychiatry, 38*, 56–63.

Lewinsohn, P. M., Rohde, P., Seeley, J. R., Klein, D. N., & Gotlib, I. H. (2000). Natural course of adolescent major depressive disorder in a community sample: Predictors of recurrence in young adults. *American Journal of Psychiatry, 157*, 1584–1591.

Murray, C. J. L., & Lopez, A. D. (Eds.). (1996). *Global burdens of disease and injury, Volume 1*. Cambridge, MA: Harvard Univeraity Press.

Pardini, D., White, H. R., & Stouthamer-Loeber, M. (2007). Early adolescent psychopathology as a predictor of alcohol use disorders by young adulthood. *Drug and Alcohol Dependence, 88*, S38.

Pettit, J. W., Lewinsohn, P. M., & Joiner, T. E., Jr. (2006). Propagation of major depressive disorder: Relationship between first episode symptoms and recurrence. *Psychiatry Research, 141*, 271–278.

Roberts, R. E., Roberts, C. R., & Xing, Y. (2007). Comorbidity of substance use disorders and other psychiatric disorders among adolescents: Evidence from an epidemiologic survey. *Drug and Alcohol Dependence, 88*, S4.

Rohde, P., Lewinsohn, P. M., & Seeley, J. R. (1991). Comorbidity of unipolar depression: II. Comorbidity with other mental disorders in adolescents and adults. *Journal of Abnormal Psychology, 100*, 214–222.

Sandler, I. N., Ayers, T. S., Wolchik, S. A., Tein, J. Y., Kwok, O. M., Haine, R. A., et al. (2003). The family bereavement program: Efficacy evaluation of a theory-based prevention program for parentally bereaved children and adolescents. *Journal of Consulting and Clinical Psychology, 71*, 587–600.

Weissman, M. M., Leaf, P. J., Holzer, C. E., III, Myers, J. K., & Tischler, G. L. (1984). The epidemiology of depression: An update on sex differences in rates. *Journal of Affective Disorders, 7*, 179–188.

Wickramaratne, P. J., Weissman, M. M., Leaf, P. J., & Holford, T. R. (1989). Age, period, and cohort effects on the risk of major depression: Results from five United States communities. *Journal of Clinical Epidemiology, 43*, 333–344.

Wittchen H.-U., Fröhlich, C., Behrendt, S., Günther, A., Rehm, J., Zimmermann, P., et al. (2007). Cannabis use and cannabis use disorders and their relationship to mental disorders: A 10-year prospective-longitudinal community study in adolescents. *Drug and Alcohol Dependence, 88*, S60–S70.

Zito, J. M., Tobi, H., de Jong-van den Berg, L. T., Fegert, J. M., Safer, D. J., Janhsen, K., et al. (2006). Antidepressant prevalence for youths: A multi-national comparison. *Pharmacoepidemiology and Drug Safety, 15*, 793–798.

CHAPTER 3

New Behavior-Genetic Approaches to Depression in Childhood and Adolescence

Gene–Environment Interplay and the Role of Cognitions

Helena M. S. Zavos, Alice M. Gregory,
Jennifer Y. F. Lau, *and* Thalia C. Eley

Depression occurs in both children and adolescents, becoming more prevalent with age, and showing considerable continuity into adulthood (Fombonne, Wostear, Cooper, Harrington, & Rutter, 2001a). The existence of depression in childhood and adolescence was, to a large extent, a controversial issue before the late 1970s, when children were deemed to be incapable of experiencing depression due to their immature personality structures (Schulterbrandt & Raskin, 1977). However, the past two decades have seen an increasing recognition of mood disorders in childhood and adolescence (Malhotra & Das, 2007), and research in this area has increased. Epidemiological studies have shown that depression affects about 0.3–1.4% of preschool children (Egger & Angold, 2006; Stalets & Luby, 2006) and about 3–8% of adolescents (Birmaher, Ryan, Williamson, Brent, & Kaufman, 1996; Zalsman, Brent, & Weersing, 2006). A number of negative outcomes are associated with depression in this age group, including diminished self-esteem, poor physical health, and perhaps most importantly, a substantial risk for morbidity and mortality across the lifespan (Fleming,

1990; Kovacs, 1997; Fombonne, Wostear, Cooper, Harrington, & Cooper, 2001b). This emphasizes the importance of research for this age group.

Genetic research into depression in childhood and adolescence has moved beyond simple estimation of heritability to consider more complex patterns of risks, such as interaction between genes and the environment. Integrative models are now able to incorporate multiple levels of risk—from genes through cognitive vulnerabilities to acute stressors. Few studies have, however, examined more than one level of risk at a time. This chapter provides an overview of quantitative and molecular genetic research in this area and presents a series of analyses that combine multiple methods and include assessment of genetic risks, cognitive vulnerability, and environmental stress with regard to the development of depression. It begins with an introduction to the methodology used and then presents the key findings from quantitative and molecular genetic studies of depression in this age group. Research from our group focuses on two samples: GENESiS1219 (G1219) and the Emotions, Cognitions, Heredity and Outcomes study (ECHO). G1219 began as the adolescent offspring (ages 12–19) of the participants of GENESiS, a large sibling-pair study (Sham et al., 2000). Just under 1,300 parents of around 1,800 adolescents from G1219 and 1,300 twin pairs of a similar age were recruited via the Office of National Statistics. ECHO consisted of 300 pairs of twins selected for high levels of mother-reported anxiety-related behaviors at age 7 (Gregory, Rijsdijk, Dahl, McGuffin, & Eley, 2006) from the Twins Early Development Study (TEDS) sample (Trouton, Spinath, & Plomin, 2002). The twins were 8 years at wave 1; this age group was chosen as this is considered by some to be approximately the youngest age that children can reliably report on internal cognitions (Merrell, McClun, Kempf, & Lund, 2002).

QUANTITATIVE GENETIC METHODOLOGY

Quantitative genetics theorizes that the influence of multiple genes together with environmental variation result in quantitative (continuous) distributions of phenotypes. Research methods include family, twin, and adoption studies (Plomin, De Fries, McClearn, & McGuffin, 2008).

Family Studies

Family studies investigate the degree of clustering of conditions, such as depression, among genetically related family members. A higher than chance incidence of depression among first-degree relatives is taken as support for heritability. Conclusions from such studies are, however, limited by the fact that first-degree relatives are also likely to share the same family environment as well as genetics. To this extent, twin and adoption studies are particularly useful in estimating the influence of genetic and environmental factors on traits.

Twin Studies

Twin and adoption studies can partition variance into genetic and environmental factors. Genetic influences do not typically account for all variance on a phenotype, and what is not assigned to genetics is assigned to environmental factors. Environmental factors are further separated into two types: shared and nonshared influences. *Shared environment* refers to influences that make members of a family similar to one another and could include factors such as family socioeconomic status. *Nonshared environmental* influences, or child-specific effects, serve to make members of a family different from one another. This component also incorporates a measure of error. It is important to note that it is not the environment itself that is shared or nonshared but the *effect* the environment has on an individual.

The twin design disentangles genetic from environmental sources of resemblance by comparing within-pair similarity for monozygotic (MZ) twins and dizygotic (DZ) twins who both have their shared environment in common but differ in their genetic relatedness. DZ twins share, on average, half their segregating genes, whereas MZ twins are genetic clones (Plomin et al., 2008). In the standard twin design, variance in a phenotype (V_p) is divided into three latent variables: additive genetics (A) effects of alleles or loci "adding up," common or shared environment (C), and nonshared environment (E). That is, $V_p = A + C + E$. Resemblance within MZ twin pairs (r_{MZ}) is due to genes as well as environment; hence $r_{MZ} = A + C$. Resemblance within DZ (r_{DZ}) pairs is expressed as $r_{DZ} = \frac{1}{2}(A) + C$, because DZ twins share only half of their segregating genes, but they share all the of the same environment. *Heritability* refers to the proportion of phenotypic variation in a population that is attributable to genetic variation among individuals. In the twin design heritability is calculated as twice the difference between MZ and DZ correlations ($A = 2(r_{MZ} - r_{DZ})$). Shared environment can be estimated as the difference between the MZ correlation and the heritability (i.e., $r_{MZ} - A = C$). Because nonshared environment is the only factor that acts to make MZ twins different from one another, it can be calculated as the total phenotypic variance minus the MZ correlation (i.e., $V_p - r_{MZ} = E$).

Twin studies have been described as "the perfect natural experiment" (Martin, Boomsma, & Machin, 1997), but as with most methodologies, they have limitations. Topics of debate include the validity of the equal environments assumption (the assumption that the environment is equally similar for MZ and DZ twins), and the effects of chorionicity and assortative mating on estimates of genetic and environmental influences on traits. Furthermore, it has been argued that it is not possible to generalize findings from twins to the nontwin population (for a discussion, see Plomin et al., 2008). Limitations, such as the ones mentioned above, are likely to have only small effects on estimates and work in different directions, some leading to inflated heritability estimates and others artificially deflating genetic estimates. As such, derived estimates of heritability and environmental influences should be taken as indicative rather than as absolute.

Adoption Studies

Adoption designs provide another way of investigating the genetic and environmental structures of a disorder. These designs separate genetic and environmental influences because adoption per force leads to pairs of genetically related individuals not sharing a common family environment and to pairs of individuals sharing common environment but not genes. Any resemblance between the latter individuals would therefore imply genetic contribution to the trait. The contribution of family environment to a trait can be examined, for example, by comparing adopted children to their adoptive siblings (with whom they share environment but not genes). Any resemblance between them would be due to environmental influences, as they are not genetically related. Three main problems are proposed when using the adoption paradigm; the significance of these for estimates of genetic and environmental influences on traits have been discussed thoroughly (see Plomin et al., 2008). The first of these problems is that families involved in adoption are unlikely to be representative of the population. Second, similarity between the biological mother and child could be increased as a function of the 9 months in which the biological mother provides the prenatal environment; this factor would inflate heritability. Third, the selective placement of adopted children into families that are matched on certain characteristics to the biological parents could artificially inflate the estimations of shared environment. Again, as with heritability estimates from twin studies, those derived from adoption studies should be seen as showing general patterns of influence rather than precise estimates.

Molecular Genetic Methodology

Quantitative designs have demonstrated that genetic influences are important for most behavioral disorders and dimensions. Using molecular genetic techniques, specific variants in DNA sequencing that contribute to this heritability can be identified.

It is now clear that, as with other complex phenotypes, depression is influenced by multiple genes of small effect. These are known as quantitative trait loci (QTLs) and refer to genes involved in determining individual differences of continuously measured traits. In contrast to single-gene disorders, whereby variation within a single gene is sufficient to cause the disorder, QTLs are neither necessary nor sufficient to cause a phenotype. This difference has meant that traditional techniques employed for the identification of genes are underpowered for identifying variants that contribute to variation in complex traits. In recent years, new study designs and analytic strategies with greater statistical power have been utilized. These developments have led to a proliferation of molecular genetic studies that aim to locate susceptibility genes for behavioral disorders, including depression.

Linkage Analysis

Linkage approaches systematically scan the genome and require only a few hundred DNA markers looking for violations of Mendel's law of independent assortment between a disorder and a marker. Genetic linkage occurs when a disease-causing variant and a marker are inherited together from parent to offspring at a level greater than expected under independent inheritance (Teare & Barrett, 2005). Linkage studies can be used to identify chromosomal regions where susceptibility genes may lie. Linkage analysis is often the first step in the genetic investigation of a trait because it can identify broad regions of the genome that may contain a disease gene, and it can be done in the absence of a hypothesis regarding specific genes.

Affected sibling pair (sib-pair) linkage designs are generally used to study complex disorders because they have a greater power to detect genes of smaller effect size. In a sib-pair design, families with two affected siblings are studied. The term *affected* can refer to a variety of factors; it can mean that both siblings meet the criteria for a diagnosis or that both siblings have an extreme score on a certain quantitative trait. The method is based on allele sharing—whether affected siblings share zero, one, or two alleles for a DNA marker (Plomin et al., 2008). Thus if a marker is linked to a gene that influences the disorder, more than 25% of the affected individuals will share the two alleles for the marker. When a marker is not linked to a gene implicated in the disorder, the probability of their co-occurrence is 25%.

Linkage approaches, although systematic, cannot detect linkage for genes of the small effect size expected for most complex disorders without vast samples (Risch, 2000). A useful analogy for viewing linkage studies is a telescope that clearly scans the horizon for distant mountains (large QTL effects) but goes out of focus when trying to detect nearby hills (small QTL effects) (Plomin et al., 2008).

Association Studies

Genetic association studies assess correlations between genetic variants and trait differences on a population scale. Association studies have the statistical power to detect QTLs of small effect size, but, unlike linkage studies, associations can be detected only if a DNA marker is itself the QTL or very close to it. As a result, the candidate gene approach has tended to be used, as tens of thousands of DNA markers would be needed to scan the genome thoroughly. Candidate genes are normally selected based on biological function and a priori evidence to suggest that this function plays a part in the expression of a trait. Therefore, candidate genes for depression are chosen based on their function. Genes involved in the regulation of the serotonin system have been the focus of much research attention because this system has been implicated in both the etiology and treatment of depression (Meltzer, 1989; Goodnick & Goldstein, 1998).

Association studies take advantage of *linkage disequilibrium*, which occurs when linkage between two alleles is so tight that it leads to an association at the population level. This is unlike simple linkage, where the two loci tend to be farther apart and the chance of recombination at any single meiosis is greater. At a population level, every time recombination occurs between the loci, linkage disequilibrium is weakened. It is only maintained if the loci are very close together. This is why association studies focus on more specific regions.

Association studies test whether the presence of a specific genetic variant is associated with an increased risk of disease. Initially, association methods depended on allelic associations between single markers (including microsatellites and single nucleotide polymorphisms [SNPs]) and disease. Markers are compared between affected and unaffected individuals from the same population. Success depends partly on the degree of genetic heterogeneity (both allelic and nonallelic) underlying a disease sample. A significant result for testing an association between a disease and marker implies one of three findings; (1) the result is due to a direct association, in that the marker directly affects disease risk; (2) there is an indirect association and the marker is in linkage disequilibrium with the true functional disease mutation; or (3) there is a population stratification or a random effect (i.e., a false-positive result). *Population stratification* refers to differences in allele frequencies between cases and controls due to systematic differences in ancestry rather than to an association of genes with disease.

Although association studies have been more successful than linkage studies in the search for risk loci involved in complex disorders such as depression, the literature is still teeming with reports of associations that cannot be replicated or that are not supported by linkage studies. Common errors in association studies include small sample size, poorly matched control group, overinterpretation of results, and positive publication bias.

Genomewide Association Studies

Genomewide association studies (GWAS) go some way in solving the conundrum that linkage is systematic but not powerful whereas allelic association is powerful but not systematic. GWAS approaches survey a large proportion of the genome for causal genetic variants (Hirschhorn & Daly, 2005). Unlike other association studies, in this approach no assumptions are made about the genomic location of the causal variants; consequently, this approach represents a fairly unbiased yet comprehensive option for identifying genes. Genomewide approaches have been made possible only as a result of the human genome project, HapMap, an international HapMap project whose goal is to develop a haplotype map of the human genome and the advent of microarrays, a tool for analyzing many genetic variants simultaneously.

There are 10 million common SNPs in the human genome. The International HapMap Project (HapMap) has been able to demonstrate that the 10 million variants cluster together in neighbourhoods of tight linkage disequilibrium (LD) called haplotypes. These can be accurately sampled by approximately 300,000 carefully chosen SNPs. This process substantially reduces the cost of scanning the genomes of large numbers of patients for a large number of variants.

In GWA studies researchers tend to compare cases (people with an illness) to controls (unaffected individuals). Highly powered GWA studies show great promise in the identification of risk alleles that are associated with psychiatric problems.

We now provide an overview of the findings from both quantitative and molecular genetic studies of child and adolescent depression.

QUANTITATIVE GENETIC STUDIES OF DEPRESSION

There are several key findings from quantitative genetic studies of child and adolescent depression. First, genetic influences on depression in this age range are generally found to be moderate, with a substantial contribution from the nonshared environment (see Rice, Harold, & Thapar, 2002). Second, genetic influences on depression appear to increase from childhood into adolescence (e.g., Scourfield et al., 2003). Third, genetic influences on child and adolescent depression are largely the same as those on trait anxiety or measures of generalized anxiety (Eley & Stevenson, 1999b; Thapar & McGuffin, 1997). These findings reflect the tendency, seen across psychopathology, for genes to have a somewhat general effect as compared to the environment, which appears to have more specific effects (Kovas & Plomin, 2006).

Developmental Effects

Cross-sectional comparisons of the magnitude of genetic and environmental indices across different-age samples have suggested larger genetic and smaller shared environmental effects in adolescents than in children (Thapar & McGuffin, 1994; Hewitt, Silberg, Neale, Eaves, & Erickson, 1992; Eley & Stevenson, 1999a; Silberg et al., 1999; Silberg, Rutter, Neale, & Eaves, 2001; Rice et al., 2002; Scourfield et al., 2003). Although these results make sense in the context of the rise in depressive symptoms in adolescents, given that this rise is largely driven by an increase in prevalence in girls, it is possible that sex effects could influence age-related changes. For example, two studies have reported larger genetic influence in adolescent females (Hewitt et al., 1992; Silberg et al., 1999, 2001). However, another has found increases in adolescent males only (Eley & Stevenson, 1999a), and a fourth study showed a greater genetic component in both males and females (Scourfield et al., 2003).

Longitudinal analyses offer an even more informative approach to the question of development. Such analyses allow for an estimation of the extent to which the same genetic and environmental factors are important to depression symptoms at different time points (continuity) and whether there are new genetic and environmental factors in operation at a later time point (change).

Early studies utilizing this design demonstrated that whereas genetic factors contributed toward the stability of symptoms over a period of 2–3 years, new environmental effects were responsible for change (O'Connor, Neiderhiser, Reiss, Hetherington, & Plomin, 1998; Silberg et al., 1999). Both of these studies focused on transitions during adolescence, whereas other studies examining different age ranges found results that deviated from this pattern. Using a sample that spanned childhood and adolescence (5–14 years), Scourfield and colleagues (2003) demonstrated an opposite pattern of effects: notably, the emergence of "new" genetic influences over a 3-year period, with shared and some nonshared environmental influences remaining stable. Similarly, in a second study of childhood (van der Valk, van den Oord, Verhulst, & Boomsma, 2003), "new" genetic factors specific to each age were observed, although some genetic influences persisted between ages 3 and 7, contributing to stability.

We explored genetic and environmental continuity and change at three time points in adolescence and young adulthood, using the G1219 sample in which the average ages of participants were 14 years, 5 months; 15 years;

and 17 years, 8 months (Lau & Eley, 2006). Results showed a fairly consistent profile of genetic effects (45%, 40%, and 45% at each time point, respectively), decreasing shared environmental (19%, 9%, and 0%) but increasing nonshared environmental (36%, 51%, and 55%) effects. Decomposing these influences into the effect of "stable" and "new" factors, genes contributed primarily toward the continuity of symptoms across time, although new genetic factors were evident at the second time point, which corresponds roughly to midadolescence. New nonshared environmental effects emerged at each time point, and overall these factors contributed to change rather than stability of symptoms.

Finally, a more recent study has investigated the development of genetic and environmental risk factors for a measure of combined anxiety–depression symptoms in a population-based cohort of Swedish twins (Kendler, Gardner, & Lichtenstein, 2008). A particular strength of this study was the tight age ranges at each assessment point, with participants assessed at four time points between 8 and 20 years old (i.e., 8–9, 13–14, 16–17, and 19–20). Analyses showed that genetic effects accounted for the continuity of symptoms, with one genetic risk factor acting at all age groups, but that new genetic factors come online in early adolescence. This is in line with the above findings from the G1219 sample. Overall, four genetic factors accounted for variation over development. Stable genetic influences were present from ages 8 to 9, with new genetic influences on depression and anxiety emerging at each of the successive ages. Genetic attenuation was also demonstrated; for example, genetic factor 1 accounted for 72% of the variance at ages 8–9 but only 12% of the variation by 19–20.

The results from the above studies demonstrate that genetic effects on depression are developmentally dynamic and that there is both genetic innovation and attenuation. The emergence of new genetic effects that "come on line" in early adolescence, late adolescence, and early adulthood has implications for molecular genetic studies of depression because it suggests that such designs should incorporate tests for gene × age interaction.

Sex Effects

In spite of the clear mean sex differences for depression, there are no consistent patterns of effect in the genetic and environmental estimates by sex. Where there is evidence of sex-related differences in the environmental and genetic estimates, the direction of effects is difficult to decipher. Four studies show greater genetic effects among adolescent females (Boomsma, van Beijsterveldt, & Hudziak, 2005; Jacobson & Rowe, 1999; Silberg et al., 1999; Scourfield et al., 2003), whereas two others report larger estimates in adolescent males (Rice et al., 2002; Eley & Stevenson, 1999a). In children, there is some consensus that females show larger genetic effects (Eley &

Stevenson, 1999a; Scourfield et al., 2003; Happonen et al., 2002; van der Valk et al., 2003), although this finding has not always been replicated (van der Valk et al., 2003; Hewitt et al., 1992). Our recent research has found no evidence of sex differences (Lau & Eley, 2006, 2008a), in line with other research in this area (Bartels et al., 2003; Gjone & Stevenson, 1997; Thapar & McGuffin, 1994). Together, these studies provide no evidence of consistent sex differences in the heritability of depression.

Gene–Environment Interplay

There are two main forms of gene–environment interplay: gene–environment correlation (rGE) and gene–environment interaction (GxE). Gene–environment correlation refers to genetic influence on individual variation in *exposure* to particular environments. There are three types of rGE: passive, evocative, and active (Plomin, De Fries, & Loehlin, 1977). *Passive* rGEs occur when parents pass both genes and environmental experiences onto their children. As an example, offspring of depressed mothers are likely to receive both a genetic predisposition for the condition and the environmental effects of a depressogenic parenting style. *Evocative* rGE occurs when the child's phenotype evokes a certain reaction from others, and this reaction could potentially influence the type and quality of the individual's interpersonal relationships. An infant who cries easily or shows irritability may be more likely to elicit negative reactions from caregivers, which may impact on parenting style, influencing the child's development. Intermediate phenotypes, such as temperament, may mediate these effects. Finally, *active* rGEs occur when an individual selects and adapts experiences according to his or her genetic propensities. A behaviorally inhibited or shy individual may be less likely to seek out friends, choosing instead to engage in solitary activities, thereby ultimately influencing social development.

Interactions refer to the differential effect of one variable at varying levels of another variable. G × E interactions occur when environmental risks change as a function of genetic risk, or indeed vice versa, when genetic risks are expressed only in the certain environments. In terms of risk mechanisms, *interactions* may refer to genetic influences on reactivity toward the environment or when a stressor elicits (latent) genetic susceptibilities.

Gene–Environment Correlations

The most compelling evidence of a gene–environment effect was initially provided by adoption studies (O'Connor et al., 1998, Riggins-Caspers, Cadoret, Knutson, & Langbehn, 2003). These studies reported that adoptees' at high genetic risk for psychopathology received more discipline and control from their adoptive parents than adoptees at low genetic risk. These findings provide robust evidence for a genetically mediated child effect, in which the causal arrow runs from the child's behavior to parenting (genes to environment).

Numerous twin studies have also been able to demonstrate the importance of gene–environment correlations (rGE) in depression. Not only are there genetic influences on a wide variety of environmental experiences associated with depression, such as negative life events (Silberg et al., 1999; Thapar, Harold, & McGuffin, 1998) and parental negativity (Pike, Reiss, Hetherington, & Plomin, 1996), but these genetic influences have been found to overlap with those on depression. Interestingly, it has been proposed that prevalence of different types of rGEs are likely to change with age; thus, as an individual gains greater opportunity to select aspects of his or her environment, there would be an increase in active rGE, accompanied a decline in passive rGE. If the rate of active rGE increase is greater than the rate of decline of passive rGE, then heritability estimates should increase over this time frame (Bergen, Gardner, & Kendler, 2007). Because heritability does tend to increase with age, this hypothesis seems plausible. Notably, one study found evidence for an increase in rGE from childhood into adolescence when analyzing life events and depression in line with this theory (Rice, Harold, & Thapar, 2003). It should also be noted that puberty is likely to act to change gene expression, with different genes turning "on" or "off," and this marker of development in itself has been shown to be under genetic influence (Pickles et al., 1998). Overall, adolescence and young adulthood thus represent a developmental period in which there is a substantial flux in gene expression and environmental opportunities.

Gene–Environment Interactions

Twin studies can be used not only to disentangle the effects of genes and environment but also to investigate the interactions between them. A study of adolescent females, for example, has shown that negative life events (an environmental risk) exacerbated genetic effects on self-reported depressive (and anxiety) symptoms (Silberg et al., 2001). This finding is evidence of differences in genetic effects across levels of environmental risk. These researchers also found that individuals at genetic risk for depression (and anxiety), indexed by the presence of parental emotional disorders, were more likely to exhibit depressive symptoms following recent negative life events. This finding demonstrates the influence of genetic factors on reactivity toward environmental risk.

It is, however, possible that studies of G × E are confounded by effects of rGE. What are recognized as interactions can also be interpreted, in certain cases, as genetic risks for depression that increase social adversity.

The validity of interactions as a construct is based on the assumption that there is no correlation between the two risks. This assumption, however, can be violated when *r*GEs are present, because these occur (by definition) when individuals with a certain genotype are more likely to be exposed to particular environmental events. Given that *r*GEs and G × E are likely to coexist, a more sophisticated approach is to simultaneously assess but differentiate these effects (Purcell, 2002).

To this end, Eaves, Silberg, and Erklani (2003) were able to demonstrate both *r*GE and G × E on the relationship between life events and adolescent depression. They found that genes for depressive symptoms first influenced the individual's exposure to negative life events (*r*GE) and that although life events did have a main effect on depression, they also interacted with genetic factors (G × E). This finding is of particular interest because both the *r*GE and G × E occurred in relation to the same environmental (life events) and genetic influences. We too explored whether genetic effects on depressive outcomes varied as a function of maternal punitive discipline and negative life events (G × E) after controlling for genetic effects on these variables (Lau & Eley, 2008b). Results for both social risk measures indicated the joint presence of *r*GE and G × E. Thus, genetic influences on adolescent depression were not only shared with those on punitive parenting or life events (*r*GE), but they were also moderated by the presence of these risks (*r*GE), such that genetic variance increased substantially with higher levels of each environmental risk. On the basis of these results, it can be concluded that adolescents with higher genetic liability are more likely to be exposed to the double disadvantage of environmental risk (*r*GE). Furthermore, under these high levels of adversity, genetic risks for depression have greater opportunity to be expressed (G × E).

Cognitive Mediators

Our cognitions or our cognitive styles are like prisms through which we interpret and attend to the world. They therefore represent a logical place to start when investigating the interplay between genes and environment. Here we discuss genetic and environmental influences on biases of attribution, interpretation, and perception.

Negative attributional style refers to the tendency to attribute negative experiences to internal (to do with oneself rather than someone else), global (i.e., applying generally rather than to this one specific instance), and stable (as an ongoing tendency rather than discrete event) causes. There is a considerable body of literature supporting the association between this cognitive bias and depression symptoms (Abramson, Seligman, & Teasdale, 1978; Gladstone & Kaslow, 1995; Hankin & Abramson, 2001). Much less is known about the origins of this cognitive style.

Research that takes a developmental approach to investigating attributional style is beneficial for several reasons. First, the marked increase in the prevalence of depression symptoms from childhood to adolescence may partially reflect the possibility that attributional style and thus its association with depression becomes fully operational only during adolescence (Hankin & Abramson, 2001). Second, the heritability of depressive symptoms increases in line with the increase in prevalence, so it would also be interesting to examine whether a similar increase in heritability is seen for attributional style across this period.

We found a similar magnitude of association between attributional style and depression in samples that span childhood and adolescence (ECHO and G1219), with correlations in the .4 region (Lau, Rijsdijk, & Eley, 2006). However, in every other way the findings were very different for the two age-ranges. In the younger sample, heritability of attributional style was less than 10%, with modest shared environment and large non-shared environment (Lau, Gregory, Goldwin, Pine, & Eley, 2007). Similarly, the association with depressive symptoms was accounted for solely by environmental influences, split evenly into shared and nonshared environments. In contrast attributional style for the adolescentshad a heritability of almost 40%, with nearly half the correlation with depressive symptoms accounted for by shared genetic effects, and the remainder almost entirely due to nonshared environmental influences that impacted on both phenotypes (Lau et al., 2006). Thus, although the association between attributional style and depression symptoms was of similar magnitude in middle childhood and in adolescence, the influence of genes on attributional style and its relationship with depression symptoms only come onboard during adolescence. This finding is likely to reflect genes that, prior to adolescence, have no or only minimal influence, but that from adolescence onward play a role in the development of depression.

In the younger ECHO sample we were able to consider variation in response to ambiguous stimuli. Children were assessed using two tasks that incorporated the interpretation of ambiguous stimuli. The first of these was a homophone word task (*homophones* are words that have two or more meanings). As in similar research, a list of homophones was obtained that was deemed to be age-appropriate and for which there was a high threat differential in the two *main* meanings of the word. The second measure was an ambiguous scenarios task in which the children were presented with 12 ambiguous scenarios, each with four possible interpretations, of which two were negative and two were neutral. Thus for both tasks the number of threat interpretations could be calculated for each child. Both of these measures were found to be specifically associated with depression rather than anxiety, in that the association with depression remained even after controlling for anxiety, whereas those with anxiety (which were more modest to start with as well) were reduced to close to zero after controlling for depression (Eley et al., 2008). Both measures had a significant heritability of around 20%, with substantial nonshared environment. Furthermore, there was a significant genetic contribution to the association between each of these variables and depression. However, it should be noted that the role of environmental factors in these relationships was of far greater effect size, indicating that this association comes about largely as a result of experiences associated with both interpretation of ambiguous information as threatening and the development of depressive symptoms.

The third aspect of cognition we considered was children's expectations and perceptions of social situations in relation to depressive symptoms (Gregory et al., 2007). Children completed two related measures. The first reflected children's *expectations* of their peers and their mothers, and the second asked about *perceptions* of themselves and their peers using real-life scenarios. Factor analyses of the expectations measure led to the creation of two scales (expectations of peers and expectations of mothers) for the task focusing on perceptions of self and their peers: positive and negative perceptions. In line with the tripartite model of anxiety and depression (Clark & Watson, 1991), negative perceptions were associated with both anxiety and depression symptoms, whereas a lack of positive perceptions was specifically associated with depressive symptoms. Expectations of both mothers and peers were also associated with depression to a much greater extent than they were to anxiety. What is particularly unusual about the results of these analyses is the virtual absence of genetic effects from both the expectation and perception scales. Modest to moderate shared environmental influences (also incorporating error) were found for positive perceptions and both mother and peer expectations, with the remainder of the variance in all four measures due to nonshared environment. Associations with depression symptoms were entirely accounted for by environmental influences (both shared and nonshared aspects)—in line with our findings regarding attributional style in the same child sample and presenting the interesting possibility that genetic influences on these types of cognitions come online only during adolescence.

MOLECULAR GENETIC STUDIES OF DEPRESSION

A review of all the molecular genetic research on depression is beyond the scope of this chapter. Instead this chapter largely focuses on genes implicated in the serotonin system, as these contribute to variation in many physiological functions; for example, food intake, sleep, motor activity, and reproductive activity, in addition to emotional states such as anxiety and depression. Furthermore, genes implicated in the serotonin system have been the focus of molecular genetic research on depression. Other genes, such as the estrogen receptor alpha gene, are also discussed in the context of sex and development.

Serotonin Pathway and Depression

Given the extensive evidence of genetic influence on depression, a more specific approach to understanding this effect is to identify specific genetic variants that are associated with depression. By far the most frequently investigated neurobiological system targeted in attempts to locate candidate genes for depression is the serotonergic (5-HT) neurotransmitter system, a choice fuelled largely by prevailing physiological theories that the activity of monoaminergic neurotransmitters is somewhat compromised in individuals with depression (for a review on the neurobiology of depression, see Hirschfeld, 2000). In short, these neurotransmitters, including serotonin, represent the chemically induced transmission mechanisms by which neurons connecting different regions of the brain, particularly those involved in emotion regulation, communicate. There are now a number of consistent findings linking abnormal serotonin levels and vulnerability to depression in adults. Among these include pharmacological studies of certain antidepressant drugs that may alleviate symptoms by altering the functioning of this system and studies of indirect markers of serotonergic activity, such as the density of receptor-binding sights or quantities of metabolites and by-products in depressed individuals, which are suggestive of abnormalities to the system (Charney, Menkes, & Heninger, 1981; Coppen, Eccleston, & Peet, 1973; Drevets et al., 1999; Lopez, Chalmers, Littler, & Watson, 1998). Yet in spite of this large body of evidence in support of the role of serotonin in depression, it is not yet known which of the multiple regulatory processes involved in chemical transmission is responsible for the deficiency in levels (Manji, Drevets, & Charney, 2001). As such, from a molecular genetic perspective, studies have had to concentrate on a number of genes known to code for different steps involved in the transmission process.

The serotonin transporter (5-HTT) includes several polymorphisms, such as a variable number tandem repeat polymorphism in the 5' region (5-HTTLPR). 5-HTTLPR has attracted much research interest because it is common in human populations of all ethnicities (Gelernter et al., 1999), and it appears to have an impact on 5-HTT gene expression and serotonergic function. The 5-HTTLPR has two common alleles: a "long" (L) allele and a "short" (S) allele. Individuals can either be homozygous for either the short form (SS) or long form (LL) or hetrozygous (SL). In vitro studies of human lymphoblastoid cells show that the S allele has lower transcriptional efficiency than the L allele at baseline and after stimulation (Bradley, Dodelzon, Sandhu, & Philibert, 2005). In vivo studies investigating the effect of *5-HTTLPR* polymorphisms on 5-HTT functioning are not as straightforward. For example, human neuroimaging studies of 5-HTT availability (e.g., Parsey et al., 2006) and postmortem studies of 5-HTT bindings and mRNA expression have not detected consistent effects (Lim, Papp, Pinsonneault, Sadee, & Saffen, 2006; Little et al., 1998).

The first major result in this area was between *5-HTTLPR* and anxiety-related traits such as neuroticism and harm avoidance (Lesch et al., 1996). In two samples, individuals with one or two copies of the S allele had higher anxiety-related personality trait scores than individuals homozygous for the L allele. In the context of adult depression, when positive, findings suggest a moderate association with bipolar disorder, suicidal behaviour (particularly violent suicidal behaviour) and depression-related trait scores (see Levinson, 2006). Less research had been conducted in younger samples but studies that have, tend to be in line with research in adults (Twitchell et al., 2000, Twitchell et al., 2001, Nobile et al., 1999, Pfeffer et al., 1998). Interestingly, one of these studies reported findings that children with the LL genotype showed significantly higher levels of behavioural inhibition and negative affect than children the SS or SL genotype (Twitchell et al., 2001). This is contrary to research in older samples which tends to show that the lower functioning s variant is associated with negative affect. Due to its sample size, however, any conclusions as to the action of the serotonin transporter in childhood should be viewed with caution.

Other genes of interest include those that code the monoamine oxidase type A (*MAOA*) and tryptophan hydroxylase (*TPH1*) enzymes. Examination of these genes has led to both positive and negative results (for more details on individual studies, the reader is referred to Huezo-Diaz, Tandon, & Aitchison, 2005, and Levinson, 2006). Thus far, there are good theoretically driven reasons for examining genetic variants involved in the release and regulation of serotonin, but the field is still within its infancy, and studies of children and adolescents have been rare.

Development and Sex

Gene action and expression are likely to be dependent on a number of factors such as development and sex. There is some evidence to support this hypothesis, both in the depression and antidepressant response literature.

Interactive effects of sex and *5-HTTLPR* on mood have been demonstrated in a recent study measuring acute tryptophan depletion (ATD) (Walderhaug et al., 2007). This intervention reduces 5-HT function in the brain. The main findings of this study were that men and women adopt opposite responses to ATD, with men tending to adopt impulsive responses without mood reduction and women adopting a cautious response style and low mood. The effect of 5-HT disturbance in women was particularly pronounced in the LL and SS groups.

The differential associations between genetic polymorphisms and antidepressant response have been reported according to the age of participants corroborating the above findings. Polymorphisms in the G protein beta$_3$ subunit, for example, have been found to predict response in younger participants only, whereas the SS genotype of the serotonin transporter has been associated with poorer response to antidepressants only in older patients (Joyce et al., 2003). In contrast, another study found that polymorphisms in *5-HTTLPR* predicted response to selective serotonin reuptake inhibitors (SSRIs) only in younger male patients (Huezo-Diaz et al., 2005). These differential pharmacogenetic predictors of antidepressant response by age may provide clues to understanding the discontinuities in pharmacological responsiveness of child/adolescent and adult depressive disorders.

Dysregulation of the hypothalamic–pituitary–adrenal (HPA) axis has been observed in around 50% of patients with depression (Watson, Gallagher, Ferrier, & Young, 2006; Parker, Schatzberg, & Lyons, 2003). The HPA axis is responsible for activating hormonal responses toward acute and chronic stressors. Developmental and sex effects have been demonstrated in HPA functioning. The primary hormones in this system are corticotropin-releasing hormones and arginine vasopressin (AVP). These work synergically to stimulate the release of pituitary corticotrophin (Scott & Dinan, 2002). The end product of the cascade is cortisol in humans, which is involved in the stress response via the HPA axis. Molecular genetic findings regarding alterations in the HPA axis have been inconsistent, especially in children and adolescents. However, a recent study of AVP found that, at least in children and adolescents, there is a relationship between the DAVPRIB gene and depression (Dempster et al., 2007). The association was, however, restricted to females.

Other receptors of interest include estrogen, especially when trying to understand the susceptibility of depression in postpubertal girls. This hormone is known to interact with the central nervous system and has been shown to influence anxiety and depressive behaviors (Walf & Frye, 2006). Moreover, as noted, after puberty, women have twice the lifetime risk of men (Kuehner, 2003). This may be in part due to hormonal changes, particularly increased estrogen levels, occurring in females during adolescence.

A recent study genotyped 11 SNPs spanning the estrogen receptor alpha gene in a large family-based child-onset mood disorder sample (Mill et al., 2008). Individual SNPs were not found to be significant; however, haplotype analysis of three SNPs in linkage disequilibrium (*rs746432*, *rs2077647*, and *rs532010*) uncovered an association, specifically in females. Results are in line with Tsai, Wang, Hong, and Chiu's (2003) strong finding that there is a female specific association with MDD. Findings such as this point to a sex-specific etiological factor in depressive disorders, related to estrogen, with onset in childhood. Only a few studies have previously investigated *ESR1*, and findings have been mixed, with some finding an association (e.g., Tsai et al., 2003) whereas others have failed to show any association (e.g., Tiemeier et al., 2005; Kravitz, Meyer, Seeman, Greendale, & Sowers, 2006). Generally, the molecular genetic studies that take a developmental approach are scarce. Results are, however, suggestive of developmental and sex effects on genetic associations.

Gene–Environment Interplay

Gene–Environment Interaction

Genetic factors have been shown to influence an individual's *susceptibility* to environmental stimuli or, put another way, the effect of genes are different depending on the environment (gene–environment interaction). A seminal paper by Caspi and colleagues (2003) neatly demonstrated this phenomenon. The authors showed that the effect of life stresses on depression were moderated by variation in the serotonin transporter gene (*5-HTT*). A similar interaction was also observed for the effect of depression on the number of positive maltreatment indices between the ages of 3 and 11 years. Their assertion was that the *5-HTTLPR* genotype does not directly "cause" depression; instead, it seems to be involved in individual variation to stress reactivity. This hypothesis has been supported by several other studies, including an association between the short alleles and depression following stress in women (Wilhelm et al., 2006); onset of depression following low-threat events for the ss genotype (Kendler, Kuhn, Vittum, Prescott, & Riley, 2005); and increased amygdalar activation in response to aversive stimuli (Hariri et al., 2005).

We tested this effect in our adolescent study. DNA samples were collected from G1219 children in the top and bottom 15% of the scores for self-reported depression. This interaction was tested using a broad parent-reported measure of background environmental risk (including parental education, social problems such as housing, and familywide negative life events) to reduce the chances of our measure of environmental risk being influenced by the child's genes. As expected, this variable was not associated with *5-HTTLPR* genotype and was included in the interaction analysis as a dichotomous variable with scores divided into low and high environmental risk at the mean of the distribution. In the adolescent girls (but not in the boys), those with two copies of the short allele, or SS for *5-HTTLPR*, who were also high for environmental risk scores were almost twice as likely to be in the severe depression group as those who had the SS genotype but were low for environmental risk (Eley et al., 2004). This effect was also upheld by another population-based adolescent sample (Aslund et al., 2009), with G × E interaction between the SS allele and maltreatment found for girls but not boys. Together these studies provide preliminary evidence of sex differences between *5-HTTLPR* polymorphism and environment measures in the prediction of adolescent depression.

Although, as noted, there have been replications of such interactions and positive results from a meta-analysis, negative findings have been reported in two large samples (for a review, see Uher & McGuffin, 2008). A recent meta-analysis has also failed to find evidence that the serotonin transporter genotype alone or in interaction with stressful life events is associated with an elevated risk of depression (Risch et al., 2009), although it should be noted that the analysis failed to include all relevant studies. This potentially paradigm-changing finding has some limitations because it fails to adequately account for differences in methodology, such as genotype definition and environmental measures, which may account for some of the discrepant findings in this literature (Uher & McGuffin, 2008).

Interestingly, age and sex have also been muted as possible reasons for nonreplication. That the interaction effect is more commonly noted in females after adolescence could be due to a number of factors, including the possibilities that (1) the depressogenic effect of life events is stronger in females than males, and (2) current instruments may not give sufficient weight to life events relevant for males. The apparent effect of age may reflect the distinction between first episode and recurrent episodes; the effect of life events decreases with number of episodes (Kendler, Thornton, & Gardner, 2000). Given that evere negative life events are relatively common, and people are likely to have experienced at least one by middle age, we might expect that with advancing age, the G × E would gradually transform into a direct gene–disorder association. However, since no direct associations have been reported in older samples (e.g., Grabe et al., 2005), it is possible that this vulnerability operates in a developmentally sensitive period comprising young adulthood (Uher & McGuffin, 2008).

Gene–Environment Correlation

The first report of a measured *r*GE found that an SNP in *GABRA2* was associated with alcohol dependence and marital status (Dick et al., 2006). Those with the high-risk variant, associated with alcohol dependence, were less likely to be married, in part due to their high risk for antisocial personality disorder.

Perhaps the strongest evidence of rGE in molecular genetic studies was in a study which found that an association between the *G1438A* polymorphism of the serotoin transporter receptor and peer relationship was mediated in part by its effects on men's rule-breaking behavior (Burt, 2009). These studies confirm the existence of rGEs in research that has measured genetic variants in addition to the environment.

There are, however, a number challenges with molecular genetic investigations of rGE. First, sample size must be large in order to detect genetic effects; second, the environments must be well specified and measured; third, researchers must balance the risks of false-positive results against false-negative (for a more detailed discussion, see Jaffee & Price, 2007). It will be important in the future for molecular genetic studies of G × E to adequately test for the presence rGEs because the existence of rGEs, however small, will inflate type I errors.

Cognitive Mediators

Molecular genetic studies of experimental and neuropsychological measures are beginning to be undertaken. Although interesting, they almost all suffer from a lack of statistical power due to very small sample sizes. There are, however, some interesting findings that hint at some directions future research might take. For example, one of the first studies in this area found an association between the *5-HTTLPR* genotype and amygdalar response to fearful stimuli (Hariri et al., 2002). A subsequent paper from this same group replicated the finding, confirmed that it applied in both males and females, and also confirmed that the result was specific to the experimental task and that there was no association between the marker and harm avoidance (Hariri, Drabant, & Weinberger, 2006). More recently this marker has been associated with negative information-processing styles following a negative mood prime in a nonclinical sample of 7-year-old children (Hayden et al., 2007). Another group has been looking at a combination of genotoype (*5-HTTLPR*), cognitive style, and environmental risks (e.g., maternal expressed emotion or experience of maternal depression) and have found evidence for three-way interactions (Gibb, Uhrlass, Grassia, Benas, & McGeary, 2009; Gibb, Benes, Grassia, & McGeary, 2009). In the first study, the role of environmental stress for children with negative cognitive style was increased when in the presence of the short allele of the *5-HTTLPR* (Gibb et al., 2009). In the second study, the association between maternal and child depression was strongest among children who carried the short allele of the *5-HTTLPR* and who exhibited attentional avoidance of negative faces (Gibb et al., 2009).

Finally, recent work with which our group was involved genotyped *5-HTTLPR* in a group of 33 psychiatrically well adolescents and 31 unmedicated adolescents with a current diagnosis of an anxiety disorder or major depressive disorder (MDD) (Lau et al., 2009). Both groups underwent a face–emotion paradigm, one component of which was to rate the level of fear felt on seeing sets of emotional facial expressions. There was a significant difference in right amygdalar activation in response to the fearful faces as a function of the *5-HTTLPR* genotype. In the healthy adolescents, as in adults, activation was greater in those with lower levels of 5-HT. In contrast, in the patients with anxiety or depressive disorder, the result was in the reverse direction: that is, greater amygdalar activation in response to fearful faces in those with higher levels of 5-HT. This difference in direction of findings between the healthy adolescents and the psychiatric patients is hard to explain, and further studies are necessary. However, it is exciting to see the findings from healthy adults extended to a younger sample.

FUTURE DIRECTIONS AND CONCLUSION

Both quantitative and molecular genetic studies have been useful in the study of depression. The challenge for the future, however, seems to be in incorporating the two approaches and producing more stringent study designs that are able to detect the potentially subtle effects of genes and environment.

Behavioral genetic studies have been able to demonstrate that both the environment and genes are important in depression. This should direct molecular studies away from simple association studies that are unlikely to elucidate the pathway from genes to phenotype. Positive steps have been taken, with gene–environment interaction studies providing some interesting results regarding genetic sensitivity to particular environments. However, as quantitative studies of depression have started to take account of *r*GEs when investigating possible G × E (Lau & Eley, 2008b; Eaves et al., 2003), so too must molecular genetic studies. This is going to require increased sample sizes, because current studies lack the power to detect gene–environment correlations.

Quantitative genetic studies have also demonstrated that genetic effects on depression are developmentally dynamic—with both genetic innovation and attenuation (Kendler et al., 2008; Lau & Eley, 2008b). Genetic mediation of exposure to different environments has also been shown to change during development. It therefore seems that genes are developmentally sensitive. However, because the vast majority of molecular studies fails to take a developmental approach to depression, an incomplete picture of the genetic architecture may be gathered.

It is clear that more work needs to be done in order to unravel the complex interplay between genes and the environment on the development of depression. Future studies should seek to examine sources of heterogeneity, such as age, sex, and environmental stress, as well as incorporating multiple levels of risk. Such interdisciplinary work is likely to be the most fruitful in moving this field forward.

REFERENCES

Abramson, L. Y., Seligman, M. E., & Teasdale, J. D. (1978). Learned helplessness in humans: Critique and reformulation. *Journal of Abnormal Psychology, 87,* 49–74.

Aslund, C., Leppert, J., Comasco, E., Nordquist, N., Oreland, L., & Nilsson, K. W. (2009). Impact of the interaction between the *5-HTTLPR* polymorphism and maltreatment on adolescent depression: A population-based study. *Behavior Genetics, 39,* 524–531.

Bartels, M., Hudziak, J. J., Boomsma, D. I., Rietveld, M. J., Van Beijsterveldt, T. C., & Van Den Oord, E. J. (2003). A study of parent ratings of internalizing and externalizing problem behavior in 12-year-old twins. *Journal of the American Academy of Child and Adolescent Psychiatry, 42,* 1351–1359.

Bergen, S. E., Gardner, C. O., & Kendler, K. S. (2007). Age-related changes in heritability of behavioral phenotypes over adolescence and young adulthood: A meta-analysis. *Twin Research on Human Genetics, 10,* 423–433.

Birmaher, B., Ryan, N. D., Williamson, D. E., Brent, D. A., & Kaufman, J. (1996). Childhood and adolescent depression: A review of the past 10 years: Part II. *Journal of the American Academy of Child and Adolescent Psychiatry, 35,* 1575–1583.

Boomsma, D. I., Van Beijsterveldt, C. E., & Hudziak, J. J. (2005). Genetic and environmental influences on anxious/depression during childhood: A study from the Netherlands Twin Register. *Genes, Brain, and Behavior, 4,* 466–481.

Bradley, S. L., Dodelzon, K., Sandhu, H. K., & Philibert, R. A. (2005). Relationship of serotonin transporter gene polymorphisms and haplotypes to mRNA transcription. *American Journal of Medical Genetics B: Neuropsychiatric Genetics, 136B,* 58–61.

Burt, A. (2009). A mechanistic explanation of popularity: Genes, rule breaking, and evocative gene–environment correlations. *Journal of Personality and Social Psychology, 96,* 783–794.

Caspi, A., Sugden, K., Moffitt, T. E., Taylor, A., Craig, I. W., Harrington, H., et al. (2003). Influence of life stress on depression: Moderation by a polymorphism in the 5-HTT gene. *Science, 301,* 386–389.

Charney, D. S., Menkes, D. B., & Heninger, G. R. (1981). Receptor sensitivity and the mechanism of action of antidepressant treatment: Implications for the etiology and therapy of depression. *Archives of General Psychiatry, 38,* 1160–1180.

Clark, L. A., & Watson, D. (1991). Tripartite model of anxiety and depression: Psychometric evidence and taxonomic implications. *Journal of Abnormal Psychology, 100,* 316–336.

Coppen, A., Eccleston, E. G., & Peet, M. (1973). Total and free tryptophan concentration in the plasma of depressive patients. *Lancet, 2*, 60–63.

Dempster, E. L., Burcescu, I., Wigg, K., Kiss, E., Baji, I., Gadoros, J., (2007). Evidence of an association between the vasopressin V1b receptor gene (*AVPR1B*) and childhood-onset mood disorders. *Archives of General Psychiatry, 64*, 1189–1195.

Dick, D. M., Agrawal, A., Schuckit, M. A., Bierut, L., Hinrichs, A., Fox, L., et al. (2006). Marital status, alcohol dependence, and GABRA2: Evidence for gene–environment correlation and interaction. *Journal of Studies on Alcohol, 67*, 185–194.

Drevets, W. C., Frank, E., Price, J. C., Kupfer, D. J., Holt, D., Greer, P. J., et al. (1999). PET imaging of serotonin 1A receptor binding in depression. *Biological Psychiatry, 46*, 1375–1387.

Eaves, L., Silberg, J., & Erkanli, A. (2003). Resolving multiple epigenetic pathways to adolescent depression. *Journal of Child Psychology and Psychiatry, 44*, 1006–1014.

Egger, H. L., & Angold, A. (2006). Common emotional and behavioral disorders in preschool children: Presentation, nosology, and epidemiology. *Journal of Child Psychology and Psychiatry, 47*, 313–337.

Eley, T. C., Gregory, A. M., Lau, J. Y., McGuffin, P., Napolitano, M., Rijsdijk, F. V., et al. (2008). In the face of uncertainty: A twin study of ambiguous information, anxiety, and depression in children. *Journal of Abnormal Child Psychology, 36*, 55–65.

Eley, T. C., & Stevenson, J. (1999a). Exploring the covariation between anxiety and depression symptoms: A genetic analysis of the effects of age and sex. *Journal of Child Psychology and Psychiatry, 40*, 1273–1282.

Eley, T. C., & Stevenson, J. (1999b). Using genetic analyses to clarify the distinction between depressive and anxious symptoms in children. *Journal of Abnormal Child Psychology, 27*, 105–114.

Eley, T. C., Sugden, K., Corsico, A., Gregory, A. M., Sham, P., McGuffin, P., et al. (2004). Gene–environment interaction analysis of serotonin system markers with adolescent depression. *Molecular Psychiatry, 9*, 908–915.

Fleming, J. E., & Offord, D. R. (1990). Epidemiology of childhood depressive disorders: A critical review. *Journal of the American Academy of Child and Adolescent Psychiatry, 29*, 571–580.

Fombonne, E., Wostear, G., Cooper, V., Harrington, R., & Rutter, M. (2001a). The Maudsley long-term follow-up of child and adolescent depression: 1. Psychiatric outcomes in adulthood. *British Journal of Psychiatry, 179*, 210–217.

Fombonne, E., Wostear, G., Cooper, V., Harrington, R., & Rutter, M. (2001b). The Maudsley long-term follow-up of child and adolescent depression: 2. Suicidality, criminality and social dysfunction in adulthood. *British Journal of Psychiatry, 179*, 218–223.

Gelernter, J., Cubells, J. F., Kidd, J. R., Pakstis, A. J., & Kidd, K. K. (1999). Population studies of polymorphisms of the serotonin transporter protein gene. *American Journal of Medical Genetics, 88*, 61–66.

Gibb, B. E., Benas, J. S., Grassia, M., & McGeary, J. (2009). Children's attentional biases and 5-HTTLPR genotype: Potential mechanisms linking mother and child depression. *Journal of Clinical Child and Adolescent Psychology, 38,* 415–426.

Gibb, B. E., Uhrlass, D. J., Grassia, M., Benas, J. S., & McGeary, J. (2009). Children's inferential styles, 5-HTTLPR genotype, and maternal expressed emotion—criticism: An integrated model for the intergenerational transmission of depression. *Journal of Abnormal Psychology, 118,* 734–745.

Gjone, H., & Stevenson, J. (1997). The association between internalizing and externalizing behavior in childhood and early adolescence: Genetics of environmental common influences? *Journal of Abnormal Child Psychology, 25,* 277–286.

Gladstone, T. R., & Kaslow, N. J. (1995) Depression and attributions in children and adolescents: A meta-analytic review. *Journal of Abnormal Child Psychology, 23,* 597–606.

Goodnick, P. J., & Goldstein, B. J. (1998). Selective serotonin reuptake inhibitors in affective disorders: I. Basic pharmacology. *Journal of Psychopharmacology, 12,* S5–S20.

Grabe, H. J., Lange, M., Wolff, B., Volzke, H., Lucht, M., Freyberger, H. J., et al. (2005). Mental and physical distress is modulated by a polymorphism in the 5-HT transporter gene interacting with social stressors and chronic disease burden. *Molecular Psychiatry, 10,* 220–224.

Gregory, A. M., Rijsdijk, F. V., Dahl, R. E., McGuffin, P., & Eley, T. C. (2006) Associations between sleep problems, anxiety, and depression in twins at 8 years of age. *Pediatrics, 118,* 1124–1132.

Gregory, A. M., Rijsdijk, F. V., Lau, J. Y., Napolitano, M., McGuffin, P., & Eley, T. C. (2007). Genetic and environmental influences on interpersonal cognitions and associations with depressive symptoms in 8-year-old twins. *Journal of Abnormal Psychology, 116,* 762–775.

Hankin, B. L., & Abramson, L. Y. (2001). Development of gender differences in depression: An elaborated cognitive vulnerability–transactional stress theory. *Psychological Bulletin, 127,* 773–796.

Happonen, M., Pulkkinen, L., Kaprio, J., Van Der Meere, J., Viken, R. J., & Rose, R. J. (2002). The heritability of depressive symptoms: Multiple informants and multiple measures. *Journal of Child Psychology and Psychiatry, 43,* 471–479.

Hariri, A. R., Drabant, E. M., Munoz, K. E., Kolachana, B. S., Mattay, V. S., Egan, M. F., et al. (2005). A susceptibility gene for affective disorders and the response of the human amygdala. *Archives of General Psychiatry, 62,* 146–152.

Hariri, A. R., Drabant, E. M., & Weinberger, D. R. (2006). Imaging genetics: Perspectives from studies of genetically driven variation in serotonin function and corticolimbic affective processing. *Biological Psychiatry, 59,* 888–897.

Hariri, A. R., Mattay, V. S., Tessitore, A., Kolachana, B., Fera, F., Goldman, D., et al. (2002). Serotonin transporter genetic variation and the response of the human amygdala. *Science, 297,* 400–403.

Hayden, E. P., Dougherty, L. R., Maloney, B., Durbin, E. C., Olino, T. M., Nurnberger, J. I., Jr., et al. (2007). Temperamental fearfulness in childhood and the serotonin transporter promoter region polymorphism: A multimethod association study. *Psychiatric Genetics, 17,* 135–142.

Hewitt, J. K., Silberg, J. L., Neale, M. C., Eaves, L. J., & Erickson, M. (1992). The analysis of parental ratings of children's behavior using LISREL. *Behavior Genetics, 22,* 293–317.

Hirschfeld, R. M. (2000). History and evolution of the monoamine hypothesis of depression. *Journal of Clinical Psychiatry, 61*(Suppl. 6), 4–6.

Hirschhorn, J. N., & Daly, M. J. (2005). Genome-wide association studies for common diseases and complex traits. *Nature Reviews: Genetics, 6,* 95–108.

Huezo-Diaz, P., Tandon, K., & Aitchison, K. J. (2005). The genetics of depression and related traits. *Current Psychiatry Reports, 7,* 117–124.

Jacobson, K. C., & Rowe, D. C. (1999). Genetic and environmental influences on the relationships between family connectedness, school connectedness, and adolescent depressed mood: Sex differences. *Developmental Psychology, 35,* 926–939.

Jaffee, S. R., & Price, T. S. (2007). Gene–environment correlations: A review of the evidence and implications for prevention of mental illness. *Molecular Psychiatry, 12,* 432–442.

Joyce, P. R., Mulder, R. T., Luty, S. E., Mckenzie, J. M., Miller, A. L., Rogers, G. R., et al. (2003). Age-dependent antidepressant pharmacogenomics: Polymorphisms of the serotonin transporter and G protein beta$_3$ subunit as predictors of response to fluoxetine and nortriptyline. *International Journal of Neuropsychopharmacology, 6,* 339–346.

Kendler, K. S., Gardner, C. O., & Lichtenstein, P. (2008). A developmental twin study of symptoms of anxiety and depression: Evidence for genetic innovation and attenuation. *Psychological Medicine, 38,* 1567–1575.

Kendler, K. S., Kuhn, J. W., Vittum, J., Prescott, C. A., & Riley, B. (2005). The interaction of stressful life events and a serotonin transporter polymorphism in the prediction of episodes of major depression: A replication. *Archives of General Psychiatry, 62,* 529–535.

Kendler, K. S., Thornton, L. M., & Gardner, C. O. (2000). Stressful life events and previous episodes in the etiology of major depression in women: An evaluation of the "kindling" hypothesis. *American Journal of Psychiatry, 157,* 1243–1251.

Kovacs, M. (1997). Depressive disorders in childhood: An impressionistic landscape. *Journal of Child Psychology and Psychiatry and Allied Disciplines, 38,* 287–298.

Kovas, Y., & Plomin, R. (2006) Generalist genes: Implications for the cognitive sciences. *Trends in Cognitive Sciences, 10,* 198–203.

Kravitz, H. M., Meyer, P. M., Seeman, T. E., Greendale, G. A., & Sowers, M. R. (2006). Cognitive functioning and sex steroid hormone gene polymorphisms in women at midlife. *American Journal of Medicine, 119,* S94–S102.

Kuehner, C. (2003). Gender differences in unipolar depression: An update of epidemiological findings and possible explanations. *Acta Psychiatrica Scandinavica, 108,* 163–174.

Lau, J. Y., & Eley, T. C. (2006). Changes in genetic and environmental influences on depressive symptoms across adolescence and young adulthood. *British Journal of Psychiatry, 189,* 422–427.

Lau, J. Y., & Eley, T. C. (2008a). Attributional style as a risk marker of genetic effects for adolescent depressive symptoms. *Journal of Abnormal Psychology, 117,* 849–859.

Lau, J. Y., & Eley, T. C. (2008b). Disentangling gene–environment correlations and interactions on adolescent depressive symptoms. *Journal of Child Psychology and Psychiatry, 49*, 142–150.

Lau, J. Y., Goldman, D., Buzas, B., Fromm, S. J., Guyer, A. E., Hodgkinson, C., et al. (2009). Amygdala function and 5-HTT gene variants in adolescent anxiety and major depressive disorder. *Biological Psychiatry, 65*, 349–355.

Lau, J. Y., Gregory, A. M., Goldwin, M. A., Pine, D. S., & Eley, T. C. (2007). Assessing gene–environment interactions on anxiety symptom subtypes across childhood and adolescence. *Developmental Psychopathology, 19*, 1129–1146.

Lau, J. Y., Rijsdijk, F., & Eley, T. C. (2006). I think, therefore I am: A twin study of attributional style in adolescents. *Journal of Child Psychology and Psychiatry, 47*, 696–703.

Lesch, K. P., Bengel, D., Heils, A., Sabol, S. Z., Greenberg, B. D., Petri, S., et al. (1996). Association of anxiety-related traits with a polymorphism in the serotonin transporter gene regulatory region. *Science, 274*, 1527–1531.

Levinson, D. F. (2006). The genetics of depression: A review. *Biological Psychiatry, 60*, 84–92.

Lim, J. E., Papp, A., Pinsonneault, J., Sadee, W., & Saffen, D. (2006). Allelic expression of serotonin transporter (SERT) mRNA in human pons: Lack of correlation with the polymorphism *SERTLPR*. *Molecular Psychiatry, 11*, 649–662.

Little, K. Y., Mclaughlin, D. P., Zhang, L., Livermore, C. S., Dalack, G. W., Mcfinton, P. R., et al. (1998). Cocaine, ethanol, and genotype effects on human midbrain serotonin transporter binding sites and mRNA levels. *American Journal of Psychiatry, 155*, 207–213.

Lopez, J. F., Chalmers, D. T., Little, K. Y., & Watson, S. J. (1998). A. E. Bennett Research Award: Regulation of serotonin1A, glucocorticoid, and mineralocorticoid receptor in rat and human hippocampus: Implications for the neurobiology of depression. *Biological Psychiatry, 43*, 547–573.

Malhotra, S., & Das, P. P. (2007). Understanding childhood depression. *Indian Journal of Medical Research, 125*, 115–128.

Manji, H. K., Drevets, W. C., & Charney, D. S. (2001). The cellular neurobiology of depression. *Nature Medicine, 7*, 541–547.

Martin, N., Boomsma, D., & Machin, G. (1997). A twin-pronged attack on complex traits. *Nature Genetics, 17*, 387–392.

Meltzer, H. (1989). Serotonergic dysfunction in depression. *British Journal of Psychiatry, 155*(8), 25–31.

Merrell, K. W., McClun, L. A., Kempf, K. K. G., & Lund, J. (2002). Using self-report assessment to identify children with internalizing problems: Validity of the Internalizing Symptoms Scale for Children. *Journal of Psychoeducational Assessment, 20*, 223–239.

Mill, J., Kiss, E., Baji, I., Kapornai, K., Daroczy, G., Vetro, A., et al. (2008). Association study of the estrogen receptor alpha gene (*ESR1*) and childhood-onset mood disorders. *American Journal of Medical Genetics B Neuropsychiatric Genetics, 147B*, 1323–1326.

Nobile, M., Begni, B., Giorda, R., Frigerio, A., Marino, C., Molteni, M., et al. (1999). Effects of serotonin transporter promoter genotype on platelet serotonin transporter functionality in depressed children and adolescents. *Journal of the American Academy of Child and Adolescent Psychiatry, 38,* 1396–1402.

O'Connor, T. G., Neiderhiser, J. M., Reiss, D., Hetherington, E. M., & Plomin, R. (1998). Genetic contributions to continuity, change, and co-occurrence of antisocial and depressive symptoms in adolescence. *Journal of Child Psychology and Psychiatry, 39,* 323–336.

Parker, K. J., Schatzberg, A. F., & Lyons, D. M. (2003). Neuroendocrine aspects of hypercortisolism in major depression. *Hormones and Behavior, 43,* 60–66.

Parsey, R. V., Hastings, R. S., Oquendo, M. A., Huang, Y. Y., Simpson, N., Arcement, J., et al. (2006). Lower serotonin transporter binding potential in the human brain during major depressive episodes. *American Journal of Psychiatry, 163,* 52–58.

Pfeffer, C. R., Mcbride, P. A., Anderson, G. M., Kakuma, T., Fensterheim, L., & Khait, V. (1998). Peripheral serotonin measures in prepubertal psychiatric inpatients and normal children: Associations with suicidal behavior and its risk factors. *Biological Psychiatry, 44,* 568–577.

Pickles, A., Pickering, K., Simonoff, E., Silberg, J., Meyer, J., & Maes, H. (1998). Genetic "clocks" and "soft" events: A twin model for pubertal development and other recalled sequences of developmental milestones, transitions, or ages at onset. *Behavior Genetics, 28,* 243–253.

Pike, A., Reiss, D., Hetherington, E. M., & Plomin, R. (1996). Using MZ differences in the search for nonshared environmental effects. *Journal of Child Psychology and Psychiatry, 37,* 695–704.

Plomin, R., DeFries, J. C., & Loehlin, J. C. (1977). Genotype–environment interaction and correlation in the analysis of human behavior. *Psychological Bulletin, 84,* 309–322.

Plomin, R., DeFries, J. C., McClearn, G. E., & McGuffin, P. (2008). *Behavioural genetics* (5th ed.). New York: Worth.

Purcell, S. (2002). Variance components models for gene–environment interaction in twin analysis. *Twin Research, 5,* 554–571.

Rice, F., Harold, G. T., & Thapar, A. (2002). Assessing the effects of age, sex and shared environment on the genetic aetiology of depression in childhood and adolescence. *Journal of Child Psychology and Psychiatry, 43,* 1039–1051.

Rice, F., Harold, G. T., & Thapar, A. (2003). Negative life events as an account of age-related differences in the genetic aetiology of depression in childhood and adolescence. *Journal of Child Psychology and Psychiatry, 44,* 977–987.

Riggins-Caspers, K. M., Cadoret, R. J., Knutson, J. F., & Langbehn, D. (2003). Biology–environment interaction and evocative biology–environment correlation: Contributions of harsh discipline and parental psychopathology to problem adolescent behaviors. *Behavior Genetics, 33,* 205–220.

Risch, N. J. (2000). Searching for genetic determinants in the new millennium. *Nature, 405,* 847–856.

Risch, N. J., Herrell, R., Lehner, T., Liang, K. Y., Eaves, L., Hoh, J., et al. (2009). Interaction between the serotonin transporter gene (*5-HTTLPR*), stressful life events, and risk of depression: A meta-analysis. *Journal of the American Medical Association, 301,* 2462–2471.

Schulterbrandt, J. G., & Raskin, A. (1977). *Depression in childhood: Diagnosis, treatment, and conceptual models*. New York: Raven Press.

Scott, L. V., & Dinan, T. G. (2002). Vasopressin as a target for antidepressant development: An assessment of the available evidence. *Journal of Affective Disorders, 72*, 113–124.

Scourfield, J., Rice, F., Thapar, A., Harold, G. T., Martin, N., & McGuffin, P. (2003). Depressive symptoms in children and adolescents: Changing aetiological influences with development. *Journal of Child Psychology and Psychiatry, 44*, 968–976.

Sham, P. C., Sterne, A., Purcell, S., Cherny, S., Webster, M., Rijsdijk, F., et al. (2000). GENESiS: Creating a composite index of the vulnerability to anxiety and depression in a community-based sample of siblings. *Twin Research, 3*, 316–322.

Silberg, J., Pickles, A., Rutter, M., Hewitt, J., Simonoff, E., Maes, H., et al. (1999). The influence of genetic factors and life stress on depression among adolescent girls. *Archives of General Psychiatry, 56*, 225–232.

Silberg, J., Rutter, M., Neale, M., & Eaves, L. (2001). Genetic moderation of environmental risk for depression and anxiety in adolescent girls. *British Journal of Psychiatry, 179*, 116–121.

Stalets, M. M., & Luby, J. L. (2006). Preschool depression. *Child and Adolescent Psychiatry Clinics of North America, 15*, 899–917, viii–ix.

Teare, M. D., & Barrett, J. H. (2005). Genetic linkage studies. *The Lancet, 366*, 1036–1044.

Thapar, A., Harold, G., & McGuffin, P. (1998). Life events and depressive symptoms in childhood: Shared genes or shared adversity?: A research note. *Journal of Child Psychology and Psychiatry, 39*, 1153–1158.

Thapar, A., & McGuffin, P. (1994). A twin study of depressive symptoms in childhood. *British Journal of Psychiatry, 165*, 259–265.

Thapar, A., & McGuffin, P. (1997). Anxiety and depressive symptoms in childhood: A genetic study of comorbidity. *Journal of Child Psychology and Psychiatry, 38*, 651–656.

Tiemeier, H., Schuit, S. C., Den Heijer, T., Van Meurs, J. B., Van Tuijl, H. R., Hofman, A., et al. (2005). Estrogen receptor, alpha gene polymorphisms and anxiety disorder in an elderly population. *Molecular Psychiatry, 10*, 806–807.

Trouton, A., Spinath, F. M., & Plomin, R. (2002). Twins early development study (TEDS): A multivariate, longitudinal genetic investigation of language, cognition, and behavior problems in childhood. *Twin Research, 5*, 444–448.

Tsai, S. J., Wang, Y. C., Hong, C. J., & Chiu, H. J. (2003). Association study of oestrogen receptor alpha gene polymorphism and suicidal behaviours in major depressive disorder. *Psychiatric Genetics, 13*, 19–22.

Twitchell, G. R., Hanna, G. L., Cook, E. H., Fitzgerald, H. E., & Zucker, R. A. (2000). Serotonergic function, behavioral disinhibition, and negative affect in children of alcoholics: The moderating effects of puberty. *Alcohol—Clinical and Experimental Research, 24*, 972–979.

Twitchell, G. R., Hanna, G. L., Cook, E. H., Stoltenberg, S. F., Fitzgerald, H. E., & Zucker, R. A. (2001). Serotonin transporter promoter polymorphism genotype is associated with behavioral disinhibition and negative affect in children of alcoholics. *Alcohol—Clinical and Experimental Research, 25*, 953–959.

Uher, R., & McGuffin, P. (2008). The moderation by the serotonin transporter gene of environmental adversity in the aetiology of mental illness: Review and methodological analysis. *Molecular Psychiatry, 13*, 131–146.

van Der Valk, J. C., van Den Oord, E. J., Verhulst, F. C., & Boomsma, D. I. (2003). Genetic and environmental contributions to stability and change in children's internalizing and externalizing problems. *Journal of the American Academy of Child and Adolescent Psychiatry, 42*, 1212–1220.

Walderhaug, E., Magnusson, A., Neumeister, A., Lappalainen, J., Lunde, H., Refsum, H., et al. (2007). Interactive effects of sex and *5-HTTLPR* on mood and impulsivity during tryptophan depletion in healthy people. *Biological Psychiatry, 62*, 593–599.

Walf, A. A., & Frye, C. A. (2006). A review and update of mechanisms of estrogen in the hippocampus and amygdala for anxiety and depression behavior. *Neuropsychopharmacology, 31*, 1097–1111.

Watson, S., Gallagher, P., Ferrier, I. N., & Young, A. H. (2006). Post-dexamethasone arginine vasopressin levels in patients with severe mood disorders. *Journal of Psychiatric Research, 40*, 353–359.

Wilhelm, K., Mitchell, P. B., Niven, H., Finch, A., Wedgwood, L., Scimone, A., et al. (2006). Life events, first depression onset and the serotonin transporter gene. *British Journal of Psychiatry, 188*, 210–215.

Zalsman, G., Brent, D. A., & Weersing, V. R. (2006). Depressive disorders in childhood and adolescence: An overview—epidemiology, clinical manifestation, and risk factors. *Child and Adolescent Psychiatry Clinics of North America, 15*, 827–841, vii.

CHAPTER 4

Integrating Affective, Biological, and Cognitive Vulnerability Models to Explain the Gender Difference in Depression

The ABC Model and Its Implications for Intervention

Amy H. Mezulis, Janet Shibley Hyde,
Jordan Simonson, *and* Anna M. Charbonneau

The gender difference in depression is among the most robust of findings in psychopathology research. Research indicates that, although girls are no more depressed than boys in childhood (Anderson, Williams, McGee, & Silva, 1987; Cohen et al., 1993), more girls than boys are depressed by ages 13–15 (Hankin et al., 1998; Kessler, McGonagle, Swartz, Blazer, & Nelson, 1993; Wade, Cairney, & Pevalin, 2002). Therefore, if we are to understand the gender difference in depression in adulthood, we must understand its development in adolescence.

Though numerous models of gender differences in depression have been posed, a truly integrated, developmental model has been lacking. The ABC model integrates affective, biological, and cognitive factors into a single model, which asserts that these vulnerability factors emerge and converge in adolescence to form an overall level of depressogenic vulnerability (Hyde, Mezulis, & Abramson, 2008). Individual differences in overall depressogenic vulnerability, in interaction with individual differences in stress, contribute to the emergence of the gender difference in depression (see Figure 4.1). Each of the main elements of the model—affective vul-

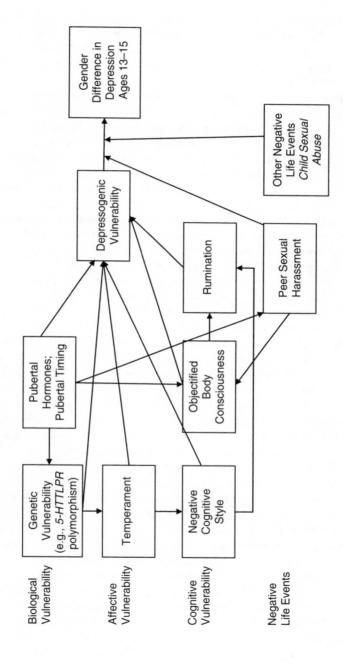

FIGURE 4.1. Graphical representation of the ABC model.

nerability, biological vulnerability, cognitive vulnerability, and stress—is detailed and evaluated below. We emphasize the ways in which these vulnerabilities emerge or intensify in early adolescence, and how each individually and/or in interaction with other vulnerabilities may contribute to the gender difference in depression.

The ABC model incorporates many elements of previous models but is also distinctive in three important ways. First, it is an *integrative model* that examines multiple domains of vulnerability and allows for relationships among vulnerability factors beyond simply additive or cumulative ones. Many of the vulnerabilities incorporated in the ABC model are hypothesized to influence each other developmentally; for example, genetic vulnerability (a biological factor) is presumed to influence temperament (an affective vulnerability); temperament is presumed to contribute to negative cognitive style (a cognitive vulnerability); and early pubertal development (a biological vulnerability) is presumed to contribute to greater objectified body consciousness (a cognitive vulnerability) as well as to evoke greater frequency of peer sexual harassment (a stressor). Many of the vulnerabilities in the ABC model are also hypothesized to influence each other reciprocally; for example, objectified body consciousness (a cognitive vulnerability) and rumination (a cognitive vulnerability) are hypothesized to be mutually facilitating over time.

Second, the ABC model is a *developmental model* of the emergence of the gender difference in depression insofar as we examine how depressogenic vulnerability across these three domains (affective, biological, and cognitive) emerges and/or increases in early adolescence to increase overall depressogenic vulnerability particularly for females and particularly during this developmental period. The ABC model proposes six hypothetical developmental models to explain the emergence of the gender difference in depression (building on models of Nolen-Hoeksema & Girgus, 1994). These models are not competing hypotheses, but rather offer heuristics with which to examine complex longitudinal data. Each individual vulnerability factor or stressor presented in the ABC model may develop in ways consistent with one or more of these developmental models.

Developmental Model 1 states that the causes of depression are the same for boys and girls, but that an important causal factor(s) becomes more prevalent for girls than boys in early adolescence. Examples of factors in our model that may fit this pattern are negative cognitive style and stress. Our *Developmental Model 2* states that the causes of depression are somewhat different for girls compared with boys, and that levels of the causes for girls rise in early adolescence. Examples of such a factor might be objectified body consciousness or gonadal hormones. *Developmental Model 3* states that girls are higher in vulnerabilities for depression even before adolescence, and that the increases in negative life events in adolescence combine with the vulnerabilities to produce depression. Our *Developmental Model 4* holds that there is greater female variability in one or more of the vulnerability factors, such that in the absence of a mean gender difference in the vulnerability factor, more girls than boys may have levels of that vulnerability that put them at risk for depression. An example in our model might be temperament, and specifically, negative emotionality. *Developmental Model 5* focuses on vulnerability–stress interactions and presents the possibility that such an interaction may be more potent for girls than for boys. Finally, our *Developmental Model 6* is a mixed model that specifies that there are multiple pathways to depression (e.g., Kendler, Gardner, & Prescott, 2002), some of which are more common in girls than boys, and that different pathways may conform to Developmental Model 1, 2, 3, 4, or 5. Each pathway explains only a small percentage of the variance in depression but, taken together, the multiple pathways can explain most cases and can explain the gender difference.

The third distinctive feature of the ABC model is the use of *multiple pathways* to explain the emergence of the gender difference in depression. As such, it is consistent with the developmental psychopathology concept of equifinality, which states that individuals with the same psychological outcome may have arrived there via different developmental origins (Cicchetti & Rogosch, 1996). It seems clear that there are multiple pathways to adolescent girls' depression (e.g., Harrington, Rutter, & Fombonne, 1996). An implication of the principle of multiple pathways is that, in empirical tests of the ABC model, any single pathway should yield significant results but the effect will not be large, because only a subset of girls may follow that pathway to depression. We believe that the ABC model provides the structure to accommodate these multiple pathways.

In following sections we describe the affective, biological, and cognitive vulnerability and stressor components of the ABC model. Following these sections, we further discuss specific developmental and integrative hypotheses deriving from the ABC model and examine the empirical support for each hypothesis. In doing so, we report data from our own longitudinal study, the Wisconsin Study of Families and Work, as well as other relevant research, when available. Finally, we conclude by examining the implications of the ABC model for prevention and intervention efforts.

A: AFFECTIVE VULNERABILITY

Definition

We define affective vulnerability as representing individual differences in emotionality—both baseline emotionality as well as emotional reactivity and recovery. A constellation composed of high baseline negative affect, high negative emotional reactivity, high intensity of negative emotional reactions, low adaptability, and low approach is typically labeled "negative emotionality" or "negative affectivity." Children high in negative emotionality typically dislike and/or avoid novel situations; show distress to novelty; become upset, fearful, sad, or tearful easily; and appear highly sensitive to negative stimuli (Buss & Plomin, 1986; Belsky, Hsieh, & Crnic, 1996). By contrast, a constellation of temperamental characteristics composed of high positive affect, high sociability, high adaptability, and high approach is typically labeled "positive emotionality." Children high in positive emotionality typically seek novel sensations and situations, are goal-oriented, sociable, easygoing, and extraverted (Rothbart & Bates, 1998).

Links to Depression

Several studies have found that both negative emotionality and positive emotionality are associated with and predictive of depression in adults, adolescents, and children (Goodyer, Ashby, Altham, Vize, & Cooper, 1993; Roberts & Kendler, 1999; Rothbart & Bates, 1998). The pattern of results indicates that low positive emotionality may be uniquely associated with depression, whereas high negative emotionality is a nonspecific factor predictive of both depression and anxiety (Clark & Watson, 1991; Phillips, Lonigan, Driscoll, & Hooe, 2002). In one of the few prospective studies examining the relationship between temperament and depression, Caspi and colleagues (1995) followed a large community sample of children from ages 3–21. They found that behavioral inhibition in early childhood predicted diagnoses of depression in adolescence. Davies and Windle (2001) found evidence for a temperament × environment interaction, with temperamental characteristics typical of negative emotionality significantly interacting with parents' marital discord to predict depression. Moreover, the relationship between temperament and depression holds even when overlap between temperament and symptom measures is removed (Lengua, West, & Sandler, 1998).

Developmental Course and the Emergent Gender Difference in Depression

Our model proposes three developmental relationships between negative emotionality and depression vulnerability in adolescence, with subsequent implications for the emergence of the gender difference in depression. First, we propose, as outlined above, a direct relationship between negative emotionality and depression that represents an underlying affective vulnerability present since childhood and continuing into the adolescent period; this vulnerability may become increasingly salient when it encounters the particular negative life events that become prominent in early adolescence. As such, gender differences in affective vulnerability may directly contribute to a gender difference in depression in adolescence; this hypothesis is discussed in detail below. Second, we propose that the normal hormonal and social changes associated with puberty and early adolescence may intensify negative emotionality for all youth, suggesting a developmental trajectory in which affective vulnerability is increased in adolescence; this hypothesis is also discussed in detail below. Finally, we suggest that negative emotionality contributes developmentally to greater cognitive vulnerability, which emerges in early adolescence; this final, integrative hypothesis is addressed in more detail in the later section on integrative hypotheses.

Gender differences in affective vulnerability may contribute to the emergence of gender differences in depression in adolescence through three potential mechanisms: (1) a gender difference in negative emotionality, with girls scoring higher, combined with an increase in negative life events in early adolescence (Developmental Model 3, described above); (2) in the absence of an average gender difference in temperament, a greater variance in scores for girls so that more girls are above the cutoff for high negative emotionality (Developmental Model 4); and/or (3) a more potent interaction between temperament and negative life events for girls than for boys (Developmental Model 2).

There is little evidence of the first mechanism, namely, that there are gender differences in mean levels of affective vulnerability. A recent meta-analysis found that, across diverse measures of negative emotionality, effect sizes for gender differences in overall emotionality, negative emotionality, sadness, and positive emotionality all indicated no meaningful gender differences (all $ds < .10$; Else-Quest, Hyde, Goldsmith, & Van Hulle, 2006).

Although these findings suggest no mean gender differences in affective vulnerability, the same study found some support for the second mechanism: greater female variability. The statistic used to evaluate this hypothesis is the variance ratio (VR), which is the ratio of the male variance to the female variance. Values > 1.0 reflect greater male variance, and values < 1.0 reflect greater female variance. For overall emotionality, VR = 0.94, indicating slightly greater female variance. For negative emotionality, VR = 0.88, again indicating somewhat greater variance among girls than among boys. This greater female variance could create a larger pool of girls at the upper tail of the distribution, that is, more girls than boys scoring high on this dimension, creating more vulnerable girls in the absence of a gender difference in mean scores.

As far as we know, there have been no published studies examining the final mechanism, which is that affective vulnerability, either directly or in interaction with stress, may be more strongly predictive of depression for girls than boys. This is an intriguing avenue for future research efforts.

Our second hypothesis regarding affective vulnerability and depression is that adolescence may bring an intensification of negative affect for most teens, which increases the number of youth for whom that vulnerability factor is sufficiently elevated as to pose a risk for the development of depression. Adolescence involves dramatic biological changes, including changes in mean levels and variability in hormones associated with stress and neurotransmitters associated with emotion regulation (pubertal hormones are reviewed in more detail below). Compared with children and adults, adolescents report more extreme negative emotions in response to stress (Larson & Richards, 1994) as well as greater physiological responses to stress (Allen & Matthews, 1997). Spear (2000) has suggested that these changes in stress sensitivity may increase adolescents' vulnerability to a host of psychopathologies, including depression. In our longitudinal study of over 350 youth from birth to age 15, we found that youths' self-reported subjective distress to stressors increased from age 11 to 15, that gender differences in self-reported subjective distress emerged by age 15 (particularly in the domain of interpersonal stress), and that early childhood negative emotionality predicted subjective distress at age 15. Most interestingly, we also found that this temperament-based index of subjective distress in adolescence moderated the relationship between stress and depression in a complex model in which stress mediated the gender difference in depression (Charbonneau, Mezulis, & Hyde, 2009). These findings suggest that one pathway from affective vulnerability to depression is via an adolescent increase in emotional reactivity to stressful events.

B: BIOLOGICAL VULNERABILITY

Definition

Biological factors that may contribute to depression include genetics, pubertal hormones, and pubertal timing. Genetic contributions to depression have long been implicated by increased rates of depression in families with affected individuals. Beyond this, research has recently begun to focus on specific genetic loci that may confer vulnerability to depression. Advances of the Human Genome Project have allowed several studies to conduct genomewide scans to detect linkage among relatives affected by depression. Findings from these studies have pointed to specific loci that may be linked to depression, including several that are involved in the serotonin system.

Another potential vulnerability to depression is puberty and its accompanying hormonal changes. Puberty is not a single event, but rather a process that occurs over several years, resulting in adult appearance and physiology. Puberty is actually preceded by adrenarche—the time of increasing secretion of adrenal androgens—which generally begins somewhat before age 8

(Grumbach & Styne, 1998; Remer, Boye, Hartmann, & Wudy, 2005). The adrenal gland secretes adrenal androgens, including dehydroepiandrosterone (DHEA) and its sulfate (DHEAS) (see Sulcová, Hill, Hampl, & Stárka, 1997, for data on gender differences in DHEA and DHEAS levels over the lifespan). Adrenarche is then followed by gonadarche, which involves the maturation of the gonads—ovaries in females, testes in males—and sharp increases in their production of the sex hormones estrogen, progesterone, and testosterone. These changes then create the other changes of puberty. We hypothesize that changes in hormone levels in interaction with other stressors of puberty may act as a vulnerability to depression.

A final biological factor is pubertal processes, particularly pubertal timing. Pubertal timing (early, on time, or late) and status (stage of development at a particular time point) are crucial to understanding the transition to adolescence and the emergence of gender differences in many domains, including depression.

Links to Depression

A number of lines of evidence points to genetic influences on depression. Sullivan, Neale, and Kendler (2000) meta-analyzed studies using genetic designs to evaluate family resemblance for major depression. Based on twin studies, depression was moderately heritable, with 37% of the variance due to additive genetic effects. Using genotyping methods, several specific loci have been identified that confer vulnerability to depression. Research has documented an association between major depression and serotonin receptor genes: *HTR1A* (Lemonde et al., 2003; Neumeister, Young, & Stastny, 2004) and *HTR2A* (Eley et al., 2004; for a review of these and hypotheses about other loci and neurotransmitters, see Levinson, 2005). Another candidate gene is *TPH2*, the tryptophan hydroxylase (TPH) gene that is active in the cental nervous system (CNS); TPH is the rate-limiting enzyme in serotonin synthesis (Li & He, 2006; Walther et al., 2003). Imaging genetics has also demonstrated a link between this polymorphism and amygdalar reactivity (Brown et al., 2005). Yet another candidate is the *MAOA* gene, located on the X chromosome (Gutierrez et al., 2004; Yu et al., 2005). Monoamine oxidase A plays a key role in the metabolism of several neurotransmitters, including serotonin.

Perhaps the most promising avenue of research linking specific loci to depression has been on genes related to the serotonin transporter (5-HT) system. The 5-HT system is an excellent candidate, given the success of the selective serotonin inhibitor (SSRI) antidepressants in treating depression (Tamminga et al., 2002). Genotyping studies have shown an association between major depression and the short variant (s allele) of *5-HTTLPR*, the promoter region of the *5-HTT* (serotonin transporter) gene located on chromosome 17, in samples of adults (Hoefgen et al., 2005) children and adolescents (Kaufman et al., 2004). Many of these studies support a vulnerability–stress model in which the s allele of *5-HTTLPR* confers a vulnerability to depression; when combined with stress, depression is a likely outcome (Caspi et al., 2003; Kaufman et al., 2004; Kendler Kuhn, Vittum, Prescott, & Riley, 2005).

Links between pubertal hormones and depression are likely to be complex, nonlinear, and interactional. For example, a study of men showed a U-shaped relationship between depressive symptoms and testosterone levels; men with low levels or high levels of testosterone reported the most depressive symptoms, compared with those with moderate levels (Booth, Johnson, & Granger, 1999). Goodyer, Herbert, Tamplin, and Altham (2000) have found a similar curvilinear relationship between DHEA levels and depression among adolescents. A curvilinear effect was also found for the relationship between estradiol and negative affect for early-adolescent girls; depressive affect was highest for girls with rapidly increasing but subadult levels of hormone (Brooks-Gunn & Warren, 1989).

Interactions have been found as well. Booth, Johnson, Granger, Crouter, and McHale (2003), with a sample of youth between the ages of 6 and 18 years, found that testosterone's positive relation to risk behavior and negative relation to depression depended on the quality of parent–child relations. Testosterone did not show simple correlations with depression for either boys or girls. But for both boys and girls, testosterone levels interacted significantly with the quality of the parent-child relationship in predicting depressive symptoms. Both boys and girls with low testosterone levels and low-quality parental relationships showed the highest levels of depressive symptoms.

Finally, extensive research has linked pubertal timing to depression; in particular, early puberty is associated with negative mental health outcomes for girls (Caspi & Moffitt, 1991; Caspi, Lynam, Moffitt, & Silva, 1993; Ge, Conger, & Elder, 1996). For example, Ge and colleagues (1996) found that early puberty was associated with psychological distress (depression and anxiety) in adolescent girls (see also, Graber, Lewinsohn, Seeley, & Brooks-Gunn, 1997; Stice, Presnell, & Bearman, 2001). In the largest study to date, Kaltiala-Heino, Kosunen, and Rimpela (2003) found that early puberty was associated with depression among girls; among boys, both very early and late puberty were associated with depression.

Developmental Course and the Emergent Gender Difference in Depression

The ABC model proposes four hypotheses regarding the relationship between biological vulnerabilities and the emergence of the gender difference in depression. First, we hypothesize that genetic vulnerability—most specifically, the *5-HTTLPR* polymorphism, but also perhaps other polymorphisms—may become a salient vulnerability factor for girls in the transition to adolescence when they encounter the increases in stress associated with this developmental period. Second, we hypothesize that, developmentally, the phenotypic expression of one or more of the serotonin genotypes implicated in depression may result in temperament-based individual differences in negative emotionality. This integrative hypothesis, linking genetics (a biological factor) with emotionality (an affective factor), is discussed in the section below on integrative hypotheses. Third, we suggest that, as a whole, puberty initiates a series of hormonal and social changes that functions to increase negative emotionality among all adolescents. For those who already have above-average levels of negative emotionality, this general increase in emotionality may serve to heighten their affective vulnerability to depression. This integrative hypothesis, again linking a biological factor with an affective factor, is discussed below. Finally, we hypothesize that a dominant biological vulnerability to depression among girls is early pubertal timing. Although there may be direct effects between early puberty and depression for girls, we suggest that it is more likely that this relationship is mediated by other psychological factors, such as greater objectified body consciousness (a cognitive vulnerability) and greater peer sexual harassment (a stressor). These integrative hypotheses are addressed in more detail in the section below on integrative hypotheses.

A number of mechanisms may explain how genetic vulnerability can contribute to gender differences in depression: more potent genotype–stress interactions for females than for males, X-linked genetic factors, gene–gene interactions, sex-specific trait loci, and hormone-induced gene expression. For example, Eley and colleagues (2004) found a significant genotype–stress interaction involving *5-HTTLPR* for female, but not male, adolescents (see also, Sjöberg et al., 2006). Two studies have found evidence that the *MAOA* gene, located on the X chromosome, conferred vulnerability to depression more in women than in men (Gutierrez et al., 2004; Yu et al., 2005).

Whatever the final outcome of the genome studies, mediating processes will need to be identified. These are likely to involve synthesis of neurotransmitters such as serotonin and structures such as the amygdala (Eley et al., 2004; Hariri, Drabant, & Weinberger, 2006). We believe that the behavioral and developmental link between these genetic factors and the phenotype of depression occurs, in part, via temperament. And, indeed, the *5-HTTLPR* region has been linked to negative emotionality in 2-month-old infants (Auerbach et al., 1999). In short, known genetic mechanisms are proposed to contribute to the adolescent upsurge in depression and specifically to the emergence of the gender difference in depression between ages 13 and 15.

Regarding the relationship between pubertal hormones and the gender difference in depression, several studies implicate the adrenal androgens in gender differences in depression (van Broekhoven & Verkes, 2003). Nottelmann and colleagues, with participants between the ages of 9 and 14, found that adjustment problems for girls were associated with low levels of DHEAS (Nottelmann et al., 1987). In various samples, Goodyer and colleagues have found that DHEA hyposecretion or hypersecretion was associated with major depression in adolescence (Goodyer et al., 2000), suggesting the possibility of a U-shaped function relating DHEA levels and depression. Moreover, administration of DHEA to women with adrenal insufficiency reduces depression and anxiety (Arlt et al., 1999; see also, Wolkowitz et al., 1999). The mechanism behind this action appears to be that DHEA protects against the negative effects of cortisol in the brain and also modulates various neurotransmitters, including raising serotonin levels (van Broekhoven & Verkes, 2003).

Numerous studies have linked estrogen to depression and the neurotransmitters known to be associated with depression, including MAO and serotonin (for reviews, see Halbreich & Kahn, 2001; Rubinow, Schmidt, & Roca, 1998; Steiner, Dunn, & Born, 2003). In brief, estrogen—like other gonadal steroid hormones—acts on intracellular estrogen receptors. When the hormone binds to the receptor, a cascade of events ensues that modulates the transcription of genes that encode the manufacture of numerous proteins. Among these are proteins necessary for the synthesis of serotonin. Estrogen also increases serotonergic postsynaptic responsivity, increases the number of serotonergic receptors, increases the transport and uptake of serotonin (Halbreich & Kahn, 2001), and operates through both genomic and nongenomic mechanisms (Sanborn & Hayward, 2003). Postpartum depression and premenstrual dysphoric disorder both occur at the time of low estrogen levels, again suggesting a link.

If low estrogen levels are associated with depression, then why would estrogen be associated with depression in pubertal girls, whose estrogen levels are rising? One hypothesis is that estrogen homeostasis is disrupted during puberty, and this disrupted homeostasis may disturb serotonin processes and thereby trigger mood disorders (Halbreich & Kahn, 2001). Altemus (2006) has argued that, more generally, women's experience of greater hormone fluxes across the lifespan plays a role in depression by destabilizing homeostatic systems. This explanation is consistent with Brooks-Gunn and Warren's (1989) finding that among pubertal girls, negative affect occurred specifically at the time of rapid increases in estradiol levels.

Finally, testosterone—both level and diurnal variation—has been associated with several forms of psychopathology in both boys and girls around ages 11–13. Angold, Costello, Erkanli, and Worthman (1999) found that testosterone levels increase substantially over the five Tanner

stages of puberty for girls, and that higher levels of testosterone were associated with higher rates of diagnosable depression. Granger et al. (2003)
also found positive correlations between testosterone levels and depressive
symptoms for girls. In addition, testosterone is known to have effects on
multiple neurotransmitter systems, including serotonin, dopamine, and
gamma-aminobutyric acid (GABA) (Rubinow & Schmidt, 1996).

In summary, the evidence suggests that DHEA, estrogen, and/or testosterone may be involved in the increase in girls' depression at ages 13–15,
although certainly these factors are not the sole cause. Current research
does not definitively identify which hormone or hormones are most potent,
but research does point to the likelihood of nonlinear and interactional
effects. In addition, pubertal development and timing are important, especially insofar as early puberty is disadvantageous for girls, in part because
they are then sexually objectified by peers. Hormone–gene interactions
are another possibility. We cannot reach a definitive conclusion regarding
the effects of hormones or pubertal development on gender differences in
depression. Our goal, instead, has been to suggest possible mechanisms and
review related research, leaving it to future researchers to test the models
against each other.

Finally, we believe that early puberty is a vulnerability factor for girls
that, when combined with stressors, leads to depression. Early puberty is
less of a vulnerability factor for depression in boys in large part because
puberty moves boys more toward the idealized masculine, muscular body
type. Several studies have found a direct relationship between pubertal timing and depression for girls (e.g., see, Caspi & Moffitt, 1991; Ge et al.,
1996). Even more promising may be the hypothesis that early puberty puts
girls at risk for the development of other vulnerabilities, such as greater
objectified body consciousness and peer sexual harassment. This hypothesis is examined below.

C: COGNITIVE VULNERABILITY

Definition

We incorporate three specific cognitive vulnerability factors. The first is
negative cognitive style, which is defined as the tendency to make negative
inferences about cause, self, and future following stressful life events. Negative cognitive style is the vulnerability factor posited by the hopelessness
theory of depression (Abramson, Metalsky, & Alloy, 1989). The second is
rumination, which is defined as the tendency to think repetitively and passively about negative events and the negative affect elicited by them. Rumination was first proposed as a cognitive vulnerability factor to depression
in the response styles theory of depression (Nolen-Hoeksema, 1991), and

its definition was limited to perseverative attention to negative affect. Since then, other researchers—the current authors included—have expanded the conceptualization of rumination to explicitly include perseverative attention to negative events, negative thoughts, and negative affect (Mezulis, Abramson, & Hyde, 2002). The third cognitive vulnerability factor is *objectified body consciousness*, defined as the tendency to view one's body as an object to be viewed and evaluated. Objectified body consciousness originates from the objectified body consciousness theory (OBC theory; McKinley & Hyde, 1996; Fredrickson & Roberts, 1997), which specifies that two processes are involved in the generation of negative beliefs about the body: (1) self-surveillance, a cognitive process in which individuals become observers and critics of their bodies and appearance; and (2) body shame, an affective component in which individuals feel shame when their bodies do not conform to cultural ideals (McKinley & Hyde, 1996; see also, Fredrickson & Roberts, 1997).

Links to Depression

Extensive research has linked all three cognitive vulnerability factors—negative cognitive style, rumination, and objectified body consciousness—with depression. Retrospective and prospective tests of the hopelessness theory in adults and adolescents have supported the hypothesis that negative cognitive style does, in fact, confer vulnerability to depression (Abramson et al., 1999; Alloy et al., 2000; Hankin, Abramson, & Siler, 2001). Perhaps the most stringent test of negative cognitive style as a vulnerability to depression came from the Temple–Wisconsin Cognitive Vulnerability to Depression (CVD) Project, which found that participants with more negative cognitive styles, when faced with stressful events, were more likely to develop depression in the subsequent 5 years of the study, even in the absence of prior depressive episodes (Alloy et al., 2000).

Numerous studies also confirm the prediction that a more ruminative response style predicts depression (see review by Nolen-Hoeksema, 2000). Although most of the theorizing on rumination has focused on the main effects of rumination on depression, Nolen-Hoeksema and Girgus (1994) briefly speculated that preexisting tendencies to ruminate may interact with an escalation in stressors at the beginning of adolescence to increase rates of depression (see also, Nolen-Hoeksema, 1994). This approach is consistent with a cognitive vulnerability–stress interaction model.

Finally, research also supports the link between objectified body consciousness and depressive symptoms (Muehlenkamp & Saris-Baglama, 2002; Tiggemann & Kuring, 2004). In at least one study, this link has been shown to be predictively significant for girls but not boys (Grabe, Hyde, & Lindberg, 2007).

Developmental Course and the Emergent Gender Difference in Depression

Our model hypothesizes four developmental relationships between cognitive vulnerabilities and the emergent gender difference in depression. First, we hypothesize that negative cognitive style emerges as a relatively new and more salient vulnerability factor in the transition to adolescence as a result of cognitive development and puberty's biological, psychological, and social impact. Second, we hypothesize that gender differences in all three cognitive vulnerability factors will emerge by early to middle adolescence. Effect sizes for the gender difference in rumination and objectified body consciousness are likely moderate to large, whereas effect sizes for the gender difference in cognitive style may be smaller. Third, we hypothesize that rumination may mediate the developmental relationships between cognitive style and depression and between objectified body consciousness and depression; in other words, tendencies to generate negative thoughts about stressful events (negative cognitive style) and about one's body (objectified body consciousness) may reinforce, developmentally, a more general tendency to attend perseveratively to negative stimuli (rumination). Fourth, we hypothesize a developmental link between pubertal development (a biological factor) and objectified body consciousness (a cognitive factor); we address this integrative hypothesis in the subsequent section on integrative hypotheses.

Our first hypothesis is that cognitive style emerges in adolescence as a relatively new vulnerability to depression, particularly in the context of a vulnerability–stress model. Several studies have failed to find that cognitive style, in interaction with stress, predicts depression in children. However, this vulnerability–stress interaction typically predicts depression in children after age 11 (Abela, 2001; Garber, Keiley, & Martin, 2002; but see Lewinsohn, Joiner, & Rohde, 2001). We hypothesize that one reason for the inconsistency in results is that children younger than 11 may not yet have formed a stable cognitive "style" that functions as a reliable vulnerability factor. Cole and colleagues found support for this hypothesis in a recent study, reporting that attributional style became more internally consistent and stable over time, all the way into middle adolescence (Cole, Ciesla, Dallaire, Jacquez, Pineda, et al., 2008).

In regards to the second hypothesis, there is evidence of emergent gender differences in all three cognitive vulnerability factors in the transition to adolescence. Research with children under 11 indicates no gender difference in negative cognitive style or that boys may have the more negative style (Abela, 2001; Mezulis, Hyde, & Abramson, 2006). However, research with adolescents shows girls having more negative styles (Hankin & Abramson, 2002; Nolen-Hoeksema & Girgus, 1994). There is some indication, in a study of high school students, that negative cognitive style is more strongly linked to depression for girls than for boys (Gladstone, Kaslow, Seeley, & Lewinsohn, 1997). Similarly, another high school study found that negative cognitive style mediated the gender difference in depressive symptoms, reducing the gender–depression association by 53% (Hankin & Abramson, 2002).

Nolen-Hoeksema (2001; Nolen-Hoeksema & Girgus, 1994) has proposed that the gender difference in depression can be accounted for, at least in part, by gender differences in the tendency to ruminate. Developmental research on gender differences in rumination has yielded mixed results, sometimes finding significant gender differences as early as fourth grade (age 9; Broderick, 1998) and sometimes not finding significant gender differences in childhood (Broderick & Korteland, 2004). Gender differences are present and significant in samples of early and middle adolescents (Compas, Malcarne, & Fondacaro, 1988) and college students (Nolen-Hoeksema, 1987).

Mezulis et al. (2002) expanded the traditional focus of rumination research from depressed mood to include domains about which individuals might ruminate. It is possible, in addition, to ruminate about negative events. Mezulis and colleagues found that college women reported more rumination than college men not only about depressed mood, but also about negative events in three domains: achievement, interpersonal, and body image/attractiveness. However, gender differences in self-reported rumination about depressed mood and about negative events in the achievement domain were small ($d = 0.24$ and 0.28, respectively). Gender differences in rumination about interpersonal and body image events were considerably larger ($d = 0.55$ and 0.68). These findings highlight the importance of considering different domains of rumination and point to the crucial importance of the interpersonal and body image domains in explaining gender differences in depression (Cyranowski, Frank, Young, & Shear, 2000; Nolen-Hoeksema & Girgus, 1994).

Research based in OBC theory has confirmed the existence of moderate gender differences in self-surveillance (McKinley, 1998; Tiggemann & Kuring, 2004, with an Australian sample). In addition, our own data confirm developmental changes in the magnitude of the gender difference in self-surveillance. Using longitudinal data, we found that the gender difference in self-surveillance was already significant in 5th grade (age 11, $d = 0.49$; Lindberg, Hyde, & McKinley, 2006). The gender difference in rumination was not significant at that age, nor was the gender difference in symptoms of depression (Grabe et al., 2007). In adolescents, we see that self-surveillance at age 11 predicts rumination at age 13 for girls but not boys, suggesting that habitual self-surveillance, particularly among girls, may be a cognitive process that contributes to the development of habitual rumination (Grabe et al., 2007).

Finally, in regard to our third hypothesis, there is a small body of evidence suggesting that cognitive style, rumination, and may be related both over time and within individuals. First, negative cognitive style may prospectively predict rumination. Negative cognitive style represents the negative content of cognitions following stress, whereas rumination primarily represents the perseveration of attention on negative emotional and cognitive content; conceptually, both are implicated in the development and maintenance of negative affect, and so one would expect a correlation between the two, at minimum. However, Abramson and colleagues (2001) suggested that rumination may mediate the relationship between negative cognitive style and depression because it may be particularly difficult to disengage attention from highly negative thoughts regarding the causes and consequences of negative events; evidence for this predicted mediation effect was found in the CVD study (Alloy et al., 2004).

Second, the self-surveillance component of OBC may prospectively predict rumination as well; self-surveillance may represent a specific example of ruminative focus on the self that is both perseverative and evaluative. Evidence from our longitudinal data supports the prospective relationship between self-surveillance and rumination. For girls, self-surveillance at age 11 was significantly correlated with depression at ages 11 and 13. Structural equation modeling confirmed that, for girls, rumination and body shame mediate the relationship between age 11 self-surveillance and age 13 depression, with age 11 depression controlled (Grabe et al., 2007). The model for boys was significantly different from that for girls; specifically, age 11 self-surveillance did not predict age 13 rumination. These data, taken together, support the notion that the gender difference in self-surveillance precedes and predicts gender differences in both rumination and depression and that self-surveillance may contribute, developmentally, to rumination.

NEGATIVE LIFE EVENTS

Definition

Negative or stressful life events are a key component of the ABC model (see Figure 4.1). The affective, biological, and cognitive components of our model of depression are predicated on interactions between these vulnerabilities and negative or stressful life events. Indeed, these vulnerability factors should not necessarily lead to depression in the absence of negative events.

Links to Depression

It is well established that stressful life events are associated with the onset of episodes of depression (e.g., Kendler, Karkowski, & Prescott, 1999) and that negative life events predict depressive symptoms specifically in adolescence (Grant et al., 2003). First episodes of depression—which are particularly relevant to the emergence of depression in adolescence—are especially likely to be triggered by negative life events (Monroe & Harkness, 2005).

Developmental Course and the Emergent Gender Difference in Depression

The ABC model asserts three salient hypotheses regarding the relationship between stress and the emergent gender difference in depression. First, we suggest that although stressful events increase for all youth in the transition to adolescence, a small gender difference in total stress emerges in adolescence as well, with larger gender differences in some specific stress domains. Second, we suggest that more significant than gender differences in the mean level of stress are gender differences in stress appraisal, or perceived stress. Finally, we suggest a developmentally integrated relationship between early puberty and one specific type of stress, namely, peer sexual harassment; we discuss this integrative hypothesis in more detail in the next section.

The evidence suggests that gender differences exist in the frequency and type of negative events during childhood and adolescence. A number of studies has found that adolescent girls report more negative events than do boys (e.g., Davies & Windle, 1997; Ge, Lorenz, Conger, Elder, & Simons, 1994; Graber, Brooks-Gunn, & Warren, 1995), particularly in early adolescence (Compas, Davis, & Forsythe, 1985). Davis, Matthews, and Twamley (1999) conducted a meta-analysis of studies of gender differences in major and minor life events. They found, overall, that females were exposed to more stress than males, by only a small amount ($d = 0.12$). The gender difference in exposure was not significant for children or young adults, but was significant for adolescents ($d = 0.12$), with girls exposed to more negative events. Research indicates that girls experience more interpersonal negative events, particularly with family and peers, than do boys (Crick, Casas, & Nelson, 2002; Larson & Ham, 1993; Stark, Spirito, Williams, & Guevremont, 1989). In research on high school students' reports of their main problems, boys reported more problems with school whereas girls reported more problems with interpersonal relationships (Stark et al., 1989). At least two studies have found that higher rates of depression in adolescent girls were explained by greater exposure to interpersonal stress (Charbonneau et al., 2009; Shih, Eberhart, Hammen, & Brennan, 2006).

These findings indicate that, consistent with the ABC model, adolescence is a time of increased gender differences in exposure to negative life events, with girls having the greater exposure. However, can these relatively modest gender differences in exposure to negative life events explain the 2:1 gender ratio for depression in adolescence and its persistence throughout adulthood? One explanation may be found in the second hypothesis that gender differences in stress appraisals may be larger than the gender differences in stress events themselves. When predicting depression, appraisals of the event are more important than simply whether the event occurred (Lazarus & Launier, 1978). One possible explanation for this discrepancy comes from our vulnerability–stress interaction model. That is, girls who score higher on some aspect of vulnerability—for example, negative emotionality in temperament—may find negative events more aversive than other girls and than most boys, and appraise them more negatively. A recently published paper from our own study finds support for this hypothesis: In addition to a gender difference in interpersonal stressful events that mediated the gender–depression relationship in adolescence, we found that gender differences in subjective emotional reactions to interpersonal stressors further moderated this relationship (Charbonneau et al., 2009).

EXAMPLES OF THE INTEGRATIVE NATURE OF THE ABC MODEL

One of the strengths of the ABC model is that it proposes specific, integrative hypotheses regarding developmental relationships among vulnerability factors across different domains. In this section, we outline three of these integrative hypotheses and identify the empirical support for each.

The first integrative hypothesis is that negative emotionality (an affective vulnerability) in childhood contributes developmentally to more cognitive style and more rumination (cognitive vulnerabilities) in adolescence. In support of this hypothesis, Rothbart and Bates (1998) argued that temperament directly affects children's perception of the aversiveness of events. Negative emotionality may be associated with a greater perception of novel events as stressful (Costa, Somerfield, & McCrae, 1996). Children high in this temperamental characteristic may be more likely to experience intense negative affect in response to negative life events than children low on this dimension. Negative emotionality is also associated with greater attention to negative events (Derryberry & Reed, 1994), an increase in self-focus which is in turn associated with increased negative expectancies for the future (Pyszczynski, Holt, & Greenberg, 1987), and more focus on negative aspects of the self, other people, and the world (Watson & Clark, 1984).

In the last few years, there has been increased empirical investigation of the hypothesized relationship between negative emotionality and cognitive vulnerability. Several studies have demonstrated that trait negative emotionality is concurrently and prospectively associated with greater trait rumination among adolescents and adults (Chang, 2004; Feldner, Leen-Feldner, Zvolensky, & Lejuez, 2006; Mezulis, Priess, & Hyde, 2010; Verstracten, Vasey, Raes, & Bijtterbier, 2009). By contrast only a few studies have examined the relationship between negative emotionality and negative cognitive styles. Lengua and colleagues found that children's cognitive appraisals of negative events mediated the relationship between negative emotionality and depression, even after controlling for children's ratings of how emotionally upset each event made them. Mezulis and colleagues (2006), using data from the Wisconsin Study of Families and Work (WSFW), found that greater mother-rated withdrawal negativity in infancy interacted with child-reported negative life events in the past year to predict negative cognitive style at age 11. Children high in negative emotionality who experienced greater numbers of negative life events had the most negative cognitive styles. In followup analyses of the WSFW data, we have found that negative emotionality in infancy predicts cognitive style trajectories from ages 11 to 15; youth high in negative emotionality in infancy demonstrated markedly greater increases in negative cognitive style across this time period than youth low in negative emotionality (Mezulis, Funasaki, & Hyde, in press). Thus, the available evidence, although limited, supports the hypothesis that negative emotionality is associated with increased negative cognitive evaluations of negative events. Over time, this pattern of negative cognitive evaluations of events then contributes to the development of a stable negative cognitive style, which confers vulnerability to depression.

Our second integrative hypothesis is that early pubertal development (a biological vulnerability) contributes to greater OBC (a cognitive vulnerability) as well as elicits greater peer sexual harassment (a stressor). Various physical changes across the span of pubertal development (e.g., breast development and menarche) reorganize the girl's body image (Brooks-Gunn & Petersen, 1983; Koff, Rierdan, & Silverstone, 1978), which may itself be a stressor and may increase OBC. In particular, the weight gain associated with puberty makes girls—but not boys—feel overweight, which makes them vulnerable to depressed mood (Ge, Elder, Regnerus, & Cox, 2001). Pubertal changes also result in a changed social environment for girls; male peers react differently. Boys are more likely to sexualize the girls, and the girls are more likely to be the object of peer sexual harassment, as discussed below. Our data from the WSFW provide support for these hypotheses. We hypothesized that, especially for girls, pubertal development would lead to increased peer sexual harassment victimization (PSHV), and that PSHV, in turn, would heighten body surveillance. As hypothesized, stage of pubertal development at age 11 predicted the extent of later PSHV for girls but not boys (Petersen & Hyde, 2009). For girls at age 11, all paths in a path model were significant, indicating that pubertal development predicted PSHV, which in turn predicted greater OBC (Lindberg, Graber, & Hyde, 2007). The boys' model was significantly different, and the path from pubertal development to PSHV was not significant.

A third integrative hypothesis is that there is a behavioral and developmental link between genetic factors, specifically the *5-HTTLPR* polymorphism, and affective vulnerability, specifically temperament-based individual differences in negative emotionality. And, indeed, the *5-HTTLPR* region has been linked to negative emotionality in 2-month-old infants (Auerbach et al., 1999). This novel hypothesis is the least researched of the integrative hypotheses, but we eagerly await further research in this domain.

IMPLICATIONS OF THE ABC MODEL FOR THE PREVENTION OF DEPRESSION IN ADOLESCENT GIRLS

The ABC model is an integrative developmental model that emphasizes (1) vulnerability factors across multiple domains that may emerge and/or strengthen in the transition to adolescence, and (2) stressors across multiple domains that may increase in the transition to adolescence for all or some adolescents. As such, this model has several implications for clinical intervention. Below we articulate the three primary clinical implications of the ABC model. We argue that prevention efforts should target the reduction of established vulnerability factors; that prevention efforts should start prior to the surge in depression at around age 13; and that prevention efforts should take an individualized, modular approach to match interventions with the unique clinical presentation of each girl.

Implication 1: Target Vulnerability Factors

To date, three main types of interventions have been developed with the goal of preventing depression in youth. *Universal interventions* include all possible participants and are typically conducted in schools in large formats. *Selective interventions* target specific children, typically those who are at some elevated risk because of family history or some other predetermined vulnerability factor(s). *Indicated interventions* are those developed for children who are already showing some symptoms of depression (Horowitz & Garber, 2006).

Research shows that selective interventions—for example, those that select participants based on the presence of empirically validated vulnerability to depression but without requiring the current presence of depression symptoms—have the most promise to prevent depression in youth (Horowitz & Garber, 2006). However, most prevention programs use an indicated selection procedure with the most common enrollment criteria being elevated current symptoms rather than elevated vulnerability. When studies such as these find significant effects of treatment, it is difficult to know whether depression has been prevented or whether relapse has been prevented (e.g., see Clarke et al., 1995). The ABC model suggests that selecting participants based on known affective, biological, and cognitive vulnerabilities is a key component to the development of effective preventive interventions.

The ABC model hypothesizes that negative emotionality is a primary affective vulnerability factor which, in interaction with stress, may lead to the development of depression among girls. We conceptualize negative emotionality as highly negative, intense, and prolonged reactions to stressful events. As reviewed above, the ABC model hypothesizes that high negative emotionality is linked to depression and depressive symptoms in adolescence, both directly and indirectly, through its influence on the development of cognitive vulnerability. As such, future studies targeted to the prevention of depression in females should consider negative emotionality both as a selection criterion and as a target of intervention efforts. Interventions that improve girls' ability to identify negative emotional states and regulate their negative emotionality may help prevent depression. Many existing cognitive-behavioral interventions for depression include emotion labeling, arousal reduction, stress reduction, breathing, meditation, and relaxation components that are designed to help individuals cope better with stress. For example, the Penn Resiliency Program, discussed by Gillham and Chaplin in Chapter 11, includes a component focused on using deep breathing and relaxation as techniques for handling difficult emotions. Dialectical Behavior Therapy (DBT), originally designed for individuals with borderline personality disorder, includes emotion regulation and distress tolerance techniques that have been adapted for use in treating depression (Harley, Sprich, Safren, Jacobo, & Fava, 2008); suicidality (Miller, Rathus, & Linehan, 2007); and for use among adolescents (e.g., see Miller et al., 2006). However, these components are typically delivered clinically in conjunction with other more cognitive (e.g., thought restructuring) or behavioral (e.g., activity scheduling) techniques, so their impact specifically on reducing negative emotionality as a mediator in the reduction or prevention of depression is not well understood.

The timing of the pubertal process for girls has emerged as one of the most salient factors in negative psychological outcomes (Angold, Costello,

& Worthman, 1998), with an early start to puberty associated with negative outcomes in girls. The ABC model hypothesizes that early timing may be associated with additional body fat, peer harassment, self-surveillance, and body shame that may render girls particularly vulnerable to developing depression. Although most of the vulnerabilities within the biological component of the ABC model are beyond the purview of psychological intervention, age and pubertal stage for girls may present the most promising selection criterion to be used in identifying girls who could benefit the most from a preventive intervention. We suggest that interventions focused on maintaining a positive body image throughout the pubertal transition may be most successful.

Without doubt, the cognitive vulnerability components of the ABC model are the most supported by previous research and are the target of most existing interventions. The ABC model specifies that cognitive style and rumination are two of the primary cognitive vulnerabilities to depression in girls. These specific cognitive vulnerabilities could serve as selection criteria for preventive efforts, and previous research suggests at least moderate success with this method. Initial studies from the Penn Resiliency Program (PRP), which targeted university students identified as at risk for depression due to elevations on measures of cognitive vulnerability, found that participation in a prevention program based on cognitive-behavioral therapy (CBT) both reduced cognitive vulnerability and prevented depression across the transition to college (Seligman, Schulman, DeRubeis, & Hollon, 1999). Downward extensions of the PRP to younger adolescents have typically selected participants based on elevated symptoms or other at-risk variables (e.g., bereavement), but the ABC model would suggest that selection based on cognitive vulnerability elevations in early to middle adolescence would be a salient criterion. Similarly, mindfulness-based cognitive therapy (MBCT) has demonstrated success in specifically reducing rumination and thus in preventing depression relapse and recurrence (Ramel, Goldin, Carmona, & McQuaid, 2004). However, to date, MBCT has been examined primarily in adult patients with treatment-resistant depression, not among at-risk adolescents.

Implication 2: Target Girls before Age 13

Age and developmental stage are crucial components of the ABC model that are woven through each of the three main vulnerabilities. The ABC model hypothesizes that vulnerabilities to depression solidify in early adolescence and that depression arises in mid to late adolescence when youth begin to experience higher rates of stress. When stress begins to increase during the adolescent transition, these vulnerabilities come into effect, and depressive symptoms increase. Taken together, all previous research on vulnerabilities to depression for girls suggests that ages 8–13 are a particular time for prevention efforts. During this time period, cognitive style is solidifying, socio-cultural influences and the peer milieu are becoming dominant, and the large majority of girls are entering puberty. These early adolescents are just beginning the process of determining their self-image and how they will relate to the outer world, and they have yet to enter the stressful world of secondary schooling, dating and sexuality maturity, and employment. This makes 8 to 13 a ripe time period for prevention efforts. Because vulnerabilities are not yet fully formed, interventions to modify these vulnerabilities have the highest chance of success. In early adolescence children are, metaphorically, getting ready to set sail into the world. It is much easier to help them board a different boat before departure than to transfer them to a different boat a few years later.

One of the most promising interventions among adolescent girls is Stark and colleagues' Taking Action program (see Stark et al., 2008). The program specifically targets currently depressed or dysthmic girls ages 9–13, and it works with girls in small groups to teach CBT-based emotion regulation, coping, and cognitive restructuring skills. We eagerly await further details about the efficacy of this intervention.

Implication 3: Tailor Interventions to the Girl

Overall, the ABC model suggests that effective prevention efforts should reflect a modular, personalized approach, with specific treatment techniques being selected to target specific individuals based on age and vulnerability. Some girls may be very high in affective vulnerability but not report OBC. Other girls may be particularly cognitively vulnerable, reporting high negative cognitive style and rumination. Yet other girls may be vulnerable to depression primarily as a result of early puberty and the accompanying OBC and sexual harassment. Each of these girls, the ABC model hypothesizes, would respond best to a different set of interventions.

For example, girls who report high negative emotionality may respond best to interventions focusing on reducing negative emotional reactivity and increasing distress tolerance, such as those discussed above within the PRP and DBT.

By contrast, girls reporting high cognitive vulnerability to depression may respond best to interventions targeting rumination and negative cognitive style. The overwhelming majority of interventions for adolescents with depression or those to prevent depression to date have focused on these cognitive vulnerabilities (e.g., the PRP, Adolescent Coping with Depression Course [CWD-A], and the ACTION program). These interventions vary in their content and delivery method, but most include mindfulness, to target rumination, and cognitive therapy, to target distorted cognitions and negative cognitive style. As we mentioned earlier, the effectiveness of these interventions for the prevention of depression among early adolescent girls has yet to be firmly established.

Furthermore, the ABC model suggests that future interventions might be developed in a modular way. Manualized treatments could be developed with sections devoted to reducing certain components of each of the three vulnerabilities within the ABC model. For example, within the domain of affective vulnerability, sections could be developed that are targeted specifically to reducing emotional reactivity and developing positive emotionality. To address biologically based challenges, chapters could focus on skills such as coping with early puberty. Other treatments could be aimed specifically toward ameliorating cognitive vulnerabilities, such as rumination. Clinicians could then select the appropriate sections of the intervention to match the needs of each individual and deliver a tailored preventive intervention. This method would also allow researchers to evaluate the effects of interventions in a more systematic and meaningful way.

REFERENCES

Abela, J. (2001). The hopelessness theory of depression: A test of the diathesis–stress and causal mediation components in third and seventh grade children. *Journal of Abnormal Child Psychology, 29,* 241–254.

Abramson, L., Alloy, L., Hankin, B., Haeffel, G., MacCoon, D., & Gibb, B. (2001). Cognitive vulnerability–stress models of depression in a self-regulatory and psychobiological context. In I. Gotlib & C. Hammen (Eds.), *Handbook of depression* (3rd ed.). New York: Guilford Press.

Abramson, L., Alloy, L., Hogan, M., Whitehouse, W., Donovan, P., Rose, D., et al. (1999). Cognitive vulnerability to depression: Theory and evidence. *Journal of Cognitive Psychotherapy, 13,* 5–20.

Abramson, L., Metalsky, G., & Alloy, L. (1989). Hopelessness depression: A theory-based subtype of depression. *Psychological Review, 96,* 358–372.

Allen, M. T., & Matthews, K. A. (1997). Hemodynamic responses to laboratory stressors in children and adolescents: The influences of age, race, and gender. *Psychophysiology, 34,* 329–339.

Alloy, L., Abramson, L., Gibb, B. E., Crossfield, A. G., Pieracci, A. M., Spasojevic, J., et al. (2004). Developmental antecedents of cognitive vulnerability to depression: Review of findings from the cognitive vulnerability to depression project. *Journal of Cognitive Psychotherapy, 18,* 115–133.

Alloy, L., Abramson, L., Hogan, M., Whitehouse, W., Rose, D., Robinson, M., et al. (2000). The Temple–Wisconsin Cognitive Vulnerability to Depression (CVD) Project: Lifetime history of Axis I psychopathology in individuals at high and low cognitive risk for depression. *Journal of Abnormal Psychology, 109,* 403–418.

Altemus, M. (2006). Sex differences in depression and anxiety disorders: Potential biological determinants. *Hormones and Behavior, 50,* 534–538.

Anderson, J., Williams, S., McGee, R., & Silva, P. (1987). DSM-III disorders in preadolescent children: Prevalence in a large sample from the general population. *Archives of General Psychiatry, 44,* 69–76.

Angold, A., Costello, E., Erkanli, A., & Worthman, C. (1999). Pubertal changes in hormone levels and depression in girls. *Psychological Medicine, 29,* 1043–1053.

Angold, A., Costello, E., & Worthman, C. (1998). Puberty and depression: The roles of age, pubertal status and pubertal timing. *Psychological Medicine, 28,* 51–61.

Arlt, W., Callies, F., van Vlijmen, C., Koehler, I., Reincke, M., Bidlingmaier, M., et al. (1999). Dehydroepiandrosterone replacement in women with adrenal insufficiency. *New England Journal of Medicine, 341,* 1013–1020.

Auerbach, J., Geller, V., Lezer, S., Shinwell, E., Belmaker, R. H., Levine, J., et al. (1999). Dopamine D4 receptor D4DR and serotonin transporter promoter (*5-HTTLPR*) polymorphisms in the determination of temperament in 2-month-old infants. *Molecular Psychiatry, 4,* 369–373.

Belsky, J., Hsieh, K., & Crnic, K. (1996). Infant positive and negative emotionality: One dimension or two? *Developmental Psychology, 32,* 289–298.

Beyer, C., Pawlak, J., Brito, V., Karolczak, M., Ivanova, T., & Kuppers, E. (2003). Regulation of gene expression in the developing midbrain by estrogen. *Annals of the New York Academy of Sciences, 1007,* 17–28.

Booth, A., Johnson, D., & Granger, D. (1999). Testosterone and men's depression: The role of social behavior. *Journal of Health and Social Behavior, 40,* 130–140.

Booth, A., Johnson, D. R., Granger, D. A., Crouter, A., & McHale, S. (2003). Testosterone and child and adolescent adjustment: The moderating role of parent–child relationships. *Developmental Psychology, 39,* 85–98.

Broderick, P. C. (1998). Early adolescent gender differences in the use of ruminative and distracting coping strategies. *Journal of Early Adolescence, 18,* 173–191.

Broderick, P. C., & Korteland, C. (2004). A prospective study of rumination and depression in early adolescence. *Clinical Child Psychology and Psychiatry, 9,* 383–394.

Brooks-Gunn, J., & Petersen, A. (Eds.). (1983). *Girls at puberty: Biological and psychosocial perspectives.* New York: Plenum Press.

Brooks-Gunn, J., & Warren, M. (1989). Biological and social contributions to negative affect in young adolescent girls. *Child Development, 60,* 40–55.

Brown, S. M., Peet, E., Manuck, S. B., Williamson, D. E., Dahl, R. E., Ferrell, R. E., et al. (2005). A regulatory variant of the human tryptophan hydroxylase-2 gene biases amygdale reactivity. *Molecular Psychiatry, 10,* 884–888.

Buss, A., & Plomin, R. (1986). The EAS approach to temperament. In R. Plomin & J. Dunn (Eds.), *The study of temperament: Changes, continuities, and challenges* (pp. 67–77). Hillsdale, NJ: Erlbaum.

Caspi, A., Henry, B., McGee, R. O., Moffit, T. E., Silva, P. A., et al. (1995). Temperamental origins of child and adolescent behavior problems: From age three to fifteen. *Child Development, 66,* 55–68.

Caspi, A., Lynam, D., Moffitt, T. E., & Silva, P. (1993). Unraveling girls' delinquency: Biological, dispositional, and contextual contributions to adolescent misbehavior. *Developmental Psychology, 29,* 19–30.

Caspi, A., & Moffitt, T. (1991). Individual differences are accentuated during periods of social change: The sample case of girls at puberty. *Journal of Personality and Social Psychology, 61,* 157–168.

Caspi, A., Sugden, K., Moffitt, T. E., Taylor, A., Craig, I. W., Harrington, H., et al. (2003). Influence of life stress on depression: Moderation by a polymorphism in the *5-HTT* gene. *Science, 301,* 386–389.

Chang, E. C. (2004). Distinguishing between ruminative and distractive responses in dysphoric college students: Does indication of past depression make a difference? *Personality and Individual Differences, 36,* 845–855.

Charbonneau, A., Mezulis, A., & Hyde, J.S. (2009). Stress and emotional reactivity as explanations for gender differences in adolescents' depressive symptoms. *Journal of Youth and Adolescence, 38,* 1050–1058.

Cicchetti, D., & Rogosch, F. A. (1996). Equifinality and multifinality in developmental psychopathology. *Development and Psychopathology, 8,* 597–600.

Clark, L. A., & Watson, D. (1991). Tripartite model of anxiety and depression: Psychometric evidence and taxonomic implications. *Journal of Abnormal Psychology, 100,* 316–336.

Clark, L. A., Watson, D., & Mineka, S. (1994). Temperament, personality, and the mood and anxiety disorders. *Journal of Abnormal Psychology, 103,* 103–116.

Clarke, G. N., Hawkins, W., Murphy, M., Sheeber, L. B., Lewinsohn, P. M., & Seeley, J. R. (1995). Targeted prevention of unipolar depressive disorder in an at-risk sample of high school adolescents: A randomized trial of a group cognitive intervention. *Journal of the American Academy of Child and Adolescent Psychiatry, 34,* 312–321.

Cohen, P., Cohen, J., Kasen, S., Velez, C., Hartmark, C., Johnson, J., et al. (1993). An epidemiological study of disorders in late childhood and adolescence: I. Age- and gender-specific prevalence. *Journal of Child Psychology and Psychiatry, 34,* 851–867.

Colder, C. R., Mott, J. A., & Berman, A. S. (2002). The interactive effects of infant activity level and fear on growth trajectories of early childhood behavior problems. *Development and Psychopathology, 14,* 1–23.

Cole, D. A., Ciesla, J. A., Dallaire, D. H., Jacquez, F. M., Pineda, A. Q., et al. (2008). Emergence of attributional style and its relation to depressive symptoms. *Journal of Abnormal Psychology, 117*(1), 16–31.

Compas, B. E., Davis, G., & Forsythe, C. (1985). Characteristics of life events during adolescence. *American Journal of Community Psychology, 13,* 677–691.

Compas, B. E., Malcarne, V. L., & Fondacaro, K. M. (1988). Coping with stressful events in older children and young adolescents. *Journal of Consulting and Clinical Psychology, 56,* 405–411.

Costa, P. T., Somerfield, M. R., & McCrae, R. R. (1996). Personality and coping: A reconceptualization. In M. Zeidner & N. Endler (Eds.), *Handbook of coping: Theory, research, applications* (pp. 44–61). New York: Wiley.

Crick, N. R., Casas, J. F., & Nelson, D. A. (2002). Toward a more comprehensive understanding of peer maltreatment: Studies of relational victimization. *Current Directions in Psychological Science, 11,* 98–101.

Cyranowski, J., Frank, E., Young, E., & Shear, K. (2000). Adolescent onset of the gender difference in lifetime rates of major depression: A theoretical model. *Archives of General Psychiatry, 57,* 21–27.

Davies, P., & Windle, M. (1997). Gender-specific pathways between maternal depressive symptoms, family discord, and adolescent adjustment. *Developmental Psychology, 33,* 657–668.

Davies, P., & Windle, M. (2001). Interparental discord and adolescent adjustment trajectories: The potentiating and protective role of intrapersonal attributes. *Child Development, 72,* 1163–1178.

Davis, M., Matthews, K., & Twamley, E. (1999). Is life more difficult on Mars or Venus?: A meta-analytic review of sex differences in major and minor life events. *Annals of Behavioral Medicine, 21,* 83–97.

Derryberry, D., & Reed, M. (1994). Temperament and attention: Orienting toward and away from positive and negative signals. *Journal of Personality and Social Psychology, 66,* 1128–1139.

De Vries, G. J. (2004). Minireview: Sex differences in adult and developing brains: Compensation, compensation, compensation. *Endocrinology, 145,* 1063–1068.

Eley, T. C., Sugden, K., Corsico, A., Gregory, A. M., Sham, P., McGuffin, P., et al. (2004). Gene–environment interaction analysis of serotonin system markers with adolescent depression. *Molecular Psychiatry, 9,* 908–915.

Else-Quest, N., Hyde, J., Goldsmith, H., & Van Hulle, C. (2006). Gender differences in temperament: A meta-analysis. *Psychological Bulletin, 132,* 33–72.

Feldner, M. T., Leen-Feldner, E. W., Zvolensky, M. J., & Lejuez, C. W. (2006). Examining the association between rumination, negative affectivity, and negative affect induced by a paced auditory serial addition task. *Journal of Behavior Therapy and Experimental Psychiatry, 37,* 171–187.

Fredrickson, B., & Roberts, T. (1997). Objectification theory: Toward understanding women's lived experiences and mental health risks. *Psychology of Women Quarterly, 21,* 173–206.

Garber, J., & Flynn, C. (2001). Predictors of depressive cognitions in young adolescents. *Cognitive Therapy and Research, 25,* 353–376.

Garber, J., Keiley, M., & Martin, N. (2002). Developmental trajectories of adolescents' depressive symptoms: Predictors of change. *Journal of Consulting and Clinical Psychology, 70,* 79–95.

Ge, X., Conger, R., & Elder, G. (1996). Coming of age too early: Pubertal influences on girls' vulnerability to psychological distress. *Child Development, 67,* 3386–3400.

Ge, X., Elder, G. H., Regnerus, M., & Cox, C. (2001). Pubertal transitions, perceptions of being overweight, and adolescents' psychological maladjustment: Gender and ethnic differences. *Social Psychology Quarterly, 64,* 363–375.

Ge, X., Lorenz, F., Conger, R., Elder, G., & Simons, R. (1994). Trajectories of stressful life events and depressive symptoms during adolescence. *Developmental Psychology, 30,* 467–483.

Gladstone, T., Kaslow, N., Seeley, J., & Lewinsohn, P. (1997). Sex differences, attributional style, and depressive symptoms among adolescents. *Journal of Abnormal Child Psychology, 25,* 297–305.

Goodyer, I. M., Ashby, L., Altham, P., Vize, C., & Cooper, P. (1993). Temperament and major depression in 11 to 16 year olds. *Journal of Child Psychology and Psychiatry, 34,* 1409–1423.

Goodyer, I. M., Herbert, J., Tamplin, A., & Altham, P. M. E. (2000). Recent life events, cortisol, dehydroepiandrosterone, and the onset of major depression in high-risk adolescents. *British Journal of Psychiatry, 177,* 499–504.

Grabe, S., Hyde, J. S., & Lindberg, S. M. (2007). Body objectification and depression in adolescents: The role of gender, shame, and rumination. *Psychology of Women Quarterly, 31,* 164–175.

Graber, J., Brooks-Gunn, J., & Warren, M. (1995). The antecedents of menarcheal age: Heredity, family environment, and stressful life events. *Child Development, 66,* 346–359.

Graber, J., Lewinsohn, P., Seeley, J., & Brooks-Gunn, J. (1997). Is psychopathology associated with the timing of pubertal development? *Journal of the American Academy of Child Adolescent Psychiatry, 36,* 1768–1776.

Granger, D., Shirtcliff, E., Zahn-Waxler, C., Usher, B., Klimes-Dougan, B., & Hastings, P. (2003). Salivary testosterone diurnal variation and psychopathology in adolescent males and females: Individual differences and developmental effects. *Development and Psychopathology, 15,* 431–449.

Grant, K., Compas, B., Stuhlmacher, A. F., Thurm, A. E., McMahon, S. D., & Halpert, J. A. (2003). Stressors and child and adolescent psychopathology: Moving from markers to mechanisms of risk. *Psychological Bulletin, 129,* 447–466.

Grumbach, M. M., & Styne, D. M. (1998). Puberty: Ontogeny, neuroendocrinology, physiology, and disorders. In J. D. Wilson et al. (Eds.), *Williams textbook of endocrinology* (9th ed., pp. 1509–1625). Philadelphia: Saunders.

Gutierrez, C., Arias, B., Gasto, C., Catalán, R., Papiol, S., Pintor, L., et al. (2004). Association analysis between a functional polymorphism in the monoamine oxidase A gene promoter and severe mood disorders. *Psychiatric Genetics, 14,* 203–208.

Halbreich, U., & Kahn, L. (2001). Role of estrogen in the aetiology and treatment of mood disorders. *CNS Drugs, 15,* 797–817.

Hankin, B., & Abramson, L. (2002). Measuring cognitive vulnerability to depression in adolescence: Reliability, validity, and gender differences. *Journal of Clinical Child and Adolescent Psychology, 31,* 491–504.

Hankin, B., Abramson, L., Moffitt, T., Silva, P., McGee, R., & Angell, K. (1998). Development of depression from preadolescence to young adulthood: Emerging gender differences in a 10-year longitudinal study. *Journal of Abnormal Psychology, 107,* 128–140.

Hankin, B., Abramson, L., & Siler, M. (2001). A prospective test of the hopelessness theory of depression in adolescence. *Cognitive Therapy and Research, 25,* 607–632.

Hariri, A. R., Drabant, E. M., & Weinberger, D. R. (2006). Imaging genetics: Perspectives from studies of genetically driven variation in serotonin function and corticolimbic affective processing. *Biological Psychiatry, 59,* 888–897.

Harley, R., Sprich, J., Sfren, S., Jacobo, M., & Fava, M. (2008). Adaptation of dialectical behavior therapy skills training group for treatment-resistant depression. *Journal of Nervous and Mental Disease, 196*(2), 136–143.

Harrington, R., Rutter, M., & Fombonne, E. (1996). Developmental pathways in depression: Multiple meanings, antecedents, and endpoints. *Development and Psychopathology, 8,* 601–616.

Hoefgen, B., Schulze, T. G., Ohlraun, S., von Widdem, O., Höfels, S., Gross, M., et al. (2005). The power of sample size and homogenous sampling: Association between the *5-HTTLPR* serotonin transporter polymorphism and major depressive disorder. *Biological Psychiatry, 57,* 247–251.

Horowitz, J. L., & Garber, J. (2006). The prevention of depressive symptoms in children and adolescents: A meta-analytic review. *Journal of Consulting and Clinical Psychology, 3,* 401–415.

Hyde, J.S., Mezulis, A., & Abramson, L.Y. (2008). The ABCs of depression: Integrating affective, biological, and cognitive models to explain the emergence of the gender difference in depression. *Psychological Review, 115,* 291–313.

Jabbi, M., Korf, J., Kema, I. P., Hartman, C., van der Pompe, G., Minderaa, R., et al. (2007). Convergent genetic modulation of the endocrine stress response involves polymorphic variations of *5-HTT*, COMT and MAOA. *Molecular Psychiatry, 12,* 483– 490.

Kaltiala-Heino, R., Kosunen, E., & Rimpela, M. (2003). Pubertal timing, sexual behaviour and self-reported depression in middle adolescence. *Journal of Adolescence, 26,* 531–545.

Kaufman, J., Yang, B. Z., Douglas-Palumberi, H., Houshyar, S., Lipschitz, D., Krystal, J. H., et al.(2004). Social supports and serotonin transporter gene moderate depression in maltreated children. *PNAS, 101,* 17316–17321.

Kazdin, A. E., & Weisz, J. R. (1998). Identifying and developing empirically supported child and adolescent treatments. *Journal of Consulting and Clinical Psychology, 66,* 19–36.

Kendler, K., Gardner, C., & Prescott, C. (2002). Toward a comprehensive developmental model for major depression in women. *American Journal of Psychiatry, 159,* 1133–1145.

Kendler, K., Karkowski, L., & Prescott, C. (1999). Causal relationship between stressful life events and the onset of major depression. *American Journal of Psychiatry, 156,* 837–841.

Kendler, K., Kuhn, J., Vittum, J., Prescott, C., & Riley, B. (2005). The interaction of stressful life events and a serotonin transporter polymorphism in the prediction of episodes of major depression. *Archives of General Psychiatry, 62,* 529–535.

Kessler, R., McGonagle, K., Swartz, M., Blazer, D., & Nelson, C. (1993). Sex and depression in the National Comorbidity Survey: I. Lifetime prevalence, chronicity, and recurrence. *Journal of Affective Disorders, 29,* 85–96.

Koff, E., Rierdan, J., & Silverstone, E. (1978). Changes of representation of body image as a function of menarcheal status. *Developmental Psychology 14,* 635–642.

Krueger, R. F., Caspi, A., Moffitt, T. E., Silva, P. A., & McGee, R. (1996). Personality traits are differentially linked to mental disorders: A multitrait–

multidiagnosis study of an adolescent birth cohort. *Journal of Abnormal Psychology, 105,* 299–312.

Larson, R. W., & Ham, M. (1993). Stress and "storm and stress" in adolescence: The relationship of negative events with dysphoric affect. *Developmental Psychology, 29,* 130–140.

Larson, R. W., & Richards, M. H. (1994). Family emotions: Do young adolescents and their parents experience the same states? *Journal of Research on Adolescence, 4,* 567–583.

Lazarus, R. S., & Launier, R. (1978). Stress-related transactions between the person and the environment. In L. A. Pervin & M. Lewis (Eds.), *Perspectives in interactional psychology* (pp. 287–327). New York: Plenum Press.

Lemonde, S., Turecki, G., Bakish, D., Du, L., Hrdina, P. D., Brown, C. D., et al. (2003). Impaired repression at a 5-hydroxytryptamine 1A receptor gene polymorphism associated with major depression and suicide. *Journal of Neuroscience, 23,* 8788–8799.

Lengua, L. J., Sandler, I. N., West, S. G., Wolchik, S. A., & Curran, P. J. (1999). Emotionality and self-regulation, threat appraisal, and coping in children of divorce. *Development and Psychopathology, 11,* 15–37.

Lengua, L. J., West, S. G., & Sandler, I. N. (1998). Temperament as a predictor of symptomatology in children: Addressing contamination of measures. *Child Development, 69*(1), 164–181.

Levinson, D. F. (2005). The genetics of depression: A review. *Biological Psychiatry, 60,* 84–92.

Lewinsohn, P., Joiner, T., & Rohde, P. (2001). Evaluation of cognitive diathesis-stress models in predicting major depressive disorder in adolescents. *Journal of Abnormal Psychology, 110,* 203–215.

Li, D., & He, L. (2006). Further clarification of the contribution of the tryptophan hydroxylase (TPH) gene to suicidal behavior using systematic allelic and genotypic meta-analyses. *Human Genetics, 119,* 233–240.

Lindberg, S. M., Grabe, S., & Hyde, J. S. (2007). Gender, pubertal development, and peer sexual harassment predict objectified body consciousness in early adolescence. *Journal of Research on Adolescence, 17,* 723–742.

Lindberg, S. M., Hyde, J. S., & McKinley, N. M. (2006). A measure of objectified body consciousness for pre-adolescent and adolescent youth. *Psychology of Women Quarterly, 30,* 65–76.

Marino, M., Galluzzo, P., & Ascenzi, P. (2006). Estrogen signaling multiple pathways to impact gene transcription. *Current Genomics, 7,* 497–508.

McKinley, N. M. (1998). Gender differences in undergraduates' body esteem: The mediating effect of objectified body consciousness and actual/ideal weight discrepancy. *Sex Roles, 39,* 113–123.

McKinley, N. M., & Hyde, J. (1996). The Objectified Body Conscious Scale: Development and validation. *Psychology of Women Quarterly, 20,* 181–215.

Mezulis, A., Abramson, L., & Hyde, J. S. (2002). Domain specificity of gender differences in rumination. *Journal of Cognitive Psychotherapy: An International Quarterly, 16,* 421–434.

Mezulis, A., Funasaki, K., & Hyde, J. S. (in press). Negative cognitive style trajectories in the transition to adolescence: Prediction from temperament, parenting, stress, and gender. *Journal of Clinical Child and Adolescent Psychology.*

Mezulis, A., Hyde, J. S., & Abramson, L. Y. (2006). The developmental origins of cognitive vulnerability to depression: Temperament, parenting, and negative life events. *Developmental Psychology, 42,* 1012–1025.

Mezulis, A. Priess, H., & Hyde, J. S. (in press). Rumination mediates the relationship between infant temperament and adolescent depressive symptoms. *Depression Research and Treatment.*

Miller, A. L., Rathus, J. H., & Linehan, M. M. (2007). *Dialectical behavior therapy with suicidal adolescents.* New York: Guilford Press.

Monroe, S. M., & Harkness, K. L. (2005). Life stress, the "kindling" hypothesis, and the recurrence of depression: Considerations from a life stress perspective. *Psychological Review, 112,* 417–445.

Muehlenkamp, J. J., & Saris-Baglama, R. N. (2002). Self-objectification and its psychological outcomes for college women. *Psychology of Women Quarterly, 26,* 371–379.

Neumeister, A., Young, T., & Stastny, J. (2004). Implications of genetic research on the role of serotonin in depression: Emphasis on the serotonin type 1A receptor and the serotonin transporter. *Psychopharmacology, 174,* 512–524.

Nobile, M., Cataldo, M. G., & Giorda, R. (1994). A case-control and family-based association study of the *5-HTTLPR* in pediatric-onset depressive disorders. *Biological Psychiatry, 56,* 292–295.

Nolen-Hoeksema, S. (1987). Sex differences in unipolar depression: Evidence and theory. *Psychological Bulletin, 101,* 259–282.

Nolen-Hoeksema, S. (1991). Responses to depression and their effects on the duration of depressive episodes. *Journal of Abnormal Psychology, 100,* 569–582.

Nolen-Hoeksema, S. (1994). An interactive model for the emergence of gender differences in depression in adolescence. *Journal of Research on Adolescence, 4,* 519–534.

Nolen-Hoeksema, S. (2000). The role of rumination in depressive disorders and mixed anxiety/depressive symptoms. *Journal of Abnormal Psychology, 109,* 504–511.

Nolen-Hoeksema, S. (2001). Gender differences in depression. *Current Directions in Psychological Science, 10,* 173–176.

Nolen-Hoeksema, S., & Girgus, J. (1994). The emergence of gender differences in depression during adolescence. *Psychological Bulletin, 115,* 424–443.

Nolen-Hoeksema, S., Girgus, J., & Seligman, M. (1992). Predictors and consequences of childhood depressive symptoms: A 5-year longitudinal study. *Journal of Abnormal Psychology, 101,* 405–422.

Nottelmann, E., Susman, E., Inoff-German, G., Cutler, G., Loriaux, D., & Chrousos, G. (1987). Developmental processes in early adolescence: Relationships between adolescent adjustment problems and chronological age, pubertal stage, and puberty-related serum hormone levels. *Journal of Pediatrics, 110,* 473–480.

Petersen, J., & Hyde, J. S. (2009). A longitudinal investigation of peer sexual harassment victimization in adolescence. *Journal of Adolescence, 32,* 1173–1188.

Phillips, B. M., Lonigan, C. J., Driscoll, K., & Hooe, E. S. (2002). Positive and negative affectivity in children: A multitrait-multimethod investigation. *Journal of Clinical Child and Adolescent Psychology, 31,* 465–479.

Pyszczynski, T., Holt, K., & Greenberg, J. (1987). Depression, self-focused attention, and expectancies for positive and negative future life events for self and others. *Journal of Personality and Social Psychology, 52*, 994–1001.

Ramel, W., Goldin, P., Carmona, P., & McQuaid, J. (2004). The effects of mindfulness meditation on cognitive processes and affect in patients with past depression. *Cognitive Therapy and Research, 28*, 433–445.

Remer, T., Boye, K. R., Hartmann, M. F., & Wudy, S. A. (2005). Urinary markers of adrenarche: Reference values in healthy subjects, aged 3–18 years. *Journal of Clinical Endocrinology and Metabolism, 90*, 2015–2021.

Rholes, W., Blackwell, J., Jordan, C., & Walters, C. (1980). A developmental study of learned helplessness. *Developmental Psychology, 16*, 616–624.

Roberts, S., & Kendler, K. (1999). Neuroticism and self-esteem as indices of the vulnerability to major depression in women. *Psychological Medicine, 29*, 1101–1109.

Rothbart, M., & Bates, J. (1998). Temperament. In W. Damon (Ed.), *Handbook of child psychology* (Vol. 3, pp. 105–176). New York: Wiley.

Rubinow, D. R., & Schmidt, P. J. (1996). Androgens, brain, and behavior. *American Journal of Psychiatry, 153*, 974–984.

Rubinow, D. R., Schmidt, P. J., & Roca, C. A. (1998). Estrogen–serotonin interactions: Implications for affective regulation. *Biological Psychiatry, 44*, 839–850.

Sanborn, K., & Hayward, C. (2003). Hormonal changes at puberty and the emergence of gender differences in internalizing disorders. In C. Hayward (Ed.), *Gender differences at puberty* (pp. 29–60). New York: Cambridge University Press.

Seligman, M. E. P., Schulman, P., DeRubeis, R. J., & Hollon, S. D. (1999). The prevention of depression and anxiety. *Prevention and Treatment, 2*(1). Available from *journals.apa.org/prevention/volume2/pre00200Ba.html*.

Shih, J. H., Eberhart, N. K., Hammen, C. L., & Brennan, P. A. (2006). Differential exposure and reactivity to interpersonal stress predict sex differences in adolescent depression. *Journal of Clinical Child and Adolescent Psychology, 35*, 103–115.

Sjöberg, R. L., Nilsson, K. W., Nordquist, N., Ohrvik, J., Leppert, J., et al. (2006). Development of depression: Sex and the interaction between environment and a promoter polymorphism of the serotonin transporter gene. *International Journal of Neuropsychopharmacology, 9*(4), 443–449.

Spear, L. P. (2000). The adolescent brain and age-related behavioral manifestations. *Neuroscience and Biobehavioral Reviews, 24*, 417–463.

Stark, K. D., Hargrave, J., Hersh, B., Greenberg, M., Herren, J., & Fisher, M. (2008). Treatment of childhood depression: The ACTION treatment program. In J. R. Z. Abela & B. L. Hankin. (Eds.), *Handbook of depression in children and adolescents*. New York: Guilford Press.

Stark, L., Spirito, A., Williams, C., & Guevremont, D. (1989). Common problems and coping strategies: I. Findings with normal adolescents. *Journal of Abnormal Child Psychology, 17*, 203–212.

Steiner, M., Dunn, E., & Born, L. (2003). Hormones and mood: From menarche to menopause and beyond. *Journal of Affective Disorders, 74*, 67–83.

Stice, E., Presnell, K., & Bearman, S. K. (2001). Relation of early menarche to depression, eating disorders, substance abuse, and comorbid psychopathology among adolescent girls. *Developmental Psychology, 37*, 608–619.

Stipek, D., & MacIver, D. (1989). Developmental change in children's assessment of intellectual competence. *Child Development, 60*, 521–538.

Sulcová, J., Hill, M., Hampl, R., & Stárka, L. (1997). Age and sex related differences in serum levels of unconjugated dehydroepiandrosterone and its sulphate in normal subjects. *Journal of Endocrinology, 154*, 57–62.

Sullivan, P., Neale, & Kendler, K. (2000). Genetic epidemiology of major depression: Review and meta-analysis. *American Journal of Psychiatry, 157*, 1552–1562.

Tamminga, C. A., Nemeroff, C. B., Blakely, R. D., Brady, L., Carter, C. S., Davis, K. L., et al. (2002). Developing novel treatments for mood disorders. *Biological Psychiatry, 52*, 589–609.

Tiggemann, M., & Kuring, J. K. (2004). The role of body objectification in disordered eating and depressed mood. *British Journal of Clinical Psychology, 43*, 299–311.

Tung, L., Abdel-Hafiz, H., Shen, T., Harvell, D., Nitao, L. K., Richer, J. K., et al. (2006). Progesterone receptors (PR)-B and -A regulate transcription by different mechanisms: AF-3 exerts regulatory control over coactivator binding to PR-B. *Molecular Endocrinology, 20*, 2656–2670.

van Broekhoven, F., & Verkes, R. (2003). Neurosteroids in depression: A review. *Psychopharmacology, 165*, 97–110.

Verstraeten, K., Vasey, M. W., Raes, F., & Bijtterbier, P. (2009). Temperament and risk for depressive symptoms in adolescence: Mediation by rumination and moderation by effortful control. *Journal of Abnormal Child Psychology, 37*, 349–361.

Wade, R. J., Cairney, J., & Pevalin, D. (2002). Emergence of gender differences in depression during adolescence: National panel results from three countries. *Journal of the American Academy of Child and Adolescent Psychiatry, 41*, 190–198.

Walther, D. J., Peter, J. U., Bashammakh, S., Hörtnagl, H., Voits, M., Fink, H., et al. (2003). Synthesis of serotonin by a second tryptophan hydroxylase isoform. *Science, 299*, 76.

Watson, D., & Clark, L. A. (1984). Negative affectivity: The disposition to experience aversive emotional states. *Psychological Bulletin, 96*, 465–490.

Wolkowitz, O. M., Reus, V., Keebler, A., Nelson, N., Friedland, M., Brizendine, L., et al. (1999). Double-blind treatment of major depression with dehydroepiandrosterone. *American Journal of Psychiatry, 156*, 646–649.

Yu, Y. W.-Y., Tsai, S.-J., Hong, C.-J., Chen, M.-C., & Yang, C.-W. (2005). Association study of a monoamine oxidase A gene promoter polymorphism with major depressive disorder and antidepressant response. *Neuropsychopharmacology, 30*, 1719–1723.

Zhao, W., Ma, C., Cheverud, J. M., & Wu, R. (2004). A unifying statistical model for QTL mapping of genotype × sex interaction for developmental trajectories. *Physiological Genomics, 19*, 218–227.

CHAPTER 5

The Public Costs of Depression in Adolescent Girls

E. Michael Foster, Brigitt Heier-Leitzell,
and the Conduct Problems Prevention Research Group

The public and societal costs of depression among adults are well documented. These costs manifest themselves in a variety of ways, including expenditures on mental health services, physical health services, and lost work time (Dewa, Lesage, Goering, & Craven, 2004; Lerner et al., 2004a, 2004b; Murray & Lopez, 1996; Pincus & Pettit, 2001; Wang et al., 2004). Data from the Global Burden of Disease study indicate that depression is now the fourth leading cause of burden among all diseases worldwide and accounts for approximately 12% of the years lived with a disability (Ustun, et al., 2004).

By comparison, the social and public costs of depression at younger ages have received virtually no attention. Depression is the most prevalent psychiatric diagnosis in girls, with about 20% experiencing depression during the second decade of life (Stice, Presnell, & Bearman, 2001). Symptoms experienced include irritability, feeling unloved, guilt, self-deprecation, perceived lack of ability, negative body image, social withdrawal, suicide attempt, reduced appetite, increased sleep, and reduced sleep (Kovacs, Obrosky, & Sherrill, 2003).

Using data from four communities, this article examines the public (or taxpayer) costs of depression—those costs that are likely to appear on public budgets. For the purpose of this paper we examined mental health, school, and juvenile justice costs. All costs were taken from years 7–13 of the study, when study participants were generally in grades 6–12, the ages at which depression usually first emerges.

PRIOR RESEARCH

Prior research demonstrates that young women suffering from depression are involved in a variety of behaviors that are costly for public agencies and taxpayers. These behaviors include the use of costly mental health services. Other research reveals that co-occurring conditions drive these costs even higher.

Use of Mental Health Services

Data from the 1996 Medical Expenditure Panel Survey (MEPS) revealed that the costs of medical and mental health services for depressed girls totaled $2,805 per year (year 2000 dollars) (Guevara, Mandell, Rostain, Zhao, & Hadley, converted to year 2000 dollars by the authors). These total costs were spread across several types of services, including office ($528), emergency room (ER) ($186), and inpatient care ($895). For children with anxiety, those costs were $2,003 per year with the breakdown of costs at $455, $272, and $466, respectively.

Glied and Neufeld (2001) also examined data from the 1996 MEPS and evaluated costs of treatment for children diagnosed with depression and manic depression (DMD). They found that these children used an average of $2,257 per year in mental health care, which was significantly greater than the $691 spent on the care of children with other mental illness. (These costs were converted to year 2000 prices.)

These analyses are limited to individuals with treatment costs. A key question yet to be answered is whether and how expenditures on mental health services reduce expenditures in other child-serving sectors, such as juvenile justice.

Other Costly Outcomes and Behaviors

Depressed girls also are at greater risk for substance abuse, suicide, and sexually transmitted disease (STD). Substance abuse is associated with depressive symptoms in girls (Kovacs et al., 2003). Smoking, alcohol use, heavy drinking, and inhalant use also are associated with depressive symptoms (Kubik, Lytle, Birnbaum, Murray, & Perry, 2003). Drug use creates a variety of public and social costs, including the costs of treatment, and, among those arrested for drug-related crime, the costs processing and incarceration.

Although less common, suicide is also an issue facing girls who are diagnosed with depression (Lewisohn, Rhode, Seeley, & Baldwin, 2001). Suicidal ideation and attempts also have been linked to high-risk behaviors, such as substance abuse (Hallfors et al., 2004).

Other risky behavior related to sexual activity creates still other costs, such as the costs of sexually transmitted disease. Shrier, Harris, Sternberg, and Beardslee (2001) found that girls with moderate, high, or very high levels of depressive symptoms were at a two to three times greater risk of contracting an STD compared to girls with low levels of depressive symptoms.

The Role of Comorbidities

The most common comorbid internalizing disorders are anxiety disorders. Overall, 25–50% of depressed children and adolescents have comorbid anxiety disorder (Axelson & Birmaher, 2001). Children and adolescents with depression and anxiety also tend to have more severe symptoms of depression than those who are diagnosed with depression alone (Axelson & Birmaher, 2001).

Conduct disorder is also common among depressed girls. The combination of anxiety and conduct disorder has been shown to increase the likelihood of substance use in adolescence (Meller & Borchardt, 1996). Children with these comorbid conditions also have been found to generate high service costs in both childhood and adulthood (Knapp, McCrone, Fombonne, Beecham, & Wostear, 2002).

MATERIALS AND METHODS

These analyses involved 283 girls from the Fast Track project, a multicohort, multisite longitudinal study of children who were at risk for emotional and/or behavioral problems. The study is being conducted at four sites across the United States (Durham, NC; Nashville, TN; Seattle, WA; and rural Pennsylvania (Conduct Problems Prevention Group, 1992, 1999a, 1999b, 2002, 2004).

Participants

The first stage in recruitment involved identifying high-poverty schools in the four-study communities. Three cohorts of at-risk children and their parents were identified in kindergarten through a multistage screening that incorporated both teacher and parent assessment (Lochman, 1995). Children who scored as "high risk" according to these assessments were invited to participate in the longitudinal study, which began with in-home interviews during the summer preceding first grade.

Since intervention included a school-based component, elementary schools were assigned to either the intervention or the control conditions. A normative sample was selected from the first cohort class rosters of kindergarten children attending the control schools (Lochman, 1995). When combined with the control group children and adjusted appropriately with probability weights, this group of children comprises a representative sample of children in the control schools.

Measures

Diagnostic and symptomatology data for depression and related conditions were collected using three measures: the NIMH Diagnostic Interview Schedule for Children (DISC), the Reynolds Child Depression Scale (RCDS), and the Seattle Personality Questionnaire for Young School-Aged Children— Revised (SPQ-R). Conduct disorder (CD) data also were obtained through the DISC. Anxiety data were obtained through two measures: The DISC and the SPQ-R. The DISC was administered during years 7 and 10 (grades 6 and 9), the RCDS was administered during years 4, 5, and 6 (grades 3, 4, and 5), and the SPQ-R was administered in year 4 (grade 3).

The measures of depression and anxiety were used to create three groups: those who were diagnosed according to the DISC or Reynolds in years 4, 5, 6, 7, or 10—a borderline group that was determined to have elevated symptoms according to the SPQ-R in year 4—and those who were neither diagnosed or considered to have elevated symptoms. The CD diagnosis contains four groups of girls: those with CD in either year 7 or 10; never CD but oppositional defiant disorder (ODD) in year 7 or 10; never CD or ODD in year 7 or 10 but elevated symptoms; and never CD or ODD or elevated symptoms.

We then took the girls who were either diagnosed with depression or showed elevated symptoms and determined who had a comorbid anxiety diagnosis or elevated symptoms and who had a comorbid CD or ODD diagnosis or elevated symptoms. All three main groups (depression, depression and anxiety, and depression and CD) were then used to analyze cost of mental health service use.

The Use of Services and Related Expenditures

Information on the use of mental health services was provided by parents on the Service Assessment for Children and Adolescents (SACA; Stiffman et al., 2000), including how many service visits or number of service days that had occurred in the last 12 months. In addition, parents provided annual information for whether or not their child required medications for emotional/behavioral problems. This information was first collected in year 7 of the project and is ongoing.

To calculate expenditures, information on service use was combined with per-unit costs (Hargreaves, Shumway, Hu, & Cuffel, 1998). This information was taken from record reviews of services being delivered to the Fast Track sample. The latter provided information on the unit costs of services included in billing records.

A limitation of these analyses is that we applied the same per-unit costs to facilities (within a given category) regardless of the diagnosis of the children involved. As a result, we may underestimate the cost of youth who are treated in more expensive or intensive settings. For this reason, our findings should be judged as conservative. Our analyses of public costs captures some aspects of broader social costs but not others. Although we are able to capture the obvious expenditures such as treatment and school costs, we do not have data on the financial impact of these behaviors on family and friends or the costs due to decreased quality of life that is ultimately the result of these negative behaviors. If we were able to measure these aspects, the costs borne by society would undoubtedly be even higher.

Note as well that our per-unit costs refer to the marginal costs incurred as a result of an additional individual. For example, the per-unit costs of detention in the juvenile justice system represent the costs of feeding and housing the detainee. We have not included related fixed costs, such as a relevant proportion of administrative costs. If depression were eliminated among adolescents, the scale of the juvenile justice system might be reduced, cutting these administrative costs. However, in this case, since girls represent only a minority of those detained, such a reduction seems unlikely.

Variables Used for Propensity–Score Matching

In the analyses described below, we matched the group of depressed young women with other young women in the study based on race, site, two reports of aggression from kindergarten teachers (Teachers Report Form [Edelbrock & Achenbach, 1984], a measure of cognitive ability [Woodcock, 1978; Woodcock, Johnson, & Mather, 1990] and a measure of behavior problems as reported by parents in the first year of the study [Chamberlain & Reid, 1987]).

We also included the demographic variables seen in Table 5.1 as well as a composite measure of each family's socioeconomic status. The measure combines information on parental education and occupational prestige.

RESULTS

Prevalence

Descriptive information on our sample is shown in Table 5.1. Out of 283 girls, 45 (16%) were either diagnosed with depression or showed elevated symptoms. Of the 45 depressed girls 60% were African American as com-

TABLE 5.1. Descriptive Information

	Depressed	Other	Total
Observations*	45	238	283
African American[†]	60%	40%	50%
Site			
Durham	14	60	74
Nashville	14	49	63
Pennsylvania	12	74	86
Seattle	5	55	60
Cohort			
1	16	145	161
2	16	52	68
3	13	41	54
No. of children in household (mean)	3.04	2.82	2.86
Mother is a high school dropout	24%	28%	28%
Biological father is present in household	24%	20%	20%
Caregiver's age at first birth (mean)	22.04	22.77	22.66
Socioeconomic status	22.73	25.05	24.68
Comorbid conduct disorder	31%	23%	24%
Comorbid anxiety disorder	58%	28%	33%

*$p < .01$ (the p-value pertains to the null hypothesis that the depressed and other girls did not differ); [†]$p < .05$.

pared to 48% of the nondepressed girls. The entire sample was divided relatively evenly by site, with the percent of depressed girls ranging from 8 (in Seattle) to 22% (in Nashville).

As one would expect, a girl's chance of experiencing depression is related to a range of risk factors. Depressed girls had slightly more children living in their household than nondepressed girls (a mean of 3.0 vs. 2.8). They were very similar in the percentage whose mother was a high school dropout (24% vs. 28%) and the percentage that had their biological father living in the household (24% for depressed girls and 20% for nondepressed girls). Caregivers' age at birth was slightly lower for depressed girls (22.0 years) than nondepressed girls (22.8).

Overall, the differences between depressed and other girls were smaller than anticipated. One explanation involves the setting of the study: By limiting data collection to poor areas, the sample was more homogeneous than would be a sample from a full range of communities. This comparability actually strengthens our analyses because the effect of depression on public costs likely was less confounded with the effect of other factors.

Table 5.2 provides a breakdown of the percentage, mean, median, and number of girls using mental health, medical, school, and juvenile justice services as well as the overall mean cost of the sample.

Mental Health Services

We first examined the entire sample and determined the percentage of the girls that used mental health services. Over the study period, the three costliest services were residential treatment center, group home, and in-home therapist with mean total costs of $8,779, $2,868, and $2,347, respectively. Of the girls who were depressed and used mental health services, the mean total cost of service use was $19,973, whereas those service users who were not depressed used only $2,790 worth of services.

Medical Services

Hospital use was the most expensive service used by depressed girls, with a mean cost of $3,845. Somewhat surprisingly, emergency room use among this population had the lowest mean cost of $615 and $479 for depressed and other girls, respectively. This finding is surprising because emergency rooms are often a frequent provider of health services for low-income populations like those represented here.

School Services

Many of the depressed girls also used school services, the costliest of which was special education ($13,510), with an overall school service cost of $18,552. Comparatively, those girls who were not depressed used, on average, only $7,708 worth of school services during the study period.

Juvenile Justice

Juvenile justice costs among depressed girls also were substantial, with a mean total cost of $1,275, of which $985 was associated with arrests. Non-depressed girls' juvenile justice costs were almost half at $582, with the majority of these costs also coming from arrests ($459). Table 5.3 provides a summary of service costs by comorbidity.

TABLE 5.2. Service Costs

	Depressed (n = 45)		Not depressed (n = 238)	
	Mean	Median	Mean	Median
Mental health services				
Day treatment center*	$701	$0	$89	$0
Drug/alcohol clinic†	$219	$0	$48	$0
Group home*	$2,868	$0	$199	$0
In-home therapist*	$2,347	$0	$205	$0
Outpatient counselor/therapist†	$773	$0	$330	$0
Outpatient mental health center*	$1,284	$0	$473	$0
Psychiatric hospital	$1,817	$0	$380	$0
Residential treatment center*	$8,779	$0	$662	$0
Family doctor	$65	$0	$26	$0
ER*	$73	$0	$16	$0
Medications†	$302	$0	$138	$0
School counseling†	$744	$58	$226	$0
Total mental health costs*	$19,973	$1,116	$2,790	$0
Medical services				
ER	$615	$413	$470	$0
Family doctor	$747	$498	$658	$581
Hospital*	$3,845	$0	$500	$0
Total medical costs*	$5,207	$1,407	$1,629	$829
School Services				
Special education*	$13,510	$0	$4,877	$0
Grade retention*	$5,042	$0	$2,831	$0
Total school service costs*	$18,552	$13,751	$7,708	$0
Juvenile justice				
Arrest	$985	$0	$459	$0
Detention center	$290	$0	$124	$0
Total juvenile justice costs	$1,275	$0	$582	$0
All costs*	$45,008	$24,647	$12,709	$5,525

*$p < .01$; †$p < .05$.

TABLE 5.3. Service Cost by Comorbidity

Expenditures	Raw difference (SE)	Adjusted difference (SE)	Doubly robust difference (SE)
Mental health	$17,182* ($4,096)	$21,280 ($15,034)	$22,211 ($14,379)
Medical	$3,578* ($1,265)	$647 ($649)	$704 ($930)
School services	$10,845* ($2,097)	$7,392 ($4,504)	$7,186 ($3,684)
Juvenile justice	$693 ($376)	$1,054 ($933)	$1,114 ($873)
All costs	$32,298* ($5,046)	$30,373 ($16,128)	$31,215 ($15,121)[†]
All costs (except mental health)	$15,116* ($2,510)	$9,093 ($4,723)	$9,005 ($3,890)[†]

*$p < .01$; [†]$p < .05$.

Are Higher Expenditures on Depressed Young Women Due to Depression Itself?

We examined this question using propensity–score matching. (In particular, we used kernel density matching [Heckman, Ichimura, & Todd, 1997, 1998]). In essence, this method estimates the counterfactual for the depressed young woman as a weighted average of women in the nondepressed group with similar propensity scores.) Our analyses were "doubly robust" in that we also included the covariates as regressors in the model predicting expenditures. Doing so ensures that differences between groups in the covariances are properly adjusted for, if either the model generating the propensity score or the linear model predicting the outcome is correct (Lee, 2005).

In general, we found that matching reduces but does not eliminate the between-group differences in expenditures. Table 5.4 presents adjusted between-group differences in expenditures for four broad categories of costs along with total expenditures. The table includes three sets of estimates: the unadjusted differences, the propensity–score adjusted difference (excluding the comorbid diagnoses), and a second set of propensity score differences that adjusted for comorbid CD and anxiety.

In general, the three sets of estimates were similar. Two broad patterns were apparent. First, comparing the unadjusted and first set of propensity–score estimates, the latter were actually larger—adjusting for the covariates increased the between-group difference in expenditures on mental health and medical expenditures. Controlling for the comorbid conditions, however, returned the estimates to levels roughly comparable to the unadjusted differences. The second pattern is that the standard errors increase sub-

TABLE 5.4. Matched and Unmatched Comparisons of Expenditures

Type of Costs	Difference	SE	p
Unadjusted			
Mental health	$ 17,183	$ 4,096	.00
Juvenile justice	$ 693	$ 376	.07
Medical	$ 3,578	$ 1,265	.00
School	$ 10,845	$ 2,097	.00
Total	$ 32,298	$ 5,046	.00
Adjusted (no comorbidities)			
Mental health	$ 22,435	$ 12,738	.08
Juvenile justice	$ 1,016	$ 777	.19
Medical	$ 5,654	$ 4,774	.24
School	$ 9,527	$ 3,403	.01
Total	$ 38,633	$ 13,764	.01
Adjusted (including comorbidities)			
Mental health	$ 22,211	$ 14,379	.12
Juvenile justice	$ 1,114	$ 873	.20
Medical	$ 704	$ 930	.45
School	$ 7,186	$ 3,684	.05
Total	$ 31,215	$ 15,121	.04

stantially across estimates. Adjusting for the covariates reduced statistical precision rather substantially.

DISCUSSION

Although aggressive boys receive more attention from policymakers and the media, our analyses demonstrate that depressed young women create substantial costs for taxpayers and other payors. In this sample, expenditures on mental health services for depressed girls were 5.0 times those for young women without a diagnosis of depression or elevated symptoms; school services, 1.8 times as large; and juvenile justice costs, 2.6 times as large. Comorbid conditions increased the costs of service use, but based on supplemental analysis we found that these comorbidites did not explain the effect of depression on these girls.

This chapter suggests that although depressed young woman may not be as disruptive in certain settings, such as the classroom, society can hardly afford to ignore them. These young women are costing taxpayers and society more generally an enormous amount of money. Although effective treatment may further inflate specialty mental health costs, these expenditures may generate cost savings in other settings (Foster, Qaseem, & Connor, 2004).

Our results show somewhat higher costs of treatment for depression than Guevara et al. (2003) and Glied and Neufeld (2001), but those authors considered both girls and boys, and the latter tend to have a lower incidence of internalizing disorders. Either way, all three studies demonstrate that treating children with depression is a significant public policy issue, and cost-effective treatment options need to be developed and implemented.

Although the project collected cost data on many services and multiple child-serving sectors, we have only scratched the surface of the potential costs to society. A full analysis of social costs would be extended in two ways. First, the outcomes considered here are associated with other costs not included in this analysis. The use of mental health services or involvement in juvenile courts, for example, creates costs beyond those appearing on public budgets. Such costs, for example, might involve time parents miss from work dealing with their children's problems. Even more generally, the crimes and offenses that lead to juvenile court involvement are associated with a range of costs experienced by victims. Those costs can be several times larger than the court and incarceration costs included here.

Secondly, some outcomes and behaviors are not included here. Those omitted include substance abuse, suicide, STDs, and teen pregnancy. Our cost estimates would no doubt increase still further if we were able to capture public and social costs related to these outcomes.

These costs would appear still larger if considered from a life course perspective. The costs of illness considered here may very likely continue into adulthood. Depression is often a chronic and sometimes debilitating illness. Although the form of the costs change (i.e., from school problems to employment problems), the societal impact remains, and the burden on taxpayers remains the same or even increases. Such a full cost of illness study is an area for future research (Kenkel, 1994)

Finally, although the current study focuses on the U.S. health system, the broader message most definitely has a cross-cultural impact: Depression, its comorbid disorders, and its potential outcomes are costly no matter where one lives. As stated earlier in the paper, the Global Burden of Disease project found that depression was the fourth leading cause of burden *worldwide*. Treatment and service costs exist in any society, although the payor facing the financial burden will vary depending on the structure of the health care system. Societal costs, such as the costs of school services and crime, also know no borders. Perhaps the most common cost that exists across cultures is the often unmeasurable price paid by the family and friends of depressed girls, who often are hardest hit by the effects of the disease. Costs associated with missed work time, stress, and overall deterioration of relationships are difficult to capture, but are nonetheless significant.

Another key finding is that the higher costs of depression are not easily explained by other risk factors associated with depression. Adjusting for an extensive list of covariates makes little difference. This finding has important implications. Unadjusted estimates of the costs of illness identify individuals who are especially costly. If illness, however, is correlated with other risk factors (as seems likely), then treatment may not produce benefits equal to the costs of illness. If the increased costs are attributable to the illness itself, then the potential cost savings accruing from treatment may be as large as the costs of illness.

Strengths and Limitations

This study has several strengths. The data are longitudinal and therefore provide us with detailed information on girls as they mature. The data also include an oversample of girls that is at greater risk of developing depression, CD, and anxiety. Therefore, because our results are directly applicable to girls who reside in high-risk environments, they will aid policymakers in determining what monies need to be set aside for treatment.

Limitations of this study include the fact that measures of service use are based on parental reports, and therefore underreporting of services may be a problem. Another limitation involves the per-unit costs to facilities. The same per-unit costs were applied regardless of the diagnosis of the girls involved, which may understate the service costs if certain girls are treated in more expensive or intensive settings.

Finally, because our results are based on the experiences of young women living in poor neighborhoods, these findings might not generalize to more affluent communities. On the other hand, our comparisons between girls with differing levels of internalizing symptomatology involve young women living within the same types of communities. For that reason, the comparisons across subgroups of young women more likely reflect the effects of depression, per se, rather than the effect of risk factors (e.g., neighborhood poverty) that represent risks for service use and for depression. In addition, the costs documented here are more likely to be public costs as the young women in the sample are likely to be enrolled in Medicaid or the State Children's Health Insurance Program.

ACKNOWLEDGMENTS

Members of the Conduct Problems Prevention Research Group include (in alphabetical order) Karen L. Bierman, Department of Psychology, Penn State University; John D. Coie, Department of Psychology, Duke University; Kenneth A. Dodge, Center for Child and Family Policy, Duke University; Mark T. Greenberg, Department of Human Development and Family Studies, Penn State University; John E. Lochman, Department of Psychology, University of Alabama; Robert J. McMahon, Department of Psychology, University of Washington; and Ellen E. Pinderhughes, Department of Child Development, Tufts University. This work was supported by National Institute of Mental Health (NIMH) Grant Nos. R18 MH48043, R18 MH50951, R18 MH50952, and R18 MH50953. The Center for Substance Abuse Prevention and the National Institute on Drug Abuse also have provided support for Fast Track through a memorandum of agreement with the NIMH. This work was also supported in part by Department of Education Grant No. S184U30002 and NIMH Grant Nos. K05MH00797 and K05MH01027. The economic analysis of the Fast Track project is supported through Grant No. R01MH62988.

REFERENCES

Axelson, D. A., & Birmaher, B. (2001). Relation between anxiety and depressive disorders in childhood and adolescence. *Depression and Anxiety, 14*(2), 67–78.

Chamberlain, P., & Reid, J. B. (1987). Parent observation and report of child symptoms. *Behavioral Assessment, 9,* 97–109.

Conduct Problems Prevention Research Group. (1992). A developmental and clinical model for the prevention of conduct disorders: The Fast Track Program. *Development and Psychopathology, 4,* 509–527.

Conduct Problems Prevention Research Group. (1999a)Initial impact of the fast track prevention trial for conduct problems: I. The High-risk sample. *Journal of Consulting and Clinical Psychology, 67*(5), 631–647.

Conduct Problems Prevention Research Group. (1999b). Initial impact of the fast track prevention trial for conduct problems: II. Classroom effects. *Journal of Cosulting and Clinical Psychology, 67*(5), 648–657.

Conduct Problems Prevention Research Group. (2002). Evaluation of the first three years of the Fast Track Prevention Trial with children at high risk for adolescent conduct problems. *Journal of Abnormal Child Psychology, 30,* 19–35.

Conduct Problems Prevention Research Group. (2004). The effects of the Fast Track program on serious problem outcomes at the end of elementary school. *Journal of Clinical Child and Adolescent Psychology, 33,* 650–661.

Dewa, C. S,, Lesage, A., Goering, P., & Craveen, M. (2004). Nature and prevalence of mental illness in the workplace. *Healthcare Papers, 5*(2), 12–25.

Edelbrock, C. S., & Achenbach, T. M. (1984). The teacher version of the Child Behavior Profile: I. Boys aged 6–11. *Journal of Consulting and Clinical Psychology, 52*(2), 207–217.

Foster, E. M., Qaseem, A., & Connor, T. (2004). Can better mental health services reduce the risk of juvenile justice system involvement? *American Journal of Public Health, 94*(5), 859–865.

Glied, S., & Neufeld, A. (2001). Service system finance: Implications for children with depression and manic depression. *Biological Psychiatry, 49*(12), 1128–1135.

Guevara, J. P., Mandell, D. S., Rostain, A. L., Zhao, H., & Hadley, T. R. (2003). National estimates of health services expenditures for children with behavioral disorders: An analysis of the medical expenditure panel survey. *Pediatrics, 112*(6, Pt. 1), 440–446.

Hallfors, D. D., Waller, M. W., Ford, C. A., Halpern, C. T., Brodish, P. H., & Iritani, B. (2004). Adolescent depression and suicide risk: Association with sex and drug behavior. *American Journal of Preventive Medicine, 27*(3), 224–231.

Hargreaves, W. A., Shumway, M., Hu, T. W., & Cuffel, B. (1999). *Cost–outcome methods for mental health.* New York: Academic Press.

Heckman, J. J., Ichimura, H., & Todd, P. E. (1997). Matching as an econometric evaluation estimator: Evidence from evaluating a job training program. *Review of Economic Studies, 64*(4), 605–654.

Heckman, J. J., Ichimura, H., & Todd, P. E. (1998). Matching as an econometric evaluation estimator. *Review of Economic Studies, 65*, 261–294.

Kenkel, D. (1994). Cost of illness approach. In D. Kenkel & R. Fabian (Eds.), *Valuing health for policy: An economic approach* (pp. 42–71). Chicago: University of Chicago Press.

Knapp, M., McCrone, P., Fombonne, E., Beecham, J., & Wostear, G. (2002). The Maudsley long-term follow-up of child and adolescent depression: 3. Impact of comorbid conduct disorder on service use and costs in adulthood. *British Journal of Psychiatry, 180*, 19–23.

Kovacs, M., Obrosky, D. S., & Sherrill, J. (2003). Developmental changes in the phenomenology of depression in girls compared to boys from childhood onward. *Journal of Affective Disorders, 74*(1), 33–48.

Kubik, M. Y., Lytle, L. A., Birnbaum, A. S., Murray, D. M., & Perry, C. L. (2003). Prevalence and correlates of depressive symptoms in young adolescents. *American Journal of Health Behavior, 27*(5), 546–553.

Lee, M.-J. (2005). *Micro-econometrics for policy, program, and treatment effects.* New York: Oxford University Press.

Lerner, D., Adler, D. A., Chang, H., Berndt, E. R., Irish, J. T., Lapitsky, L., et al. (2004a). The clinical and occupational correlates of work productivity loss among employed patients with depression. *Journal of Occupational and Environmental Medicine, 46*(Suppl. 6), S46–S55.

Lerner, D., Adler, D. A., Chang, H., Lapitsky, L., Hood, M. Y., Perissinotto, C., et al. (2004). Unemployment, job retention, and productivity loss among employees with depression. *Psychiatric Services, 55*(12), 1371–1378.

Lewinsohn, P. M., Rohde, P., Seeley, J. R., & Baldwin, C. L. (2001). Gender differences in suicide attempts from adolescence to young adulthood. *Journal of the American Academy of Child and Adolescent Psychiatry, 40*(4), 427–434.

Lochman, J. E. (1995). Screening of child behavior problems for prevention programs at school entry: The Conduct Problems Prevention Research Group. *Journal of Consulting and Clinical Psychology, 63*(4), 549–559.

Meller, W. H., & Borchardt, C. M. (1996). Comorbidity of major depression and conduct disorder. *Journal of Affective Disorders, 39*(2), 123–126.

Murray, C., & Lopez, A. (Eds.). (1996). *The global burden of disease: A comprehensive assessment of mortality and disability from diseases, injuries, and risk factors in 1990 and projected to 2020.* Cambridge, MA: Harvard School of Public Health.

Pincus, H. A., & Pettit, A. R. (2001). The societal costs of chronic major depression. *Journal of Clinical Psychiatry, 62*(Suppl. 6), 5–9.

Shrier, L. A., Harris, S. K., Sternberg, M., & Beardslee, W. R. (2001). Associations of depression, self-esteem, and substance use with sexual risk among adolescents. *Preventive Medicine, 33*(3), 179–189.

Stice, E., Presnell, K., & Bearman, S. K. (2001). Relation of early menarche to depression, eating disorders, substance abuse, and comorbid psychopathology among adolescent girls. *Developmental Psychology, 37*(5), 608–619.

Stiffman, A. R., Horwitz, S. M., Hoagwood, K., Compton, W., 3rd, Cottler, L., Bean, D. L., et al. (2000). The Service Assessment for Children and Adolescents (SACA): Adult and child reports. *Journal of the American Academy of Child and Adolescent Psychiatry, 39*(8), 1032–1039.

Ustun, T. B., Ayuso-Mateos, J. L., Chatterji, S., Mathers, C., & Murray, C. J. (2004). Global burden of depressive disorders in the year 2000. *British Journal of Psychiatry, 184,* 386–392.

Wang, P. S., Beck, A. L., Berglund, P., McKenas, D. K., Pronk, N. P., Simon, G. E., et al. (2004). Effects of major depression on moment-in-time work performance. *American Journal of Psychiatry, 161*(10), 1885–1891.

Woodcock, R. W. (1978). *Development and standardization of the Woodcock–Johnson Psycho-Educational Battery.* Hingham, MA: Teaching Resources.

Woodcock, R. W., Johnson, M. B., & Mather, N. (1990). *Woodcock–Johnson Tests of Cognitive Ability: Standard and supplemental batteries.* Allen, TX: DLM Teaching Resources.

CHAPTER 6

The Role of Rumination in Promoting and Preventing Depression in Adolescent Girls

Katie McLaughlin *and* Susan Nolen-Hoeksema

Any successful preventive intervention must target the important causal risk factors for the disorder that it is attempting to prevent (e.g., Kraemer, Stice, Kazdin, Offord, & Kupfer, 2001). An identification of those risk factors that are malleable and most predictive of the disorder in question is therefore the first step in designing an effective preventive intervention. Cognitive factors have long been implicated in depression (Abramson et al., 2002; Beck, 1967), and have been the focus of several preventive intervention programs (Clarke et al., 2001; Gillham, Reivich, Jaycox, & Seligman, 1995). One cognitive factor that has been strongly linked to depression is rumination, the tendency to repetitively and passively focus on symptoms of distress and the possible causes and consequences of these symptoms (Mor & Winquist, 2002; Nolen-Hoeksema, Wisco, & Lyubomirsky, 2008). The content of ruminative thought in depressed people is typically negative in valence, similar to the negative thoughts that have been studied extensively in other cognitive theories. We conceptualize rumination, however, as a process of perseverative thinking about one's feelings and problems rather than in terms of the specific content of thoughts. People prone to ruminating tend to rehash negative events from the past, worry about the future, and remain fixated on their current problems without moving into active problem solving.

A number of studies has shown that people who tend to ruminate in response to distress have longer and more severe periods of depressive symptoms and are more likely to develop major depressive disorder (see Nolen-Hoeksema et al., 2008). Moreover, women and girls are more likely to ruminate in response to distress than men or boys, and rumination has been shown to mediate the gender difference in depression in some studies (Nolen-Hoeksema & Hilt, 2009). Thus, rumination represents a good target for preventive intervention programs for girls at risk for depression.

In this chapter, we briefly review the evidence for rumination as a risk factor for depression, and the gender differences in rumination. We then discuss how existing preventative intervention programs may affect rumination, and how new interventions specifically target ruminative tendencies. Finally, we suggest ways that preventive intervention programs can be tailored particularly for girls with a tendency to ruminate.

RUMINATION, DEPRESSION, AND GENDER

Much of the research on rumination in depression has used the Ruminative Responses Scale of the Response Styles Questionnaire (Nolen-Hoeksema & Morrow, 1991). This scale asks respondents how often they engage in each of 22 ruminative thoughts or behaviors when they feel sad, blue, or depressed. These include responses that are self-focused (e.g., "I think 'Why do I react this way?'"), symptom-focused (e.g., "I think about how hard it is to concentrate"), and focused on the possible consequences and causes of one's mood (e.g., "I think 'I won't be able to do my job if I don't snap out of this'").

Prospective longitudinal studies of adults have shown that people who engage in rumination when distressed have more prolonged periods of depression and are more likely to develop depressive disorders (Just & Alloy, 1997; Kuehner & Weber, 1999; Nolan, Roberts, & Gotlib, 1998; Nolen-Hoeksema, 2000; Nolen-Hoeksema, Morrow, & Fredrickson, 1993; Nolen-Hoeksema, Parker, & Larson, 1994; Nolen-Hoeksema, Larson, & Grayson, 1999; Roberts, Gilboa, & Gotlib, 1998; Sarin, Abela, & Auerbach, 2005; Segerstrom, Tsao, Alden, & Craske, 2000; Spasojevic & Alloy, 2001; Wood, Saltzberg, Neale, Stone, & Rachmiel, 1990). Similarly, longitudinal studies of children and adolescents find that rumination predicts longer and more severe periods of depression (Abela, Brozina, & Haigh, 2002; Nolen-Hoeksema, Stice, Wade, & Bohon, 2007; Schwartz & Koenig, 1996).

Rumination appears to maintain and exacerbate depression through at least three mechanisms (for a review, see Nolen-Hoeksema et al., 2008). First, rumination leads depressed people to think more negatively about the past, the present, and the future. Dysphoric participants induced to ruminate recall more negative events from the past (Lyubomirsky, Caldwell,

& Nolen-Hoeksema, 1998), make more negative inferences about ongoing events (Lyubomirsky & Nolen-Hoeksema, 1995; Lyubomirsky, Tucker, Caldwell, & Berg, 1999), and are more hopeless about the future (Lyubomirsky & Nolen-Hoeksema, 1995), compared to dysphoric people distracted from their ruminations. Similarly, studies using people meeting criteria for major depressive disorder have found that those induced to ruminate subsequently show more negative thinking about themselves and the future than those in comparison induction conditions (Lavender & Watkins, 2004; Rimes & Watkins, 2005). Thus, rumination exercises enhances negative thinking, which in turn can exacerbate depression.

Second, even though depressed people often engage in rumination as an attempt to solve their problems, rumination appears to interfere with good problem solving. Dysphoric or clinically depressed people induced to ruminate generate less effective solutions to interpersonal problems compared to those distracted from their ruminations (Donaldson & Lam, 2004; Lyubomirsky et al., 1999; Lyubomirsky & Nolen-Hoeksema, 1995; Watkins & Baracaia, 2002; Watkins & Moulds, 2005). Even when they generate reasonable solutions to problems, depressed people who ruminate lack confidence in their solutions and are more hesitant about implementing them (Ward, Lyubomirsky, Sousa, & Nolen-Hoeksema, 2003). Thus, the problems of depressed ruminators may persist and worsen, further exacerbating their depression.

Third, people who persistently ruminate may annoy and drive away others (Schwartz & McCombs, 1995). A study of bereaved adults found that ruminators reached out for social support more than nonruminators, but reported more friction in their social networks (Nolen-Hoeksema & Davis, 1999), and that family and friends became frustrated with their continued need to talk about their loss (Nolen-Hoeksema & Larson, 1999). In addition, rumination is associated with the tendency to assume undue responsibility for the well-being of others (Nolen-Hoeksema & Jackson, 2001), dependency, neediness (Spasojevic & Alloy, 2001), and sociotropy (Gorski & Young, 2002). People who ruminate over anger-provoking events show greater desire for revenge after an interpersonal transgression or slight (e.g., "I want to see her hurt and miserable"; McCullough et al., 1998; McCullough, Bellah, Kilpatrick, & Johnson, 2001), as well as increased aggression following a provocation (Collins & Bell, 1997). Thus, ruminators may have interpersonal styles that drive away social support, further exacerbating their tendency toward depression.

Adult women are more likely to engage in rumination than adult men (Butler & Nolen-Hoeksema, 1994; Nolen-Hoeksema et al., 1993, 1999; Nolen-Hoeksema & Larson, 1999; Roberts et al., 1998; Ziegart & Kistner, 2002), and this gender difference in rumination mediates the gender difference in depression (Nolen-Hoeksema et al., 1999; Roberts et al., 1998). In children and adolescence, gender differences in rumination are also found in studies with larger sample sizes (Grant et al., 2004; Hampel & Petermann, 2005; Hilt, McLaughlin & Nolen-Hoeksema, 2010; Schwartz & Koenig, 1996), although not in studies with smaller sample sizes (Abela et al., 2002; Broderick & Korteland, 2004), suggesting that the magnitude of the gender difference in rumination is smaller in younger age groups than in adults. Thus, girls appear to have a somewhat greater tendency than boys to ruminate, and this gender difference may grow with age.

RATIONALE FOR INCLUDING RUMINATION AS A TARGET FOR PREVENTION PROGRAMS

Given the robustness of rumination as a risk factor for depressive symptoms and major depression in youth as well as adults (e.g., Abela et al., 2002; Nolen-Hoeksema et al., 2007; Schwartz & Koenig, 1996), rumination represents an excellent intervention target for prevention programs aimed at reducing the incidence of depression. Whereas many similarly robust risk factors for adolescent depression, such as maternal depression (Hammen, 1991; Hammen & Brennan, 2003) and early pubertal onset (e.g., Ge, Conger, & Elder, 2001; Hayward, Gotlib, Schraedly, & Litt, 1999), are more difficult to target with prevention programs, rumination represents a risk factor that may be malleable and thus amenable to intervention efforts. Moreover, decreasing rumination represents a particularly important goal for preventive interventions aimed at reducing the onset of depression among female adolescents, because rumination has been demonstrated to occur more commonly in this group (Grant et al., 2004; Hampel & Petermann, 2005) and to mediate the gender difference in depression in adolescents (Grant et al., 2004). As such, interventions aimed at preventing the onset of depression among adolescent females should include techniques designed to reduce engagement in rumination.

RUMINATION AND CURRENT PREVENTION PROGRAMS

The majority of preventive interventions for adolescent depression has been cognitive-behavioral in nature. The two effective prevention programs that have been most thoroughly evaluated are both cognitive-behavioral interventions: the Penn Resiliency Program (PRP; Jaycox, Reivich, Gillham, & Seligman, 1994; Gillham et al., 1995; Seligman, Schulman, DeRubeis, & Holland, 1999) and the Coping with Stress Course (Clarke et al., 1995, 2001). These interventions each include classic cognitive restructuring techniques borrowed from cognitive therapy for depression, and the PRP also includes a social problem-solving component. Classic cognitive therapy identifies core negative beliefs, dysfunctional attitudes, and the negative automatic thoughts that result from such beliefs and attitudes and attempts to replace them with alternatives that are more functionally adaptive (Beck, Rush, Shaw, & Emery, 1979). The social problem-solving techniques used in the PRP involve a multistep approach that includes identifying goals prior to acting, generating multiple solutions to problem situations, evaluating the positive and negative consequences of each solution, and choosing the most appropriate course of action (e.g., Gillham et al., 1995). Other prevention programs for adolescent depression, such as the Resourceful Adolescent Program (RAP; Shochet et al., 2001) and the Problem Solving for Life Program (PSLP; Spence, Sheffield, & Donovan, 2003), also utilize similar cognitive-behavioral techniques.

Techniques included in preventive interventions are typically adapted from effective treatments for the disorder being targeted. Consistent with this practice, the intervention techniques used in the aforementioned prevention programs form the basis of effective cognitive-behavioral therapy (CBT) for depression, including treatment of adolescent depression (e.g., Lewinsohn, Clarke, Hops, & Andrews, 1990; Clarke, DeBar, & Lewinoshn, 2003). In fact, the Coping with Stress course (Clarke et al., 1995) was adapted directly from the Adolescent Coping with Depression Course, a CBT intervention that has been found to be effective at treating adolescent depression (Lewinsohn et al., 1990; Clarke, Rohde, Lewinsohn, Hops, & Seeley, 1999). Although rumination may be indirectly affected by cognitive restructuring and social problem solving, these CBT techniques do not target rumination directly. Because cognitive restructuring addresses automatic negative thoughts and beliefs, some of the *content* of ruminative thinking may be influenced by this therapeutic approach. For example, individuals who are ruminating about the causes of their dysphoria may think that they are feeling distressed because they can never do anything right. Cognitive restructuring will identify that negative thought and attempt to replace it with one that is more adaptive. However, the *process* of rumination is not necessarily affected by cognitive restructuring. Because the process of abstract self-focus on symptoms and their meaning may be what leads rumination to be depressogenic in nature (e.g., Watkins & Moulds, 2005), the impact of cognitive restructuring on rumination may not lead to an improvement in depressive symptoms. Moreover, altering a specific negative thought likely does little to prevent the occurrence of future episodes of rumination about the causes and consequences of distress, given that the content of ruminative thought, and not the process itself, is affected. Future episodes of rumination are therefore just as likely to lead to the generation of other negative thoughts and beliefs about the self. Similarly, problem-solving training may ameliorate some of the specific contents of ruminative thought. For example, an individual whose rumination includes thoughts that he or she can never get things done at work may be able to utilize problem solving to develop better work habits and organization skills. But problem solving will not influence the extent to which that individual is likely to ruminate about other causes or consequences of his or her depressive symptoms.

Given that adolescent depression programs have primarily involved cognitive restructuring and problem-solving training, rumination has not been specifically targeted in such interventions. Existing prevention programs utilizing these techniques have been demonstrated to be effective at reducing depressive symptoms among samples of adolescents selected to be at high risk for developing depression (e.g., Clarke et al., 1995, 2001; Gillham et al., 1995). However, the efficacy of current prevention programs could be greatly improved. Recent meta-analyses examining the efficacy of preventive interventions targeting adolescent depression have concluded that targeted/indicated prevention programs are effective but that treatment effect sizes are small, and preventive effects are not maintained once the intervention ends; additionally, the results indicated that universal programs have not been effective at reducing depressive symptoms or onset of depressive episodes in study participants (Garber, Webb, & Horowitz, 2009; Merry, McDowell, Hetrick, Bur, & Muller, 2004). Moreover, no existing programs have been demonstrated to have significant preventive effects on the incidence of major depressive disorder. As such, the efficacy of prevention programs may be improved by including techniques that go beyond the cognitive restructuring and social problem-solving approaches that have formed the basis of current interventions. Specifically, inclusion of techniques targeting emotion regulation processes, particularly rumination, may lead to increased efficacy.

INTERVENTION TECHNIQUES
TARGETING RUMINATION

Rumination has only recently become the focus of specific therapeutic techniques in interventions for depressed individuals. Watkins and colleagues (2007) have created a cognitive-behavioral treatment for depression, rumination-focused cognitive-behavioral therapy (RFCBT), that was developed specifically to address depressive rumination as a residual symptom of depression and harbinger of future relapse. This intervention utilizes traditional CBT techniques for depression but also includes techniques specifically targeting rumination. The first of these techniques involves a functional-analytic and contextual approach to behavioral activation (see Jacobson, Martell, & Dimidjian, 2001). This intervention technique specifically targets rumination by attempting to improve the identification of maladaptive ruminative thoughts and their associated behaviors as well as triggers and warning signs of rumination. Further, this intervention strategy involves identification of and engagement in "counter-rumination behaviors" (Watkins et al., 2007) that represent adaptive alternatives to rumination (e.g., relaxation, problem solving) as well as changing environmental contingencies that maintain rumination.

The second technique included in RFCBT that specifically targets rumination involves the use of directed imagery. Exercises are designed to help individuals recall and relive past experiences in which they engaged in adaptive thinking. Specific examples provided by Watkins and colleagues (2007) of adaptive thinking experiences include being compassionate to others or being totally engrossed in an activity. The adaptive thinking occurrences that are recalled during imagery exercises are used as counter-rumination behaviors in which individuals can engage to prevent future episodes of rumination. RFCBT demonstrated initial efficacy in a group of individuals who met criteria for medication-refractory residual depression.

Kovacs and colleagues (2006) have developed an intervention for depression that specifically targets maladaptive emotion regulation strategies and responses to dysphoria that exacerbate negative mood. The intervention, contextual emotion regulation therapy (CERT) for depression, was developed for the treatment of childhood depression and is thus particularly relevant for prevention work targeting adolescent depression. CERT for depression was specifically designed to address children's self-regulation of distress and dysphoria; in particular, regulatory difficulties during periods of stress are conceptualized as direct precursors to the onset of depressive symptoms and represent the primary intervention target. The therapy focuses on identifying children's typical responses to distressing situations and categorizing them along important dimensions (e.g., behavioral vs. social/interpersonal; adaptive vs. maladaptive). A particular emphasis is placed on identifying the contexts that elicit maladaptive management of distress.

The focus of CERT for depression involves replacing habitual maladaptive responses to distress with alternative responses from the child's own repertoire of emotion regulation responses that ameliorate negative mood (Kovacs et al., 2006). If a child does not possess an adequate reserve of adaptive responses that can be substituted for those that maintain or worsen negative mood, instruction in the use of emotion regulation strategies occurs. Additional strategies are chosen from the category of responses that the child feels most comfortable using (e.g., cognitive strategies). Preliminary efficacy of CERT for depression was found in a pilot study examining the intervention among children with dysthymia, some of whom also met criteria for major depressive disorder. Treatment led to significant symptomatic improvement of both dysthymia and major depression for the majority of participants who completed the intervention protocol (Kovacs et al., 2006). Rumination is not specifically the focus of CERT for depression. However, given that rumination is a maladaptive response to distress that maintains and exacerbates dysphoria (e.g., Nolen-Hoeksema & Morrow, 1991; Nolen-Hoeksema et al., 1993, 1994; Just & Alloy, 1997), ruminative responses to depressed mood would undoubtedly be included as targets of this intervention.

Intervention techniques targeting rumination have only recently begun to appear in the depression treatment literature. The two existing treatments that include rumination as a focus of the intervention differ in important ways, including the target population (adults vs. children) and the target disorder (refractory major depression vs. dysthymia). Nonetheless, similarities in the techniques used in these interventions are evident. Both interventions utilize the basic CBT framework that has been demonstrated to be effective at treating depression, but they apply the therapeutic strategies specifically to rumination, rather than to other dysfunctional thoughts, attitudes, and behaviors. For example, both treatments utilize a functional behavioral analysis approach to help individuals identify instances when they engage in rumination and the contextual triggers/antecedents of rumination episodes. Additionally, both emphasize the identification of adaptive emotion regulation strategies and behaviors that can be engaged in instead of rumination. Finally, an individualized approach is utilized such that the types of adaptive responses that have worked for an individual in the past are identified to replace rumination, rather than dictating a "one-size-fits-all" approach to adaptive emotion regulation.

INCLUDING TECHNIQUES TARGETING RUMINATION IN PREVENTIVE INTERVENTIONS

The intervention techniques targeting rumination used in recent treatments for depressive disorders (Kovacs et al., 2006; Watkins et al., 2007) provide an excellent starting point for the development of approaches that incorporate rumination as a target of preventive interventions for adolescent depression. The functional behavioral analysis approach to rumination utilized by each of these treatments holds much promise for improving the efficacy of prevention programs. This traditional CBT approach aims to improve identification of the environmental and organismic antecedents, emotional and behavioral responses, and consequences (interpersonal, health, etc.) of a specific maladaptive behavior (see Goldfried & Davison, 1994). Application of this behavioral analysis to rumination specifically could easily be incorporated into preventive interventions for adolescent depression. The general approach of functional analysis is already included in the majority of interventions that use cognitive restructuring (PRP, Coping with Stress Course, etc.), meaning that the groundwork for using this therapeutic strategy is already in place. The only necessary change to such existing interventions would involve incorporating rumination as a specific target of this therapeutic technique. This would require inclusion of psychoeducation regarding rumination, its consequences, and methods for identifying rumination episodes. Similar to the approach used by Watkins and colleagues (2007), the goals of this technique include improved identification of moments of self-focus on feelings of dysphoria and their associated causes and consequences, identification of the triggers and contexts in which rumination occurs, and improved awareness of the consequences of rumination. These goals are rooted firmly within a contextual approach in which importance is placed on understanding the environmental and social contingencies that are associated with rumination. Furthermore, the development of planned alternatives to replace rumination, chosen from the individual's repertoire of existing adaptive behaviors and mood management techniques, represents a critical goal of this approach. This final goal likely requires the use of other techniques (discussed below) to identify adaptive behaviors and emotion regulation strategies that can be used as alternatives to engagement in rumination.

Behavioral activation intervention strategies are another avenue for targeting rumination specifically in preventive interventions. Behavioral activation has been demonstrated to be an effective strategy for treating major depression (e.g., Jacobson et al., 1996, 2001) and may also ameliorate rumination (see Nolen-Hoeksema et al., 2008). Moreover, recent intervention work has utilized this approach for targeting rumination specifically (Watkins et al., 2007). Additionally, behavioral activation may prevent the onset of depressive symptoms both by increasing positive reinforcement and reducing avoidance patterns *and* by helping individuals to generate adaptive behaviors that can be substituted for rumination—the final goal of the functional behavior analysis/behavior change strategies described above. However, preventive interventions for adolescent depression have largely not included behavioral activation components.

Current approaches to behavioral activation involve increasing both short-term positive reinforcement, by distracting individuals from negative moods with engagement in positive activities identified by them as functional and enjoyable, and long-term reinforcement, by helping individuals to break maladaptive avoidance patterns and to solve problems in their lives by generating alternative coping methods (Jacobson et al., 1996, 2001). Behavioral activation represents a feasible approach to use in prevention programs for adolescents. This approach entails, first, psychoeducation regarding the cycle between depressed mood, lowered activation/ engagement, and subsequently worsened mood. Generation of adaptive and enjoyable behaviors for individual participants follows, with a particular emphasis on activities being goal-directed (e.g., going to a movie with friends to increase social support) rather than mood-directed (e.g., going to a movie to feel less depressed; see Jacobson et al., 2001). Finally, a focus on incorporating positive activities into individual participants' lives in a way that will prevent depression, rather than random, nonscheduled engagement in activities, should be emphasized. For example, engagement in activities that are thought to be universally pleasurable (e.g., watching a favorite movie) may not necessarily have preventive effects for depressed mood. Rather, engagement in activities identified to be related to depressed mood for the individual participant is preferable (e.g., calling a friend when feeling lonely or isolated).

RUMINATION INTERVENTION STRATEGIES TARGETING FEMALES

The previously discussed intervention strategies represent approaches that are equally applicable to male and female adolescents. Because they target rumination, these techniques may be more effective at preventing depression for females than for males, but they are not exclusively applicable to females. In addition to these strategies, several intervention techniques that target female-specific risk factors related to rumination, co-rumination, and body dissatisfaction are discussed.

Co-rumination, a variant of depressive rumination that occurs in dyadic relationships, is another potential target for preventive interventions aimed specifically at female adolescents. Specifically, co-rumination involves extensive discussion and perseveration on problems, repeated speculation about problems, and focus on the negative feelings associated with problems in the context of conversations between friends or acquaintances (Rose, 2002). Co-rumination has been demonstrated to occur more often in female versus male friendships, particularly among adolescents, and to be related to concurrent increased closeness and positive friendship quality as well as to increased symptoms of anxiety and depression (Rose, 2006). Moreover, longitudinal evidence suggests that co-rumination leads to increased symptoms of depression and anxiety only among female friends (Rose, Carlson, & Walker, 2007), indicating that this risk factor for internalizing problems is gender-specific.

Targeting co-rumination among friends is another potentially effective strategy for preventing depression onset among female adolescents; however, intervention techniques targeting co-rumination are absent in the treatment literature. As such, the possible strategies suggested for reducing co-rumination are preliminary in nature. Unlike depressive rumination, co-rumination is associated with both positive and negative outcomes. Although risk for internalizing symptoms is increased among females who engage in this behavior, co-rumination also leads to improved friendship quality and closeness. Techniques targeting this behavior should thus aim to maintain the positive consequences of co-rumination while eliminating the deleterious ones. Maintaining the positive social adjustment outcomes associated with co-rumination is an important goal, given the salience of peer relationships during adolescence (e.g., Buhrmester & Furman, 1987; Larson & Richards, 1991; Eccles, 1999), and given the importance of social support deficits as a risk factor for the development of depression during this time period (e.g., Lewinsohn et al., 1994). The first step in reducing co-rumination likely involves psychoeducation regarding the negative effects of this behavior. Further directed examination of the specific aspects of co-rumination that are associated with positive social adjustment, such as self-disclosure (Camarena, Sarigiani, & Peterson, 1990) and social support (e.g., DuBois et al., 2002), may help adolescents identify the active ingredients that lead to positive social outcomes but do not require engagement in co-rumination, per se. Identification of methods that maintain self-disclosure and social support in dyadic relationships but do not involve repetitive focus on problems and negative feelings should also be encouraged. Another strategy that may ameliorate co-rumination involves problem-solving training. If active problem-solving occurs between members of the dyad to attempt to resolve the issues that are the focus of co-rumination, discussion of problems may be continued in an adaptive way. Encouragement of engagement in active problem solving, using traditionally effective approaches (e.g., Gillham et al., 1995) instead of repetitive speculation with no subsequent attempts to solve the problem, is thus another potentially effective strategy for reducing co-rumination.

A final intervention approach that may be helpful in preventing depression among adolescent females involves reducing rumination triggered by body image concerns and body dissatisfaction. Body dissatisfaction in adolescent females has been prospectively associated with the development of depressive symptoms over time (e.g., Graber, Brooks-Gunn, Paikoff, & Warren, 1994; Stice, Hayward, Cameron, Killen, & Taylor, 2000a; Stice & Bearman, 2001). Body dissatisfaction is also both a likely trigger for ruminative thoughts (e.g., negative mood triggered by body dissatisfaction may lead to rumination specifically about shape and weight concerns) and an identified cause of dysphoria during ruminative episodes (e.g., an adolescent ruminating about the causes of negative mood may identify body dissatisfaction as the culprit). Recent evidence suggests that symptoms of bulimia, including shape and weight concerns, prospectively predict increases in rumination among adolescent females (Nolen-Hoeksema et al., 2007). Rumination was also associated with the development of bulimic symptoms over time in this study, suggesting that body image concerns and rumination are strongly associated with one another, as well as with the development of depression, among adolescent females (Nolen-Hoeksema et al., 2007).

As such, targeting body dissatisfaction in female-specific preventive interventions will likely lead to reductions in rumination as well as in depressive symptoms. A dissonance preventive intervention, in which participants engage in exercises critiquing the thin ideal, has been shown to be effective at reducing body dissatisfaction and eating pathology in randomized trials (Stice, Chase, Stormer, & Appel, 2001; Matusek, Wendt, & Wiseman, 2004; Stice, Trost, & Chase, 2003). Utilization of these intervention procedures, outlined in detail elsewhere (Stice, Mazotti, Weibel, & Agras, 2000b; Stice et al., 2001), will likely improve the efficacy of preventive interventions for adolescent depression among females. Moreover, targeting body dissatisfaction along with rumination will likely increase the spectrum of pathology (e.g., depression, eating disorders) affected by such interventions. Given the expense associated with implementation of prevention programs, bundling intervention techniques that are applicable to more than one type of psychopathology will help to broaden the impact and justify the costs associated with these programs.

CONCLUSIONS

Rumination appears to be an important target for programs designed to prevent depression in adolescent girls. Existing cognitive-behavioral interventions may reduce rumination somewhat, but newer programs specifically targeting rumination hold promise of reducing this maladaptive mood regulation response even further. These new programs could be further adapted to focus specifically on behaviors and issues pertinent to adolescent girls, including co-rumination among friends and rumination about body image.

The reduction of depression risk in adolescent girls is a critical focus for future research and public health policy. Depression is the leading cause of disease-related disability in women worldwide (Murray & Lopez, 1996). The upsurge in depression for females occurs in early adolescence (Twenge & Nolen-Hoeksema, 2002). If we can prevent this upsurge, we can save women from lifetimes of recurrent depressive episodes, improving both their lives and the lives of those around them.

REFERENCES

Abela, J. R. Z., Brozina, K., & Haigh, E. P. (2002). An examination of the response-styles theory of depression in third- and seventh-grade children: A short-term longitudinal study. *Journal of Abnormal Child Psychology, 30,* 515–527.

Abramson, L. Y., Alloy, L. B., Hankin, B. L., Haeffel, G. J., MacCoon, D. G., & Gibb, B. E. (2002). Cognitive vulnerability–stress models of depression in a self-regulatory and psychobiological context. In I. H. Gotlib & C. L. Hammen (Eds.), *Handbook of depression* (pp. 268–294). New York: Guilford Press.

Beck, A. T. (1967). *Depression: Clinical, experimental and theoretical aspects.* New York: Harper & Row.

Beck, A. T., Rush, A. J., Shaw, B. F., & Emery, G. (1979). *Cognitive therapy of depression.* New York: Guilford Press.

Broderick, P. C., & Korteland, C. (2004). A prospective study of rumination and depression in early adolescence. *Clinical Child Psychology and Psychiatry, 9,* 383–394.

Buhrmester, D., & Furman, W. (1987). The development of companionship and intimacy. *Child Development, 58,* 1101–1113.

Butler, L. D., & Nolen-Hoeksema, S. (1994). Gender differences in responses to depressed mood in a college sample. *Sex Roles, 30,* 331–346.

Camarena, P. M., Sarigiani, P. A., & Peterson, A. C. (1990). Gender-specific pathways to intimacy in early adolescence. *Journal of Youth and Adolescence, 19,* 19–32.

Clarke, G. N., DeBar, L. L., & Lewinsohn, P. M. (2003). Cognitive-behavioral group treatment for adolescent depression. In A. E. Kazdin & J. R. Weisz (Eds.), *Evidence-based psychotherapies for children and adolescents* (pp. 120–134). New York: Guilford Press.

Clarke, G. N., Hawkins, W., Murphy, M., Sheeber, L. B., Lewinsohn, P. M., & Seeley, J. R. (1995). Targeted prevention of unipolar depressive disorder in an at-risk sample of high school adolescents: A randomized trial of a group cognitive intervention. *Journal of the American Academy of Child and Adolescent Psychiatry, 34,* 312–321.

Clarke, G. N., Hornbrook, M., Lynch, F., Polen, M., Gale, J., Beardslee, W., et al. (2001). A randomized trial of a group cognitive intervention for preventing depression in adolescent offspring of depressed parents. *Archives of General Psychiatry, 58,* 1127–1134.

Clarke, G. N., Rohde, P., Lewinsohn, P. M., Hops, H., & Seeley, J. R. (1999). Cognitive-behavioral treatment of adolescent depression: Efficacy of acute group treatment and booster sessions. *Journal of the American Academy of Child and Adolescent Psychiatry, 38,* 272–279.

Collins, K., & Bell, R. (1997). Personality and aggression: The Dissipation–Rumination Scale. *Personality and Individual Differences, 22,* 751–755.

Donaldson, C., & Lam, D. (2004). Rumination, mood and social problem-solving in major depression. *Psychological Medicine, 34,* 1309–1318.

DuBois, D. L., Burk-Braxton, C., Swenson, L. P., Tevendale, H. D., Lockerd, E. M., & Moran, B. L. (2002). Getting by with a little help from self and others:

Self-esteem and social support as resources during early adolescence. *Developmental Psychology, 38,* 822–839.

Eccles, J. S. (1999). The development of children ages 6 to 14. *Future of Children, 9,* 30–44.

Garber, J., Webb, C. A., & Horowitz, J. L. (2009). Prevention of depression in adolescents: A review of selective and indicated programs. In S. Nolen-Hoeksema & L. M. Hilt (Eds.), *Handbook of depression in adolescents* (pp. 619–660). New York: Taylor & Francis.

Ge, X., Conger, R. D., & Elder, H., Jr. (2001). Pubertal transition, stressful life events, and the emergence of gender differences in adolescent depressive symptoms. *Developmental Psychology, 37,* 401–417.

Gillham, J. E., Reivich, K. J., Freres, D. M., Chaplin, T. M., Shatté, A. J., Samuels, B., et al. (2007). School-based prevention of depressive symptoms: A randomized controlled study of the effectiveness and specificity of the Penn Resiliency Program. *Journal of Consulting and Clinical Psychology, 75,* 9–19.

Gillham, J. E., Reivich, K. J., Jaycox, L. H., & Seligman, M. E. P. (1995). Prevention of depressive symptoms in schoolchildren: Two-year follow-up. *Psychological Science, 6,* 343–351.

Goldfried, M. R., & Davison, G. C. (1994). *Clinical behavior therapy.* New York: Wiley.

Gorski, J., & Young, M. A. (2002). Sociotropy/autonomy, self-construal, response style, and gender in adolescents. *Personality and Individual Differences, 32,* 463–478.

Graber, J. A., Brooks-Gunn, J., Paikoff, R. L., & Warren, M. P. (1994). Prediction of eating problems: An 8-year study of adolescent girls. *Developmental Psychology, 30,* 823–834.

Grant, K. E., Lyons, A. L., Finkelstein, J. S., Conway, K. M., Reynolds, L. K., O'Koon, J. H., et al. (2004). Gender differences in rates of depressive symptoms among low-income, urban, African American youth: A test of two mediational hypotheses. *Journal of Youth and Adolescence, 33,* 523–533.

Hammen, C. L. (1991). *Depression runs in families: The social context of risk and resilience in children of depressed mothers.* New York: Springer-Verlag.

Hammen, C. L., & Brennan, P. A. (2003). Severity, chronicity, and timing of maternal depression and risk for adolescent offspring diagnoses in a community sample. *Archives of General Psychiatry, 60,* 253–258.

Hampel, P., & Petermann, F. (2005). Age and gender effects on coping in children and adolescents. *Journal of Youth and Adolescence, 34,* 73–83.

Hayward, C. L., Gotlib, I. H., Schraedley, P. K., & Litt, I. F. (1999). Ethnic differences in the association between pubertal status and symptoms of depression in adolescent girls. *Journal of Adolescent Health, 25,* 143–149.

Hilt, L., McLaughlin, L., & Nolen-Hoeksema, S. (2010). *Examination of the response styles theory in a community sample of young adolescents. Journal of Abnormal Child Psychology, 38*(4), 545–556.

Jacobson, N. S., Dobson, K. S., Truax, P. A., Addis, M. E., Koerner, K., Gollan, J. K., et al. (1996). A component analysis of cognitive-behavioral treatment for depression. *Journal of Consulting and Clinical Psychology, 64,* 295–304.

Jacobson, N. S., Martell, C. R., & Dimidjian, S. (2001). Behavioral activation treatment for depression: Returning to contextual roots. *Clinical Psychology: Science and Practice, 8,* 255–270.

Jaycox, L. H., Reivich, K. J., Gillham, J. E., & Seligman, M. E. P. (1994). Prevention of depressive symptoms in school children. *Behaviour Research and Therapy, 32,* 801–816.

Just, N., & Alloy, L. B. (1997). The response styles theory of depression: Tests and an extension of the theory. *Journal of Abnormal Psychology, 106,* 221–229.

Kovacs, M., Sherrill, J., George, C. J., Pollack, M., Tumuluru, R. V., & Ho, V. (2006). Contextual emotion-regulation therapy for childhood depression: Description and pilot testing of a new intervention. *Journal of the American Academy of Child and Adolescent Psychiatry, 45,* 892–903.

Kraemer, H. C., Stice, E., Kazdin, A., Offord, D., & Kupfer, D. (2001). How do risk factors work together?: Mediators, moderators, and independent, overlapping, and proxy risk factors. *American Journal of Psychiatry, 158,* 848–856.

Kuehner, C., & Weber, I. (1999). Responses to depression in unipolar depressed patients: An investigation of Nolen-Hoeksema's response styles theory. *Psychological Medicine, 29,* 1323–1333.

Larson, R., & Richards, M. H. (1991). Daily companionship in late childhood and early adolescence: Changing developmental contexts. *Child Development, 62,* 284–300.

Lavender, A., & Watkins, E. (2004). Rumination and future thinking in depression. *British Journal of Clinical Psychology, 43,* 129–142.

Lewinsohn, P. M., Clarke, G. N., Hops, H., & Andrews, J. (1990). Cognitive-behavioral group treatment of depression in adolescents. *Behavior Therapy, 21,* 385–401.

Lewinsohn, P. M., Roberts, R. E., Seeley, J. R., Rohde, P., Gotlib, I. H., & Hops, H. (1994). Adolescent psychopathology: II. Psychosocial risk factors for depression. *Journal of Abnormal Psychology, 103,* 302–315.

Lyubomirsky, S., Caldwell, N. D., & Nolen-Hoeksema, S. (1998). Effects of ruminative and distracting responses to depressed mood on retrieval of autobiographical memories. *Journal of Personality and Social Psychology, 75,* 166–177.

Lyubomirsky, S., & Nolen-Hoeksema, S. (1993). Self-perpetuating properties of dysphoric rumination. *Journal of Personality and Social Psychology, 65,* 339–349.

Lyubomirsky, S., & Nolen-Hoeksema, S. (1995). Effects of self-focused rumination on negative thinking and interpersonal problem solving. *Journal of Personality and Social Psychology, 69,* 176–190.

Lyubomirsky, S., Tucker, K. L., Caldwell, N. D., & Berg, K. (1999). Why ruminators are poor problem solvers: Clues from the phenomenology of dysphoric rumination. *Journal of Personality and Social Psychology, 77,* 1041–1060.

Matusek, J. A., Wendt, S. J., & Wiseman, C. V. (2004). Dissonance thin-ideal and didactic healthy behavior eating disorder prevention programs: Results from a controlled trial. *International Journal of Eating Disorders, 36,* 376–388.

McCullough, M. E., Bellah, C. G., Kilpatrick, S. D., & Johnson, J. L. (2001). Vengefulness: Relationships with forgiveness, rumination, well-being, and the Big Five. *Personality and Social Psychology Bulletin, 27,* 601–610.

McCullough, M. E., Rachal, K. C., Sandage, S. J., Worthington, E. L., Jr., Brown, S. W., & Hight, T. L. (1998). Interpersonal forgiving in close relationships: II. Theoretical elaboration and measurement. *Journal of Personality and Social Psychology, 75,* 1586–1603.

Merry, S., McDowell, H., Hetrick, S., Bir, J., & Muller, N. (2004). Psychological and/or educational interventions for the prevention of depression in children and adolescents. *Cochrane Database of Systematic Reviews, 2,* Article No. CD003380.

Mor, N., & Winquist, J. (2002). Self-focused attention and negative affect: A meta-analysis. *Psychological Bulletin, 128,* 638–662.

Murray, C., & Lopez, E. (Eds.). (1996). *The global burden of disease, injuries and risk factors in 1990 and projected to 2020.* Cambridge, MA: Harvard University Press.

Nolan, S. A., Roberts, J. E., & Gotlib, I. H. (1998). Neuroticism and ruminative response style as predictors of change in depressive symptomatology. *Cognitive Therapy and Research, 22,* 445–455.

Nolen-Hoeksema, S. (1991). Responses to depression and their effects on the duration of depressive episodes. *Journal of Abnormal Psychology, 100,* 569–582.

Nolen-Hoeksema, S. (2000). The role of rumination in depressive disorders and mixed anxiety/depressive symptoms. *Journal of Abnormal Psychology, 109,* 504–511.

Nolen-Hoeksema, S., & Davis, C. G. (1999). "Thanks for sharing that": Ruminators and their social support networks. *Journal of Personality and Social Psychology, 77,* 801–814.

Nolen-Hoeksema, S., & Hilt, L. (2009). Gender differences in depression. In I. H. Gotlib & C. L. Hammen (Eds.), *Handbook of depression* (Vol. 2, pp. 386–404). New York: Guilford Press.

Nolen-Hoeksema, S., & Jackson, B. (2001). Mediators of the gender difference in rumination. *Psychology of Women Quarterly, 25,* 37–47.

Nolen-Hoeksema, S., & Larson, J. (1999). *Coping with loss.* Mahwah, NJ: Erlbaum.

Nolen-Hoeksema, S., Larson, J., & Grayson, C. (1999). Explaining the gender difference in depressive symptoms. *Journal of Personality and Social Psychology, 77,* 1061–1072.

Nolen-Hoeksema, S., & Morrow, J. (1991). A prospective study of depression and posttraumatic stress symptoms after a natural disaster: The 1989 Loma Prieta earthquake. *Journal of Personality and Social Psychology, 61,* 115–121.

Nolen-Hoeksema, S., Morrow, J., & Fredrickson, B. L. (1993). Response styles and the duration of episodes of depressed mood. *Journal of Abnormal Psychology, 102,* 20–28.

Nolen-Hoeksema, S., Parker, L. E., & Larson, J. (1994). Ruminative coping with depressed mood following loss. *Journal of Personality and Social Psychology, 67,* 92–104.

Nolen-Hoeksema, S., Stice, E., Wade, E., & Bohon, C. (2007). Reciprocal relations between rumination and bulimic, substance abuse, and depressive symptoms in female adolescents. *Journal of Abnormal Psychology, 116,* 198–207.

Nolen-Hoeksema, S., Wisco, B., & Lyubomirsky, S. (2008). Rethinking rumination. *Perspectives on Psychological Science 3,* 400–424.

Rimes, K. A., & Watkins, E. (2005). The effects of self-focused rumination on global negative self-judgments in depression. *Behaviour Research and Therapy, 43,* 1673–1681.

Roberts, J. E., Gilboa, E., & Gotlib, I. H. (1998). Ruminative response style and vulnerability to episodes of dysphoria: Gender, neuroticism, and episode duration. *Cognitive Therapy and Research, 22,* 401–423.

Rose, A. (2002). Co-rumination in the friendships of girls and boys. *Child Development, 73,* 1830–1843.

Rose, A., Carlson, W., & Walker, E. M. (2007). Prospective associations of co-rumination with friendship and emotional adjustment: Considering the socioemotional trade-offs of co-rumination. *Developmental Psychology, 43*(4), 1019–1031.

Sarin, S., Abela, J. R. Z., & Auerbach, R. P. (2005). The response styles theory of depression: A test of specificity and causal mediation. *Cognition and Emotion, 19,* 751–761.

Schwartz, J. A. J., & Koenig, L. J. (1996). Response styles and negative affect among adolescents. *Cognitive Therapy and Research, 20,* 13–36.

Schwartz, J. L., & McCombs, T. A. (1995). Perceptions of coping responses exhibited in depressed males and females. *Journal of Social Behavior and Personality, 10,* 849–860.

Segerstrom, S. C., Tsao, J. C. I., Alden, L. E., & Craske, M. G. (2000). Worry and rumination: Repetitive thought as a concomitant and predictor of negative mood. *Cognitive Therapy and Research, 24,* 671–688.

Seligman, M. E. P., Schulman, P., DeRubeis, R. J., & Holland, S. P. (1999). The prevention of depression and anxiety. *Prevention and Treatment, 2,* Article 8.

Shochet, I., Dadds, M. R., Holland, D., Whitefield, K., Harnett, P. H., & Osgarby, H. M. (2001). The efficacy of a universal school-based program to prevent adolescent depression. *Journal of Clinical Child Psychology, 30,* 303–315.

Spasojevic, J., & Alloy, L. B. (2001). Rumination as a common mechanism relating depressive risk factors to depression. *Emotion, 1,* 25–37.

Spence, S. H., Sheffield, J. K., & Donovan, C. L. (2003). Preventing adolescent depression: Evaluation of the Problem Solving for Life Program. *Journal of Consulting and Clinical Psychology, 71,* 3–13.

Stice, E., & Bearman, S. K. (2001). Body image and eating disturbances prospectively predict growth in depressive symptoms in adolescent girls: A growth curve analysis. *Developmental Psychology, 37,* 597–607.

Stice, E., Chase, A., Stormer, S., & Appel, A. (2001). A randomized trial of a dissonance-based eating disorder prevention program. *International Journal of Eating Disorders, 29,* 247–262.

Stice, E., Hayward, C., Cameron, R., Killen, J. D., & Taylor, C. B. (2000a). Body-image and eating disturbances predict onset of depression in female adolescents: A longitudinal study. *Journal of Abnormal Psychology, 109,* 438–444.

Stice, E., Mazotti, L., Weibel, D., & Agras, W. S. (2000b). Dissonance prevention program decreases thin-ideal internalization, body dissatisfaction, dieting, negative affect, and bulimic symptoms: A preliminary experiment. *International Journal of Eating Disorders, 27,* 206–217.

Stice, E., Trost, A., & Chase, A. (2003). Healthy weight control and dissonance-based eating disorder prevention programs: Results from a controlled trial. *International Journal of Eating Disorders, 33,* 10–21.

Twenge, J. M., & Nolen-Hoeksema, S. (2002). Age, gender, race, SES, and birth cohort differences on the Children's Depression Inventory: A meta-analysis. *Journal of Abnormal Psychology, 111,* 578–588.

Ward, A., Lyubomirsky, S., Sousa, L., & Nolen-Hoeksema, S. (2003). Can't quite commit: Rumination and uncertainty. *Personality and Social Psychology Bulletin, 29,* 96–107.

Watkins, E., & Baracaia, S. (2002). Rumination and social problem-solving in depression. *Behaviour Research and Therapy, 40,* 1179–1189.

Watkins, E., & Moulds, M. (2005). Distinct modes of ruminative self-focus: Impact of abstract versus concrete rumination on problem solving in depression. *Emotion, 5,* 319–328.

Watkins, E., Scott, J., Wingrove, J., Rimes, K., Bathurst, N., Steiner, H., et al. (2007). Rumination-focused cognitive behaviour therapy for residual depression: A case series. *Behaviour Research and Therapy, 45,* 2144–2154.

Wood, J. V., Saltzberg, J. A., Neale, J. M., Stone, A. A., & Rachmiel, T. B. (1990). Self-focused attention, coping responses, and distressed mood in everyday life. *Journal of Personality and Social Psychology, 58,* 1027–1036.

Ziegert, D. I., & Kistner, J. A. (2002). Response styles theory: Downward extension to children. *Journal of Clinical Child and Adolescent Psychology, 31,* 325–334.

CHAPTER 7

A Contextual Model of Gender Differences in the Development of Depression after the Death of a Parent

Michelle Little, Irwin N. Sandler,
Erin Schoenfelder, *and* Sharlene A. Wolchik

The death of a parent constitutes a major life stressor for children that has been associated with increased risk for mental health problems in childhood and adolescence (Cerel, Fristad, Verducci, Weller, & Weller, 2006; Worden & Silverman, 1996) as well as adulthood (Reinherz, Giaconia, Carmola Hauf, Wasserman, & Silverman, 1999). Bereaved youth are especially vulnerable to depression and are more likely than nonbereaved children to experience high levels of internalizing problems (Gersten, Beals, & Kallgren, 1991). An elevated risk of depression among bereaved children persists for up to 12 years following the death of a parent (Kendler, Sheth, Gardner, & Prescott, 2002).

Girls show higher rates of internalizing symptoms after parental death than boys (Reinherz et al., 1999; Rotheram Borus, Weiss, Alber, & Lester, 2005; Schmiege, Khoo, Sandler, Ayers, & Wolchik, 2006; Worden & Silverman, 1996). For example, Worden and Silverman (1996) found that a gender difference in internalizing problems emerged around 2 years following the loss, with girls exhibiting more depressive and anxiety symptoms. Schmiege and colleagues (2006) found gender differences in the trajectory of depressive symptoms of parentally bereaved youth over a 45-month period following the death: Boys showed a decrease in depressive symptoms over time, whereas girls' depressive symptoms remained stable over the 45-month period. Long-term risk for the development of adult major depression is also greater among bereaved females compared to bereaved males (McLeod, 1991; Reinherz et al., 1999).

CONTEXTUAL FRAMEWORK OF GENDER DIFFERENCES IN DEPRESSION AFTER THE DEATH OF A PARENT

Understanding the pathways that lead to gender differences in depressive symptoms following parental death has important implications for a broader understanding of gender differences in adaptation to other losses and consequent depression. In this chapter, we describe a theoretical framework of the contextual and psychological processes underlying gender differences in risk for the development of depression after parental death. This framework integrates current understanding of the developmental precursors of gender differences in depression as well as research on gender differences in adaptation to parental bereavement (Sandler et al., 2008b). Along the way, we present analyses that test three theoretical mechanisms articulated in this model. Finally, implications for how this framework might be used in future research on understanding children's adaptation to parental death and in the development of prevention programs are discussed.

CONTEXTUAL THEORY OF ADAPTATION TO PARENTAL DEATH

Our theoretical framework assumes that the loss of an attachment figure is an extraordinarily stressful experience for a child or adolescent (Thompson, Kaslow, Price, Williams, & Kingree, 1998). Beyond being a source of grief and distress, the loss of an attachment figure disrupts emotional security of youth and thereby reduces their threshold of perceived threat (Kobak, 1999; Shear & Shair, 2005). Increases in perceived threat and fear have the potential to alter individuals' sense of relatedness, reduce their sense of control and esteem, and thereby undermine their management of stress and competence motivation and increase their risk for the development of depression (Armsden, McCauley, Greenberg, Burke, & Mitchell, 1990; Hammen et al., 1995; Shear & Shair, 2005).

Parentally bereaved adolescents' sense of interpersonal relatedness may be especially vulnerable because internal working models of attachment relationships are believed to guide expectations of relationships and established styles of responding in relationships (Kobak, 1999). The abrupt loss of an attachment figure therefore holds the potential to disrupt the security of the youth's relationships with caregivers and other social relations (Hammen et al., 1995; Herzberg et al., 1999; Shear & Shair, 2005).

The death of an attachment figure also leads to many secondary stressors that affect multiple contexts of a child's life. Within the family context, the surviving parent typically experiences both emotional and financial strains that often interfere with effective parenting and family communication. It is not uncommon for the death of a parent to engender new caregiving arrangements and new strains within the family, including physical and mental health problems of the surviving caregiver. These changes can lead to the child's perceived loss of support, which further disrupts his or her emotional security. Beyond the family context, bereaved youth may face multiple stressful changes, including moving, disruption in peer networks and school environments, falling behind academically, and decreases in opportunities to pursue personally meaningful activities (e.g., sports, hobbies) (Abdelnoor & Hollins, 2004).

Individual vulnerability, in terms of risk and resilience, plays an important role in adolescents' ongoing adaptation to the enduring changes inherent to parental death (Sandler, Wolchik, & Ayers, 2008a). Although multiple risk and resilience factors affect youth's relative vulnerability to bereavement stress, a few factors are particularly salient in predicting their adaptation to bereavement as well as their development of depression. These include: the surviving parent/caregiver's depression, the surviving parent/caregiver's quality of parenting, and the security of attachment with the surviving parent/caregiver. Parental depression substantially raises youth's likelihood of developing a serious depressive disorder. Plausible pathways through which this risk is transmitted include heightened interpersonal stress in the family, modeling of a depressogenic coping style in response to bereavement and other stressors, impairment in the surviving parent/caregiver's ability to parent effectively, and disruption in the security of attachment to the surviving parent/caregiver (Hops, 1995, 1996; Kwok et al., 2005; Sheeber, Davis, & Hops, 2002). Although not well examined in bereaved populations of youth (Shear & Shair, 2005; Stroebe, Schut, & Stroebe, 2005), the importance of attachment security in successful adaptation during times of extraordinary stress is indicated by developmental studies. Security of attachment with their parents facilitates youth's adaptation through its impact on perceived parental support, emotional regulation, and interpersonal functioning (Abela et al., 2005; Armsden, McCauley, Greenberg, Burke, & Mitchell, 1990; Blain, Thompson, & Whiffen, 1993; Cooper, Shaver, & Collins, 1998; Hammen et al., 1995; Herzberg et al., 1999; Kobak & Sceery, 1988). Not surprisingly, adults who report having had a secure attachment relationship with a deceased parent are less likely to report depression when mourning their loss (Wayment & Vierthaler,

2002). Finally, positive parenting by the surviving parent/caregiver, characterized by high levels of support and consistent discipline, plays a critical role in buffering youth from the adverse effects of accumulated stressors in the postdeath environment and in protecting them from the development of mental health problems during adolescence (Haine, Wolchik, Sandler, Millsap, & Ayers, 2006; Kwok et al., 2005).

We propose that bereaved youth's maladaptive response to the loss of an attachment figure as well as to the cascade of associated stressors that are set in motion by the death contributes to continuity of depressive symptoms following the death (Dowdney, 2000; Sandler, 2001; Sandler et al., 2008a). Bereaved youth's encounters with cumulative stressful events that challenge fulfillment of their needs for relatedness, control, and esteem contribute to the persistence of depressive symptoms after parental death (Haine, Ayers, Sandler, Wolchik & Weyer, 2003; Wolchik, Tein, Sandler, & Ayers, 2006). One pathway by which this may occur is through a lowered threshold of perceived threat that is often the result of repeated encounters with stressful events, particularly when they are not successfully resolved. Bereaved youth are therefore more likely to appraise new stressors as involving greater threat to their need satisfaction. Youth actively construe themselves in relation to their experience in their social context (Skinner & Wellborn, 1994), which is reflected in their internal belief systems or self-system processes. As a consequence of their repeated experience with these stressful transactions, youth are also likely to develop depressogenic attributions that events are likely to be more stable (repeatedly occur), internal (reflect something about them as people), and global (affect more aspects of their lives).

Our research with bereaved youth has focused on three self-system processes reflecting three basic needs—social relatedness, control or efficacy, and self-esteem—although we recognize that other needs and their related belief systems may be particularly salient for some children (e.g., need for physical safety). From this perspective, adverse changes in youth's environment threaten these self-system processes, whereas supportive resources mitigate these efforts through compensatory factors that bolster self-systems processes. For example, negative changes in the parent–child relationship threaten social relatedness needs, and adjusting to academic or peer problems or criticism from a depressed parent may threaten self-esteem. In addition, repeated experiences of uncontrollable stressors following the death threaten control needs.

Coping in the postdeath environment is an integral facet of our contextual framework. Our framework emphasizes the *ability* of the coping effort to enable the person to adapt, both behaviorally and cognitively, to environmental and social stressors and to feelings of loss in ways that satisfy motivational needs and facilitate developmental competencies. For example, if events are uncontrollable, adaptive coping may involve the use of strategies to establish a sense of secondary control (e.g., allying with powerful others or obtaining interpretive control by developing an effective understanding of the stressors) (Rothbaum, Weisz, & Snyder, 1982). If the deceased was a primary source of intimate connection, effective coping may involve thinking about the deceased in ways that maintain a positive sense of continued connection, and seeking social support that provides a sense of secure intimate connections with others. Ineffective coping, such as withdrawal from others, dwelling on the negative consequences of the loss, or ruminating on distress can lead to increased negative affect, a negative cycle of secondary stressors, and feelings of inefficacy that converge to raise the likelihood of developing depression.

DEVELOPMENTAL FACTORS RELATED TO GENDER DIFFERENCES IN DEPRESSION

We conceptualize gender as an important marker of individual differences in the processes of adapting to parental death as well as in the likelihood of developing depression after the death (Kraemer, Kazdin, Offord, & Kessler, 1997). From a developmental perspective, one explanation for gender differences in risk for depression following parental death is that grief potentiates girls' developmental proneness for depressive symptoms during and after the adolescent transition (Angold, Costello, & Worthman, 1998). Alternative theoretical mechanisms are also plausible, however. It may be that gender-linked differences in psychological processes related to adaptation to the death itself, or gender differences in exposure and reactivity to secondary stressors, account for females' greater risk for depression compared to males (Harris, Brown, & Bifulco, 1990b). Consistent with these hypotheses, we discuss developmental precursors of gender differences in adolescent depression that may influence differential adaptation to bereavement.

A wealth of literature establishes that biological and socialization factors enhance gender differences in social adaptation during the transition to adolescence (Zahn-Waxler, 1993). Most notably, in the context of pubertal hormonal and endocrinal changes as well as rapid changes in the breadth and depth of social relationships, females' affiliative orientation in social relationships intensifies (Cyranowski, Frank, Young, & Shear, 2000). In contrast to adolescent males' focus on agency and personal autonomy, female adolescents show an increasing preference for close emotional communication, intimacy, and responsiveness within social relationships (i.e., peer, romantic, and caregiving relationships) (Allgood-Merten, Lewinsohn, & Hops, 1990). An important potential liability of female youth's affiliative style is an associated increase in exposure and sensitivity to interpersonal stress, which heightens their risk for depression relative to males (Brooks-Gunn & Warren, 1989; Ge, Conger, & Elder, 2001; Ge, Lorenz, Conger, Elder, & Simons, 1994; Rudolph & Flynn, 2007). Further, pubertal changes in level of specific neurohormones are believed to potentiate female youth's increased emotional sensitivity to interpersonal stress, thus further heightening their propensity for depression (Cyranowski et al., 2000).

Maladaptive cognitions reflecting low perceived control over events also play a potential role in explaining female vulnerability to depression. However, direct tests of gender differences in links between perceived control and adolescent depression are rare (Harris, Brown, & Bifulco, 1990a). Finally, self-esteem is also implicated as a mediator of gender differences in adolescent depression. Female youth show lower levels of self-esteem than male youth in multiple studies, and females' lower self-esteem mediates gender differences in adolescent depression (Allgood-Merten et al., 1990; Brage & Meredith, 1994; Kling, Hyde, Showers, & Buswell, 1999; Ohannessian, Lerner, Lerner, & Eye, 1999).

Differential cognitive vulnerability to stress is another factor related to gender differences in the risk for depressive symptoms and depression (Hankin & Abramson, 2001). *Cognitive vulnerability* is defined by a tendency to make negative inferences about the causes and consequences of an event (i.e., global and stable attributions) and negative inferences about the implications of the event for oneself (Hankin & Abramson, 2001, 2002). Emerging research supports girls' increased cognitive vulnerability to stress both as a partial explanation of their increased levels of depressive symptoms, as well as a potential moderator of gender differences in adolescent depression (Hankin, 2009; Hankin & Abramson, 2001, 2002; Nolen-Hoeksema, Girgus, & Seligman, 1992).

Finally, differential coping styles are also linked with gender differences in depression. Specifically, there is considerable evidence that female children and adolescents are more likely to use a ruminative coping style characterized by persistent, negative, intrusive thoughts focusing on negative affect (Abela, Brozina & Haigh, 2002; Grant et al., 2004). Focusing passively on negative affect (e.g., "Why don't I want to get out of bed? There must be something wrong with me") and self-focused negative consequences of those symptoms ("If I don't get out of bed, I'll never get my work done") rather than on active problem solving or distraction leads to greater stability in child and adolescent depression (Abela et al., 2002; Broderick & Korteland, 2004). Research suggests that females' tendency to use a ruminative coping style maintains and exacerbates depressive symptoms. As a result, females who characteristically show a ruminative coping style are also more likely to show persistent depressive symptoms and are at greater risk for the development of major depression (Hankin, 2009; Hankin & Abramson, 2001). Further, females' increased anxiety and depression are also associated with their tendency to rely less on instrumental coping strategies than males (Galambos, Almeida, & Petersen, 1990; Nolen-Hoeksema & Girgus, 1994)

In summary, in the context of rapid pubertal maturation, new social demands, and heightened affiliative needs, females are more likely than males to encounter and be sensitized to interpersonal stress that potentially threatens their sense of social relatedness, control, and esteem. In the context of increasing interpersonal stress, adolescent females are more likely to make negative inferences about negative events—a tendency that is linked to depressive symptoms. Finally, gender-related coping styles, including ruminative coping and low instrumentality, exacerbate depressive symptoms, leading to a greater persistence of negative affect and increased likelihood of the development of major depression.

GENDER AND ADAPTATION TO BEREAVEMENT

In this next section, we present an integrative model of the contextual and developmental precursors of gender differences in the persistence of depressive symptoms and the development of adolescent depression among parentally bereaved youth (see Figure 7.1).

Gender and Loss of an Attachment Figure

From a social–developmental perspective, female youth may be particularly threatened by loss of an attachment figure, given their increased affiliative orientation during and after the transition to adolescence. As social and hormonal changes intensify female adolescent affiliative needs, the loss of an attachment figure represents a greater loss of emotional and relationship support for females than males during a time when the development of intimate social relationships is a central developmental task. The loss of an attachment figure, therefore, represents a crucial disruption in both emotional security and interpersonal adaptation (Hammen et al., 1995; Rudolph & Flynn, 2007). This disruption may affect female youth's motivational needs directly by undermining their sense of secure social relations. The effects of this undermined security may be manifested in increasing fears of not being taken care of by their primary caregivers and in a reduced sense of perceived control over life events due to the uncontrollable nature of their loss. Further, females' sense of self-esteem may be depleted as the positive feedback from others is reduced.

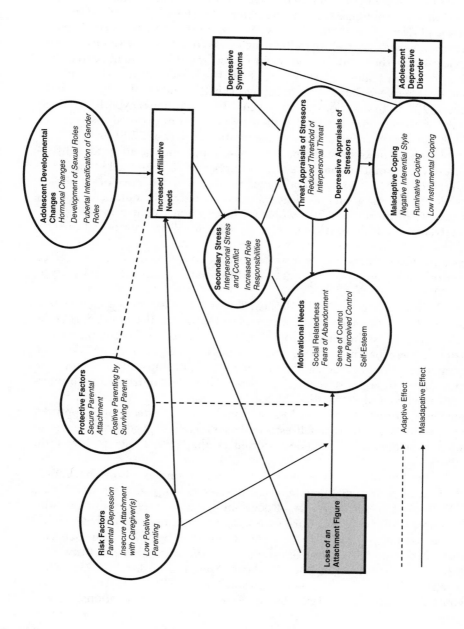

FIGURE 7.1. Contextual model of gender differences in the development of depression after the death of a parent.

137

Our current research with bereaved youth supports the notion that loss of an attachment figure has a stronger impact on females' perceived security of social relatedness than on males'. We found that bereaved female youth reported greater fear of abandonment (measured by a self-report of their concern that they may not be taken care of by their primary caregivers) than bereaved males in a sample of 8- to 16-year-old youth whose parent had died between 3 and 29 months ago (Little, Sandler, Wolchik, Tein, & Ayers, 2009). In addition, we found that bereaved female youth's elevated fears of abandonment mediated their higher level of depressive symptoms 14 months later as compared to male youth (Little et al., 2009).

To date, links between parental death and adolescent gender differences in other motivational needs have not been well examined in the literature. However, Harris and colleagues showed that a history of childhood helplessness after a parent's death was associated with adult depression in a sample of more than 200 women whose parents died prior to age 17 (Harris et al., 1990a). Although perceived control was not tested directly in this study, helplessness behaviors provide a good proxy for this contrast, because helplessness is a crucial behavioral component of low perceived control (Seligman, 1975; Seligman, Abramson, Semmel, & Von Baeyer, 1979).

Loss of a parent also holds clear implications for female youth's self-esteem. Given that parents are a crucial source of social support during the adolescent transition, female youth's esteem may be particularly threatened after losing a parent. Indeed, current research suggests that females take greater emotional responsibility for close relationships and therefore are more likely to appraise themselves negatively when confronted with interpersonal loss and/or conflict (Nolen-Hoeksema & Jackson, 2001). Potential implications of parental loss on female youth's esteem are supported by research showing that self-esteem deficits mediate gender differences in adolescent depression (Allgood-Merten et al., 1990; Brage & Meredith, 1994).

Attachment loss also affects youth's motivational needs by challenging their passage through the adolescent developmental transition (see Figure 7.1). Because of the centrality of developing intimate relationships in adolescence, losing a parent during this time period may exacerbate affiliative needs during the adolescent transition, thus leading to an increased dependency in other close or intimate relationships (Harris, Brown, & Bifulco, 1987; Prinstein, Borelli, Cheah, Simon, & Aikins, 2005). When positive alternative caregiving relationships are not available, female youth's increased dependency on either peer or romantic relationships and their choice of intimate partners who also have poor social connections with their own caregivers may then lead to rejection by their partners or to developmentally premature sexuality and/or early parenthood (Harris et al., 1987; Prinstein et al., 2005).

Gender, Risk, Stress, and Coping

Some of the most robust risk predictors of depression from a developmental perspective may also promote gender differentiated adaptation to bereavement. As shown in Figure 7.1, we propose that parent/caregiver-related variables, including depression, security of parent/caregiver–youth attachment, and quality of parenting, may have a particularly strong influence on females' adaptation to parental bereavement during the adolescent transition. Beyond affecting the likelihood that youth will develop depression in general, these risk and protective factors may play a particularly important role during times of increased affiliative needs (Cyranowski et al., 2000). A secure caregiver relationship, characterized by high levels of responsiveness, warmth, and open communication, buffers the threat that parental loss presents to satisfaction of motivational needs by reassuring youth that their emotional needs will be taken care of, in the midst of increasing social pressures inherent to the adolescent transition. As noted earlier, a positive parenting relationship also reduces female youth's exposure to familial stressors, thereby encouraging an adaptive response to interpersonal stress (Tein, Sandler, Ayers, & Wolchik, 2006). Parental depression may be particularly disruptive of the adaptation process for bereaved female adolescents because of the links between parental depression and reduced parental support for affiliative needs, increased interpersonal problems in the family, and a depressogenic model of interpersonal coping (Hops, 1995, 1996; Sheeber et al., 2002).

Researchers have suggested that the postdeath environment is more stressful for female children and adolescents as compared to males, although there are few studies that have addressed this issue (Sandler et al., 2003). As depicted in Figure 7.1, our model proposes that (1) bereaved females are exposed to a higher level of interpersonal stressors in the postdeath environment; (2) this gender differential is potentially exacerbated by increasing adolescent affiliative needs; and (3) increased exposure to interpersonal stress is related to the persistence of depressive symptoms. The salience of interpersonal postdeath stressors as factors influencing depression in females was proposed in a series of retrospective longitudinal studies of adult females who lost a parent during childhood (Bifulco, Brown, Moran, Ball, & Campbell, 1998; Harris et al., 1987, 1990a). Bifulco and colleagues (1998) found that inadequate parental care by the surviving parent and premarital pregnancy were important intervening factors in females' risk for clinical levels of depression in adulthood.

Our recent empirical work supports the hypothesis that bereaved female youth face a higher level of interpersonal stress in the postdeath environment than bereaved males, and this increased stress is associated with increased persistence of depressive symptoms in females. Using a sample of 8- to 16-year-old youth whose parent had died between 3 and 29 months earlier, we found that females reported greater exposure to stressors than males. However, we also found that females' greater exposure to *interpersonal* stressors was a particularly robust mediator of gender differences in depressive symptoms 14 months later (Little et al., 2009). That is, female youth reported significantly higher levels of interpersonal stress than males at baseline, and, in turn, baseline interpersonal stressors predicted depressive symptom levels 14 months later. Although we had speculated that bereaved girls' assumption of added caregiving responsibilities and roles within the family might account for gender differences in depression (Sandler et al., 2003), analyses showed that role stressors, including added responsibilities and changes in environment, did not differ by gender.

Our framework further proposes that bereaved females' increased exposure to interpersonal stressors may lead to negative appraisals of interpersonal events, which not only serve to maintain their distress, but may engender maladaptive coping strategies that further reduce satisfaction of motivational needs (see Figure 7.1; Hankin & Abramson, 2001, 2002; Rudolph & Flynn, 2007). To examine the possibility that gender differences in depression after parental death are related to threat appraisals of interpersonal stressors, we examined gender differences in links between exposure to interpersonal stress, threat appraisals, and depression (see Figure 7.2). We used baseline data from 112 parentally bereaved 12- to 16-year-old youth who were part of an experimental trial of a preventive intervention for bereaved families, the Family Bereavement Program, for these analyses (Sandler et al., 2003). Exposure to interpersonal stress in the prior month was assessed using four items on a measure of negative life events (Little et al., 2009). Threat appraisals were measured using 12 items assessing degree of negative self and other appraisals of two events. As shown in Figure 7.2, we found that threat appraisals mediated the effect of interpersonal stress on depressive symptoms for females only (indirect effect = 0.75, $p < .05$). Interpersonal threat appraisals were not associated with level of depressive symptoms among males. We also tested a longitudinal model using the youth in the control group ($n = 109$; see Figure 7.3) to examine this mediation path. Results partially supported cross-sectional findings; baseline threat appraisals marginally mediated links between females' baseline exposure to interpersonal stressors and depressive symptoms 14 months later (indirect effect = 0.21, $p < .10$), though this was not true for males. These findings provide support for the role of gender dif-

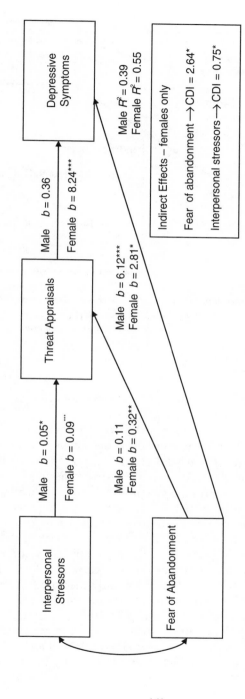

FIGURE 7.2. Cross-sectional gender differences in the mediation of interpersonal stress and fear of abandonment effects on bereaved youth's depressive symptoms. Adolescents only in model, $N = 112$; 64 males and 48 females. Months since death covaried. Effect of interpersonal stressors on symptoms of depression was included in model. Every path is significantly moderated by gender.

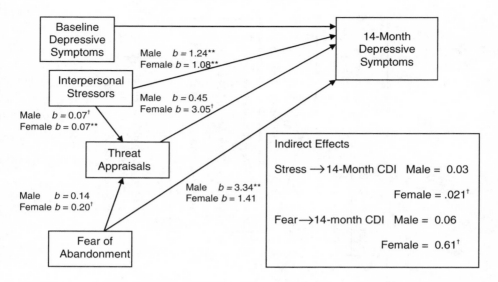

FIGURE 7.3. Longitudinal gender differences in the mediation of interpersonal stress and fear of abandonment effects on bereaved youth's depressive symptoms. $N = 109$ control group participants; 57 males, 52 females. Age covaried on fear of abandonment and interpersonal stressors. Independent variables covaried. $^†p < .10$; $^*p < .05$; $^{**}p < .01$; $^{***}p < .001$.

ferences in threat appraisals of interpersonal stressors in bereaved female youth's depressive symptoms.

In the same analyses, we examined a second potential risk path for gender differences in depressive symptoms: one involving fears of abandonment. We hypothesized that adolescents' loss of an attachment figure would engender abandonment fears that, in turn, heighten threat appraisals, leading to increased depressive symptoms. Given heightened affiliative needs in adolescence, we expected that females' threat appraisals would be particularly affected by abandonment fears. As shown in Figure 7.2, baseline cross-sectional analysis revealed that the effect of fear of abandonment on depressive symptoms was mediated by threat appraisals among females (indirect effect = 2.64, $p < .05$), but not among males. Similarly, female youth's threat appraisals at baseline marginally mediated the association between baseline scores on fear of abandonment and depressive symptoms 14 months later (indirect effect = 0.61, $p < .10$; see Figure 7.3). By contrast, although fear of abandonment was related to male youth's depression, the relation between their baseline scores on fear of abandonment and subsequent depressive symptoms was not mediated by their interpersonal appraisals (indirect effect = 0.06, $p > .10$). This pattern of findings suggests that pathways to depressive symptoms in bereaved youth differ across gender.

We also tested a third potential path by which gender may differentially affect vulnerability to depression following parental death: through its impact on youth's internal control beliefs. Control beliefs may impact appraisals of stressful events, such that the less youth believe that they have control over events, the more likely they are to make depressive appraisals of stressors in their lives (e.g., event is likely to recur in the future or always happen to them) (Hilsman & Garber, 1995). Internal control was measured using four items from the Connell Locus of Control Scale (e.g., "I can pretty much control what happens in my life"). Our measure of depressive appraisals consisted of items related to global (e.g., "You thought that nothing ever goes right for you") and stable (e.g., "You thought that things like this would always keep happening.") appraisals of two stressful events that occurred in the past month. We found that although females' depressive appraisals mediated the links between internal control and level of depressive symptoms (indirect effect = -3.46, $p < .05$), this was not true for males. Although males' depressive appraisals were related to depressive symptoms, internal control beliefs did not predict depressive appraisals. Taken together, results of these models suggest several pathways that may explain why girls are more at risk for depression following parental death than are boys. Females' fear of abandonment, which we conceptualize as an indicator of insecurity in their sense of social relatedness to caregivers, and internal control beliefs impacted their appraisals for stressful events, which in turn affected their depressive symptoms. It is notable that the same mediation relations were not detected for boys, suggesting an important direction for future research on gender differences in response to stress.

As noted in Figure 7.1, our model proposes that maladaptive coping also plays an important role in bereaved females' development of depressive disorders. We suggest that female youth's increased exposure to secondary interpersonal stressors may lead to a more entrenched negative inferential style of coping with new stressors that are encountered (Hankin, 2009; Hankin & Abramson, 2001). In addition, female youth's increased tendency to use a ruminative coping style focused on the negative consequences of depressive affect as well as noninstrumental coping strategies may serve not only to maintain depressive affect, but to engender depressive disorders in interaction with interpersonal stress (Hankin & Abramson, 2001, 2002). Notably, however, although these links are supported by current developmental theory, they have not been tested formally in research with bereaved youth, and this is therefore an important area for further investigation

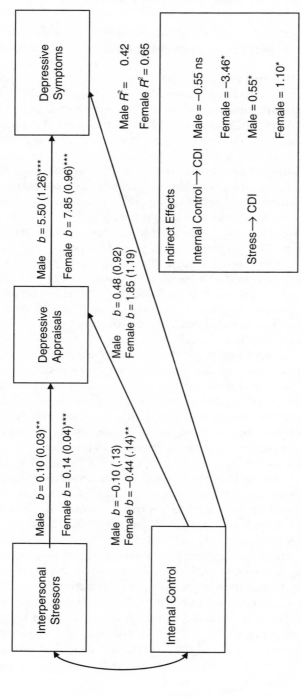

FIGURE 7.4. Cross-sectional gender differences in the mediation of interpersonal stress and perceived control effects on bereaved youth's depressive symptoms. Adolescents only in model, $N = 112$; 64 males and 48 females. Months since death covaried. Effect of negative interpersonal events on symptoms of depression was included in model and was nonsignificant in both gender groups.

IMPLICATIONS AND FUTURE DIRECTIONS FOR PREVENTION AND INTERVENTION PROGRAMMING

This chapter's model presents one theoretical starting point to explore the contribution of both bereavement adaptation and developmental factors in explanations of gender differences in adolescent depression. From our reading of the literature, however, there are many avenues of research that have yet to be examined to further our understanding of these links. We currently have limited understanding of how developmental differences in biological, psychological, and self-system processes influence gender differences in bereavement-related depression because children and youth have not been systematically compared on these variables. In addition, the contribution of differential coping processes to gender differences in bereavement-related depression has not been well examined. Finally, alternative mechanisms that promote the persistence of distress in bereaved males after losing a parent have yet to be explored.

Experimental studies of bereavement interventions for youth can also inform our understanding of gender differences in recovery needs. For example, the Family Bereavement Program was found to reduce internalizing problems for girls but not boys (Tien et al., 2006). Analysis of the mediators of the program effects of depression on girls can be seen as an important tool to test theoretical propositions of the development of depression in bereaved girls. Within the context of a randomized experimental trial, mediation analysis provides a test of whether an experimentally induced change in the mediator explains experimentally induced change in depression, thus increasing the strength of causal inference about the effects of the mediators on depression as compared to a correlational study. Findings from mediation analyses of the Family Bereavement Program provide evidence to support several propositions concerning factors that influence bereaved girls' internalizing problems. That is, girls' improvement in mental health problems at the 11-month follow-up in the intervention group was mediated by improvements in positive parenting, reductions in negative appraisals of interpersonal events and beliefs that control over events is unknown as well as improved coping efficacy (Tien et al., 2006).

Although these findings contribute directly to our understanding of the development of internalizing problems following parental death, they also provide hypotheses concerning girls' response to other major stressors that involve loss or disruption of parent–child relations within the family, such as physical or mental illness of a parent or parental divorce. Future research should extend these models to see whether they generalize to a broader class of stressors that affect the development of internalizing problems in children, including gender differences in these pathways. Understanding the pathways by which these stressors affect the development of internalizing problems in children should inform the development and testing of interventions to promote resilience in children exposed to these high-risk situations.

ACKNOWLEDGMENTS

Support for this research was provided by National Institute of Mental Health Grant No. P30 M439246-15 to establish a Preventive Intervention Research Center at Arizona State University, Grant No. 1R01 MH49155-05 to evaluate a preventive intervention for bereaved families, Grant No. 2R01 MH49155-06 to conduct a 6-year follow-up of this intervention, and Grant No. T32 MH 018387 to support postdoctoral trainees in prevention science.

REFERENCES

Abdelnoor, A., & Hollins, S. (2004). The effect of childhood bereavement on secondary school performance. *Educational Psychology in Practice, 20*(1), 43–54.

Abela, J. R. Z., Brozina, K., & Haigh, E. P. (2002). An examination of the response styles theory of depression in third- and sixth-grade children: A short-term longitudinal study. *Journal of Abnormal Child Psychology, 30,* 517–527.

Abela, J. R. Z., Hankin, B. L., Haigh, E. A. P., Adams, P., Vinokuroff, T., & Trayhern, L. (2005). Interpersonal vulnerability to depression in high-risk children: The role of insecure attachment and reassurance seeking. *Journal of Clinical Child and Adolescent Psychology, 34*(1), 182–192.

Allgood-Merten, B., Lewinsohn, P. M., & Hops, H. (1990). Sex differences and adolescent depression. *Journal of Abnormal Psychology, 99*(1), 55–63.

Angold, A., Costello, E. J., & Worthman, C. M. (1998). Puberty and depression: The role of age, pubertal status and pubertal timing *Psychological Medicine, 28,* 51–61.

Armsden, G. C., McCauley, E., Greenberg, M. T., Burke, P. M., & Mitchell, J. R. (1990). Parent and peer attachment in early adolescent depression. *Journal of Abnormal Child Psychology, 18*(6), 683–697.

Bifulco, A., Brown, G. W., Moran, P., Ball, C., & Campbell, C. (1998). Predicting depression in women: The role of past and present vulnerability. *Psychological Medicine, 28*(1), 39–50.

Blain, M. D., Thompson, J. M., & Whiffen, V. E. (1993). Attachment and perceived social support in late adolescence: The interaction between working models of self and others. *Journal of Adolescent Research, 8*(2), 226–241.

Brage, D., & Meredith, W. (1994). A causal model of adolescent depression. *Journal of Psychology: Interdisciplinary and Applied, 128*(4), 455–468.

Broderick, P. C., & Korteland, C. (2004). A prospective study of rumination and depression in early adolescence. *Clinical Child Psychology and Psychiatry, 9,* 383–394.

Brooks-Gunn, J., & Warren, M. P. (1989). Biological and social contributions to negative affect in young adolescent girls. *Child Development, 60*, 40–55.

Cerel, J., Fristad, M. A., Verducci, J., Weller, R. A., & Weller, E. B. (2006). Childhood bereavement: Psychopathology in the two years post parental death. *Journal of the American Academy of Child and Adolescent Psychiatry, 45*(6), 681–690.

Cooper, M. L., Shaver, P. R., & Collins, N. L. (1998). Attachment styles, emotion regulation, and adjustment in adolescence. *Journal of Personality and Social Psychology, 74*(5), 1380–1397.

Cyranowski, J. M., Frank, E., Young, E., & Shear, M. K. (2000). Adolescent onset and the gender difference in lifetime rates of major depression. *Archives of General Psychiatry, 57*, 21–27.

Dowdney, L. (2000). Child bereavement following parental death. *Journal of Child Psychology and Psychiatry and Allied Disciplines, 41*, 819–830.

Galambos, N. L., Almeida, D. M., & Petersen, A. C. (1990). Masculinity, femininity, and sex role attitudes in early adolescence: Exploring gender intensification. *Child Development, 61*(6), 1905–1914.

Ge, X., Conger, R. D., & Elder, G. H., Jr. (2001). Pubertal transition, stressful life events, and the emergence of gender differences in adolescent depressive symptoms. *Developmental Psychology, 37*(3), 404–417.

Ge, X., Lorenz, F. O., Conger, R. D., Elder, G. H., Jr., & Simons, R. L. (1994). Trajectories of stressful life events and depressive symptoms during adolescence. *Developmental Psychology, 30*, 467–483.

Gersten, J., Beals, J., & Kallgren, C. (1991). Epidemiology and preventive interventions: Parental death in childhood as a case example. *American Journal of Community Psychology, 19*, 481–499.

Grant, K. E., Lyons, A. L., Finkelstein, J.-A. S., Conway, K. M., Reynolds, L. K., O'Koon, J. H., et al. (2004). Gender differences in rates of depressive symptoms among low-income, urban, African American youth: A test of two mediational hypotheses. *Journal of Youth and Adolescence, 33*(6), 523–533.

Haine, R. A., Ayers, T. S., Sandler, I. N., Wolchik, S. A., & Weyer, J. L. (2003). Locus of control and self-esteem as stress moderators or stress mediators in parentally bereaved children. *Death Studies, 27*, 619–640.

Haine, R. A., Wolchik, S. A., Sandler, I. N., Millsap, R. E., & Ayers, T. S. (2006). Positive parenting as a protective resource for parentally bereaved children. *Death Studies, 30*(1), 1–28.

Hammen, C. L., Burge, D., Daley, S. E., Davila, J., Paley, B., & Rudolph, K. D. (1995). Interpersonal attachment cognitions and prediction of symptomatic responses to interpersonal stress. *Journal of Abnormal Psychology, 104*(3), 436–443.

Hankin, B. L. (2009). Development of sex differences in depressive and co-occurring anxious symptoms during adolescence: Descriptive trajectories and potential explanations in a multiwave prospective study. *Journal of Clinical Child and Adolescent Psychology, 38*, 460–472.

Hankin, B. L., & Abramson, L. Y. (2001). Development of gender differences in depression: An elaborated cognitive vulnerability–transactional stress theory. *Psychological Bulletin, 127*(6), 773–796.

Hankin, B. L., & Abramson, L. Y. (2002). Measuring cognitive vulnerability to depression in adolescence: Reliability, validity, and gender differences. *Journal of Clinical Child and Adolescent Psychology, 31*(4), 491–504.

Harris, T. O., Brown, G. W., & Bifulco, A.T. (1987). Loss of parent in childhood and adult psychiatric disorder: The role of social class position and premarital pregnancy. *Psychological Medicine, 17*(1), 163–183.

Harris, T. O., Brown, G. W., & Bifulco, A. T. (1990a). Depression and situational helplessness/mastery in a sample selected to study childhood parental loss. *Journal of Affective Disorders, 20*(1), 27–41.

Harris, T. O., Brown, G. W., & Bifulco, A. T. (1990b). Loss of parent in childhood and adult psychiatric disorder: A tentative overall model. *Development and Psychopathology, 2*(3), 311–328.

Herzberg, D. S., Hammen, C., Burge, D., Daley, S. E., Davila, J., & Lindberg, N. (1999). Attachment cognitions predict perceived and enacted social support during late adolescence. *Journal of Adolescent Research, 14*(4), 387–404.

Hilsman, R., & Garber, J. (1995). A test of the cognitive diathesis–stress model of depression in children: Academic stressors, attributional style, perceived competence, and control. *Journal of Personality and Social Psychology, 69*(2), 370–380.

Hops, H. (1995). Age- and gender-specific effects of parental depression: A commentary. *Developmental Psychology, 31*(3), 428–431.

Hops, H. (1996). *Intergenerational transmission of depressive symptoms: Gender and developmental considerations.* London: Gaskell/Royal College of Psychiatrists.

Kendler, K. S., Sheth, K., Gardner, C. O., & Prescott, C. A. (2002). Childhood parental loss and risk for first onset of major depression and alcohol dependence: The time-decay of risk and sex differences. *Psychological Medicine, 32*(7), 1187–1194.

Kling, K. C., Hyde, J. S., Showers, C. J., & Buswell, B. N. (1999). Gender differences in self-esteem: A meta-analysis. *Psychological Bulletin, 125*(4), 470–500.

Kobak, R. R. (1999). The emotional dynamics of disruptions in attachment relationships: Implications for theory, research, and clinical intervention. In J. Cassidy & P. R. Shaver (Eds.), *Handbook of attachment: Theory, research, and clinical applications* (pp. 21–43). New York: Guilford Press.

Kobak, R. R., & Sceery, A. (1988). Attachment in late adolescence: Working models, affect regulation, and representations of self and others. *Child Development, 59*(1), 135–146.

Kraemer, H. C., Kazdin, A. E., Offord, D. R., & Kessler, R. C. (1997). Coming to terms with the terms of risk. *Archives of General Psychiatry, 54*(4), 337–343.

Kwok, O.-M., Haine, R. A., Sandler, I. N., Ayers, T. S., Wolchik, S. A., & Tein, J.-Y. (2005). Positive parenting as a mediator of the relations between parental psychological distress and mental health problems of parentally bereaved children. *Journal of Clinical Child and Adolescent Psychology, 34*(2), 260–271.

Little, M., Sandler, I. N., Wolchik, S. A., Tein, J., & Ayers, T. S. (2009). Comparing cognitive, relational and stress mechanisms underlying gender differences in recovery from bereavement-related internalizing problems following the death of a parent. *Journal of Clinical Child and Adolescent Psychology, 38,* 486–500.

McLeod, J. D. (1991). Childhood parental loss and adult depression. *Journal of Health and Social Behavior, 32*(3), 205–220.

Nolen-Hoeksema, S., & Girgus, J. S. (1994). The emergence of gender differences in depression during adolescence. *Psychological Bulletin, 115*(3), 424–443.

Nolen-Hoeksema, S., & Jackson, B. (2001). Mediators of the gender difference in rumination. *Psychology of Women Quarterly, 25,* 37–47.

Nolen-Hoeksema, S., Girgus, J. S., & Seligman, M. E. (1992). Predictors and consequences of childhood depressive symptoms: A five-year longitudinal study. *Journal of Abnormal Psychology, 101*(3), 405–422.

Ohannessian, C. M., Lerner, R. M., Lerner, J. V., & Eye, A. V. (1999). Does self-competence predict gender differences in adolescent depression and anxiety? *Journal of Adolescence, 22*(3), 397–411.

Prinstein, M. J., Borelli, J. L., Cheah, C. S. L., Simon, V. A., & Aikins, J. W. (2005). Adolescent girls' interpersonal vulnerability to depressive symptoms: A longitudinal examination of reassurance-seeking and peer relationships. *Journal of Abnormal Psychology, 114*(4), 676–688.

Reinherz, H. Z., Giaconia, R. M., Carmola Hauf, A. M., Wasserman, M. S., & Silverman, A. B. (1999). Major depression in the transition to adulthood: Risks and impairments. *Journal of Abnormal Psychology, 108,* 500–510.

Rothbaum, F., Weisz, J. R., & Snyder, S. S. (1982). Changing the world and changing the self: A two-process model of perceived control. *Journal of Personality and Social Psychology, 42*(1), 5–37.

Rotheram Borus, M. J., Weiss, R., Alber, S., & Lester, P. (2005). Adolescent adjustment before and after HIV-related parental death. *Journal of Consulting and Clinical Psychology, 73*(2), 221–228.

Rudolph, K. D., & Flynn, M. (2007). Childhood adversity and youth depression: Influence of gender and pubertal status. *Development and Psychopathology, 19*(2), 497–521.

Sandler, I. N. (2001). Quality and ecology of adversity as common mechanisms of risk and resilience. *American Journal of Community Psychology, 29,* 19–61.

Sandler, I. N., Ayers, T. S., Wolchik, S. A., Tein, J.-Y., Kwok, O.-M., Haine, R. A., et al. (2003). The Family Bereavement Program: Efficacy evaluation of a theory-based prevention program for parentally bereaved children and adolescents. *Journal of Consulting and Clinical Psychology, 71*(3), 587–600.

Sandler, I. N., Wolchik, S. A., & Ayers, T. S. (2008a). Resilience rather than recovery: A contextual framework on adaptation following bereavement. *Death Studies, 32,* 59–73.

Sandler, I. N., Wolchik, S. A., Ayers, T. S., Tein, J.-Y., Coxe, S., & Chow, W. (2008b). Linking theory and intervention to promote resilience of children following parental bereavement. In M. S. Stroebe, R.O. Hansson, H. Schut, W. Stroebe, & E. Van den Blink (Eds.), *Handbook of bereavement research and practice: Advances in theory and intervention* (pp. 531–550). Washington, DC: American Psychological Association.

Schmiege, S. J., Khoo, S.-T., Sandler, I. N., Ayers, T. S., & Wolchik, S. A. (2006).

Symptoms of internalizing and externalizing problems: Modeling recovery curves after the death of a parent. *American Journal of Preventive Medicine, 31*(6, Suppl. 1), S152–S160.

Seligman, M. E. (1975). *Helplessness: On depression, development and death.* San Francisco: Freeman.

Seligman, M. E., Abramson, L. Y., Semmel, A., & Von Baeyer, C. (1979). Depressive attributional style. *Journal of Abnormal Child Psychology, 88,* 242–247.

Shear, K., & Shair, H. (2005). Attachment, loss, and complicated grief. *Developmental Psychobiology, 47*(3), 253–267.

Sheeber, L., Davis, B., & Hops, H. (2002). Gender-specific vulnerability to depression in children of depressed mothers. In S. H. Goodman & I. H. Gotlib (Eds.), *Children of depressed parents: Mechanisms of risk and implications for treatment* (pp. 253–274). Washington, DC: American Psychological Association.

Skinner, E. A., & Wellborn, J. G. (1994). Coping during childhood and adolescence: A motivational perspective. In D. Featherman, R. Lerner, & M. Permutter (Eds.), *Life-span development and behavior* (pp. 91–133). Hillsdale, NJ: Erlbaum.

Stroebe, M., Schut, H., & Stroebe, W. (2005). Attachment in coping with bereavement: A theoretical integration. *Review of General Psychology, 9*(1), 48–66.

Tien, J.-Y., Sandler, I. N., Ayers, T. S., & Wolchik, S. A. (2006). Mediation of the effects of the Family Bereavement Program on mental health problems of bereaved children and adolescents. *Prevention Science, 7,* 179–195.

Thompson, M. P., Kaslow, N. J., Price, A. W., Williams, K., & Kingree, J. B. (1998). Role of secondary stressors in the parental death–child distress relation. *Journal of Abnormal Child Psychology, 26,* 357–366.

Wayment, H. A., & Vierthaler, J. (2002). Attachment style and bereavement reactions. *Journal of Loss and Trauma, 7*(2), 129–149.

Wolchik, S. A., Tien, J.-Y., Sandler, I. N., & Ayers, T. S. (2006). Stressors, quality of the child–caregiver relationship, and children's mental health problems after parental death: The mediating role of self-system beliefs. *Journal of Abnormal Child Psychology, 34*(2), 221–238.

Worden, J. W., & Silverman, P. R. (1996). Parental death and the adjustment of school-age children. *Omega: Journal of Death and Dying, 33,* 91–102.

Zahn-Waxler, C. (1993). Warriors and worriers: Gender and psychopathology. *Development and Psychopathology, 5,* 79–90.

CHAPTER 8

Stress, Coping, Socialization, and Goals

A Self-Regulation Perspective on Gender and Depression in Adolescence

Alison A. Papadakis *and* Timothy J. Strauman

Traditionally, adolescence has been viewed as a developmental phase marked by "storm and stress" (Hall, 1904). Although that characterization has colored perspectives on the teenage years, it is not supported by the empirical literature (Brooks-Gunn, 1991; Petersen, 1988). Most adolescents of both genders pass through that developmental period without suffering a major psychological disorder (Petersen et al., 1993). However, the prevalence of unipolar depression increases substantially as children move into adolescence, particularly among girls (Hankin et al., 1998). Consequently, depression in adolescence is a significant public health problem that should not be construed as a transient by-product of a normative developmental process. Indeed, epidemiological data indicate that depression in adolescence predicts of later psychological difficulty in adulthood (Gotlib & Hammen, 1992) and that girls whose first depressive episode occurs during childhood or adolescence have greater risk for future episodes than women who have a later onset (Kovacs, 1997). In this chapter we seek to contribute to the growing body of knowledge regarding the causes and consequences of depression in adolescents, particularly adolescent girls, by proposing an integrative conceptual framework intended to identify potential pathways to depression that may help account for the emergence of gender differences in depression among teens.

THE EMERGENCE OF A GENDER DIFFERENCE IN DEPRESSION

The development of gender differences in vulnerability to depression during adolescence is a robust epidemiological phenomenon. Most studies that include rates of depression during childhood indicate that boys and girls have similar rates (Kovacs, 1996) or that boys have slightly higher rates compared to girls (Anderson, Williams, McGee, & Silva, 1987; Hankin et al., 1998; Lopez, Driscoll, & Kistner, 2009; Nolen-Hoeksema, Girgus, & Seligman, 1991; Twenge & Nolen-Hoeksema, 2002; Wade, Cairney, & Pevalin, 2002). However, between the ages of 13 and 15, gender differences in rates of depression emerge, such that girls have approximately twice the rate of boys, both in terms of depressive symptoms and clinical depression (Angold, 1990; Angold, Costello, & Worthman, 1998; Costello, Mustillo, Erkanli, Keeler, & Angold, 2003; Ge, Lorenz, Conger, Elder, & Simons, 1994; Hankin et al., 1998; Kandel & Davies, 1982, 1986; Lewinsohn, Hops, Roberts, Seeley, & Andrews, 1993; Petersen, Sarigiani, & Kennedy, 1991; Wichstrom, 1999). This gender difference persists into adulthood (for a review, see Cyranowski, Frank, Young, & Shear, 2000), with the results from one large-scale epidemiological study of 38,000 community participants from 10 countries indicating that the rates for women are consistently higher than those for men (Weissman et al., 1996). This gender difference appears to be maintained throughout adulthood (Barry, Allore, Guo, Bruce, & Gill, 2008; Sonnenberg, Beekman, Deeg, & van Tilburg, 2000), although there is some suggestion that the rates may converge again in late adulthood (Barefoot, Mortensen, Helms, Avlund, & Schroll, 2001; Kessler, McGonagle, Swartz, & Blazer, 1993). Further the gender difference appears to be a true difference, rather than a artifactual finding due to differential treatment seeking, differences in openness to reporting symptoms or other measurement problems, including thresholds for caseness, or recall biases (Cyranowski et al., 2000; Nolen-Hoeksema, 1987; Nolen-Hoeksema et al., 1991; Piccinelli & Wilkinson, 2000).

PROMINENT MODELS OF THE EMERGENCE OF GENDER DIFFERENCES IN DEPRESSION

There is great interest in understanding the reasons for girls' differential vulnerability to depression during adolescence, and it has been the focus of much study and theorizing. Researchers have explored many factors to explain the gender difference in depression, including genetics (Kendler, Gardner, Neale, & Prescott, 2001; Kendler, Kessler, Neale, Heath, &

Eaves, 1993; Silberg et al., 1999; Zubenko et al., 2002), ovarian and adrenal hormonal changes at puberty (Goodyer, Herbert, Tamplin, & Altham, 2000; Halbreich & Kahn, 2001; Steiner, Dunn, & Born, 2003), childhood and adolescent sexual abuse (Kendler, Gardner, & Prescott, 2002; Nolen-Hoeksema, 1994), cognitive vulnerability (Hankin & Abramson, 2001), dependent personality style (Allgood-Merten, Lewinsohn, & Hops, 1990), ruminative coping (Nolen-Hoeksema, 1994), negative life events (Kendler et al., 1993; Silberg et al., 1999), gender role intensification (Aubé, Fichman, Saltaris, & Koestner, 2000), and lower levels of assertiveness and instrumentality in girls (Galambos, Almeida, & Petersen, 1990). Four particularly influential reviews (Cyranowski et al., 2000; Hankin & Abramson, 2001; Hyde, Mezulis, & Abramson, 2008; Nolen-Hoeksema & Girgus, 1994) have proposed models of the emergence of gender differences in depression that have guided research. Because these articles are widely cited, we summarize them only briefly here before exploring elaborations on their contributions.

In their landmark review, Nolen-Hoeksema and Girgus (1994) proposed multiple general explanatory models and concluded that the empirical literature at the time lent the most support to one of those models. According to that model, girls have more risk factors for depression that are present before adolescence, but those risk factors become more salient and lead to vulnerability when they combine with interpersonal challenges in adolescence, which are proposed to be greater for girls than for boys. The interaction between greater risk factors and greater interpersonal challenges is postulated to lead to more depression for girls. There is support for this model for specific risk factors (e. g., rumination; Jose & Brown, 2008).

Similar to the Nolen-Hoeksema and Girgus's model, Cyranowski and colleagues (2000) proposed a model in which girls are postulated to have multiple vulnerabilities that, when combined with negative life events, increase depression. Their model was particularly innovative in that it incorporated sociocultural (e. g., intensified gender role socialization), psychosocial (e. g., anxious temperament, insecure attachment, poor coping), and biological (e. g., oxytocin levels) factors. Cyranowski and colleagues' integrative perspective led to an increase in empirical studies attempting to link contributory causal factors for adolescent depression across traditional levels of analysis.

Hankin and Abramson (2001) also postulated a general vulnerability–stress mechanism, along with a complex web of associated vulnerability factors. Specifically, they suggested that classic cognitive vulnerability combines with other cognitive vulnerabilities, such as rumination and genetic vulnerabilities, as well as with developmental factors such as pubertal onset. Those vulnerabilities, in the presence of stress, are hypothesized to lead to depression. There is both cross-sectional and longitudinal support for the predictions of their model (e. g., Hankin, 2010; Hankin, Abramson, Miller, & Haeffel, 2004; for reviews, see Ingram, Miranda, & Segal, 1998; Abramson et al., 2002).

Building upon the three previous reviews and models, Hyde and colleagues (2008) proposed an integrative model of depression in adolescent girls that includes affective (i. e., temperament), biological (i. e., timing and development of genetic and pubertal hormones), and cognitive (i. e., negative cognitive style, objectified body consciousness, and rumination) vulnerabilities. Those vulnerabilities are postulated to affect girls more than boys. Hyde and colleagues also suggest that those vulnerabilities interact with stressors, especially negative life events such as peer sexual harassment and child sexual abuse. Together the vulnerabilities and stressors result in negative emotional experiences and consequently more depression among adolescent girls than boys.

In a comprehensive review, Nolen-Hoeksema (2001) concluded that three decades of research in this area had not fully explained the emergence of gender differences in depression. At that time, Nolen-Hoeksema attributed the limited explanatory power of previous work to a tendency for investigators to focus on single-variable models, as well as to the challenges of linking etiological research with emerging knowledge regarding child and adolescent development. Kendler (2005) articulated persuasively the need for theories of psychopathology to move beyond "main effect," or statistical interaction conceptualizations, and to identify the mediating and moderating roles of multiple contributory factors at multiple levels of analysis. The perspective offered in this chapter draws upon the aforementioned models, but in addition, attempts to integrate several heretofore distinct and independent models of depressive vulnerability—self-discrepancy theory and regulatory focus theory (Higgins, 1987, 1997), theories of depressive coping (e. g., Nolen-Hoeksema, 1994), and theories of gender role ideals as a source of vulnerability to depression (e. g., Aubé et al., 2000)—into a broad psychosocial approach focused on the emergence of gender differences during adolescence.

One commonality among the four major reviews and models (Cyranowski et al., 2000; Hankin & Abramson, 2001; Hyde et al., 2008; Nolen-Hoeksema & Girgus, 1994) is their general framework. Each model uses a vulnerability–stress framework (or the similar stress and coping framework) to account for the translation of life experiences into psychopathology. These frameworks provide clear and testable hypotheses, which have been supported by both experimental and correlational studies. Nonetheless, we suggest that recent developments in social psychology and psychopathology research, pertaining to the development and dysfunction of *self-regulation* (Carver & Scheier, 1998), represent a useful organizational and conceptual framework. That framework can integrate previous models with emerging knowledge regarding changes in self content and processes due to developmental changes during adolescence. Many well-established psychosocial vulnerability factors present in the other models can be understood within a self-regulatory framework (Karoly, 1999), and we suggest that doing so has the potential to add substantially to our understanding of the factors that underlie the increase in vulnerability to depression among adolescent girls.

To our knowledge, there are currently no models of gender differences in adolescent depression that focus primarily on personal goals and self-evaluative standards as potential contributory factors in risk versus resilience. Although self-regulatory perspectives on adult depression have emerged over the past decade (e. g., Strauman, 2002), such a perspective has yet to be applied systematically to the vexing problem of gender differences in depressive vulnerability as it emerges during adolescence. We suggest that such a perspective could include both similarities and differences in the content of girls' versus boys' goals—itself already documented in the developmental literature—as well as the processes by which individuals pursue those goals and evaluate their progress toward them.

How might a theoretical perspective focusing on personal goals and self-regulatory processes be relevant, and complementary, to the more well-established perspective concerning vulnerabilities, stress, and coping? In the remaining sections we suggest that there are at least four ways in which self-regulatory *processes* and goal *content* can help to explain girls' differential vulnerability to depression. First, the content of individuals' goals and standards influences the type and level of stressors that they encounter in the course of both ordinary and extraordinary life events (Shah & Higgins, 2001). Second, the content of individuals' goals and standards also influences how they respond to stress, particularly because many life events are likely to be interpreted from a goals–self-regulatory perspective (Karoly, 1999). Third, there is a substantial experimental literature indicating that when individuals perceive themselves as unable to attain a salient personal goal, they are likely to experience chronic negative affect that increases vulnerability to depression and other psychological disorders (Scott & O'Hara, 1993). To these three postulates drawn from the existing literature, we would add a fourth, more exploratory one: that the consequences of self-regulatory failure are likely to be more affectively significant during adolescence compared to childhood, due to a combination of neurobiological and psychosocial factors (Higgins, 1989; Steinberg, 2010).

A SELF-REGULATORY PERSPECTIVE ON STRESS, COPING, DEPRESSION, AND GENDER

Self-Regulation in the Context of Development

The developmental context that surrounds children as they move into adolescence is an important backdrop to the emergence of gender differences in depression. Throughout childhood, parents help children to develop and internalize behavioral guides that lead them toward being a certain kind of person, under the assumption that certain personal qualities and characteristics will lead to enhanced well-being as the children move into adolescence and adulthood (Maccoby & Martin, 1983; Manian, Papadakis, Strauman, & Essex, 2006). Although this socialization process is ongoing, it takes on new meaning and content during adolescence, a time when individuals take on more adult-like responsibilities and have greater accountability (Graber & Brooks-Gunn, 1996). Important figures such as parents and peers, as well as the broader culture and community, shift their expectations and standards for adolescents' characteristics and behavior (Higgins, 1989). Adolescents internalize those expectations and regulate their behavior relative to them. This process, which is critical to development itself, is likely to play a critical role in emotional resilience versus vulnerability. How might theories of self-regulation, as originally developed with an emphasis on adults, provide useful insights for models of vulnerability to adolescent depression?

Theories of Self-Regulation

Theories of the self have identified positive reference values important for self-regulation, such as potential or possible selves (Markus & Nurius, 1986), the type of person individuals would like to be (Cooley, 1964; Rogers, 1961), or the type of person individuals believe they should be (James, 1948). In contrast to the developmental psychology literature (e. g., Kochanska, Murray, & Harlan, 2000), social and personality psychologists use the term *self-regulation* to refer to the ongoing process in which an individual compares a current behavior or personal attribute with a salient goal or standard and then either maintains the behavior/attribute or attempts to modify it to make it more similar to the reference value (Carver & Scheier, 1990). Psychologists have long known that people are motivated to make their current behavior or attributes (their "actual self") as similar as possible to a desired reference point, and a discrepancy between the actual self and a self-standard is postulated to induce a state in which the individual is motivated to change the behavior/attribute to meet the standard (Duval & Wicklund, 1972).

Self-discrepancy theory (Higgins, 1987) specifies how two types of self-beliefs, called *self-guides*, operate as goals within the self-regulation process. *Ideal guides* are individuals' representations of their own or someone else's hopes, wishes, or aspirations for themselves. They are one's ultimate aspirations or accomplishments, the best that one could be. *Ought guides* are individuals' representations of their own or someone else's beliefs regarding their duties or obligations. They are one's responsibilities, what one is supposed to be. In both adolescents and adults, individual differences in the strength of ideal and ought guides predict a broad range of behaviors and are stable across periods of years (Shah & Higgins, 2001; Strauman, 1996).

Self-discrepancy theory (SDT) has been expanded into a broader theory of self-regulation, namely, regulatory focus theory (RFT; Higgins, 1997). RFT predicts that children acquire self-regulatory goals based on contingent interactions with parents. According to Bowlby (1973), children must establish and maintain relationships with caretakers in order to obtain the nurturance and security they need to survive. This basic need requires that children learn how their behaviors influence caretakers' responses to them (Cooley, 1964). As the hedonic principle suggests, children are motivated to learn how to behave in order to maximize pleasure and minimize pain. Consequently, children learn that certain behaviors affect the likelihood of positive outcomes, whereas other behaviors affect the likelihood of negative outcomes (Bornstein, 1995; Chamberlain & Patterson, 1995). At the same time, the ways in which parents interact with their children convey messages about what is important. Parenting behaviors are critical in the development of self-regulation, particularly as "parents begin to convey and enforce standards for behavior, and . . . children begin to adopt and internalize parental rules, values, and standards" (Kochanska, Clark, & Goldman, 1997, p. 388).

According to RFT, childhood exposure to different patterns of parenting behaviors will lead to the emergence of individual differences in self-guide strength. Consider how children could come to possess strong ideal guides. When parents show affection to a child for behaving in a desired manner, encourage the child to overcome difficulties, or set up opportunities for the child to engage in rewarding activities, the child experiences a particular kind of pleasure—the presence of a positive outcome. The parent's message is that attaining accomplishments and fulfilling hopes and aspirations ("making good things happen") is important. In contrast, when parents stop reading a story when the child is not paying attention or withhold praise because the child buttoned his or her shirt wrong, the child experiences a particular kind of pain—the absence of a positive outcome. Once again the parent's message is that what matters is attaining accomplishments and fulfilling hopes and aspirations, but this message is communicated in reference to the absence of a desired state. Either way, the message involves advancement, growth, aspiration, and accomplishment, or what Higgins (1989) called a *promotion focus.*

How might children come to possess strong ought guides? According to RFT, a child experiences a different kind of pleasure—the absence of a negative outcome—when parents child-proof the house, train the child to be alert to potential dangers, or teach the child to mind his or her manners. The parent's message is that what matters is ensuring safety, being responsible, following rules, and meeting obligations ("keeping bad things from happening"). Similarly, a child experiences a different kind of pain—the presence of a negative outcome—when parents yell at the child when he or she doesn't listen, criticize the child when he or she makes a mistake, or punish the child for being irresponsible. Once again, the parent's message is that what matters is ensuring safety, being responsible, and meeting obligations, but the message is communicated in reference to an undesired state. In both situations, the message involves protection, safety, and responsibility, or what Higgins (1989) called a *prevention focus.*

One of the key postulates of both SDT and RFT is that individual differences in strength of orientation to promotion and prevention goals emerge over time (and hypothetically begin to stabilize by the start of adolescence) through the process of socialization and carry both costs and benefits to the individual. That is, at any given time pursuit of a promotion or prevention goal, or use of a promotion-oriented or prevention-oriented strategy in social interactions, may be more or less adaptive depending upon the circumstances (Higgins, 1989). In addition, both theories propose that the perception of discrepancy between one's actual state and a desired end state can have positive or negative consequences, depending on factors such as the individual's overall emotional state, his or her chronic magnitude of self-discrepancy, and the extent to which he or she can switch goals or goal pursuit strategies to increase the likelihood of success.

According to SDT, discrepancies between the actual self and different self-guides lead to distinct negative emotional states. The self-guide involved in a particular self-discrepancy could represent either the individual's own standpoint or that of a significant other (for children, most notably a parent; for adolescents, typically a peer). An actual-self/ideal-self discrepancy is hypothesized to lead to dejection-related emotions (e. g., sadness or disappointment) because such a perceived discrepancy signifies a failure to attain a hoped-for state. In contrast, an actual-self/ought-self discrepancy is hypothesized to lead to agitation-related emotions (e. g., anxiety, worry, or guilt) because such a perceived discrepancy signifies a failure to live up to one's responsibilities or obligations. There is consistent support for the theory's predictions in both correlational and experimental studies. In correlational studies, interview or free-response questionnaire methods are used to elicit individual's self-guides (from their own standpoint as well as the standpoint of parents or peers) as well as their beliefs about their actual attributes and behaviors. Many experimental studies (e. g., Higgins, Bond, Klein, & Strauman, 1986) of self-discrepancy have used a "priming" technique in which each participant is incidentally exposed to his or her own ideal or ought guides (as identified previously). The participant's self-guides are coded as congruent or discrepant with the actual self (i. e., "the kind of person you believe you actually are"). The priming attributes used in these experimental studies are positively valenced (e. g., "intelligent,", "successful," "attractive," and "popular"). When participants are exposed to these attributes, specific negative motivational and emotional states are hypothesized to result, even though the priming attributes are literally positive. According to SDT, it is the self-regulatory significance of these stimuli that accounts for their motivational and emotional impact (Higgins, 1997).

The predictions of SDT regarding the affective consequences of self-evaluation have important clinical implications. The theory asserts that the negative affect produced by discrepancies initially triggers self-regulatory processes aimed at reducing the discrepancies. However, when individuals are unable to reduce a discrepancy, they experience more intense and prolonged distress, which, in turn, increases vulnerability to disorders such as depression, generalized anxiety, and eating disorders (e. g., Scott & O'Hara, 1993; Strauman, 1989, 1992). There have been only a few applications of self-discrepancy theory to adolescent depression, but those applications hold promise. As in adults, self-discrepancy is associated with depression in adolescents, particularly among girls (Hankin, Roberts, & Gotlib, 1997; Moretti & Wiebe, 1999; Papadakis, Prince, Jones, & Strauman, 2006). In addition, Hankin and colleagues (1997) found that girls have higher levels of actual-ideal self-discrepancy than do boys and that that difference mediates the gender difference in depression.

We theorize that there are many possible connections between the processes of self-regulation and self-discrepancy that increase vulnerability to depression and the factors of stress and coping (present in current models of the emergence of gender differences in depression) that also increase vulnerability to depression. First, self-discrepancy can be thought of as similar to, or even a specific type of, life stress. Stress can be defined as "a particular relationship between the person and the environment that is appraised by the person as taxing or exceeding his or her resources and endangering his or her well-being" (Lazarus & Folkman, 1984, p. 19). Under many circumstances, stress could be reconceptualized as the inability to meet goals or as a reaction to a perceived self-discrepancy that occurs when an individual is unable to attain a goal. Therefore, as levels of self-discrepancy increase, we expect levels of stress to increase as well.

Second, self-regulatory processes can be viewed as cognitive processes that underlie behavior, including coping responses to stress. That is, one self-regulates in reference to goals, and therefore, the specific goal content influences the behavior in which a person engages. For example, if an adolescent girl holds strongly the goals of being a good friend and being nice, she will be more likely to respond to stress in a friendship (e. g., a disagreement) by avoiding conflict and ruminating about the disagreement rather than problem-solving or confronting the friend.

Third, one mechanism that may explain how discrepancy leads to depression is by affecting coping responses. That is, individuals cope with discrepancies in particular ways. Specifically, the inability to meet goals is associated with more catastrophizing, self-blame, and rumination; in turn those coping strategies are associated with higher levels of depression (Schroevers, Kraaij, & Garnefski, 2007).

Fourth, we suggest that the consequences of self-discrepancy may become more affectively significant during adolescence. Cognitive development, increasingly complex peer interactions and social networks, changing expectations from the social environment, and individual neurobiological changes, may lead to changes in adolescents' goals and goal structures. During this time period, adolescents themselves and those around them expect them to develop and pursue more complex goals. Those more complex goals may be associated with longer-term goals such as attending college and initiating a successful career. The goals and one's pursuit of them may also take on more significance as the goals become more central to one's identity, which gains increasing solidification during adolescence. Therefore, we suggest that as self-regulatory content and processes solidify, intensify, and generalize in adolescence, the increasing number, complexity, and importance of adolescents' goals will have greater implications for the emotional consequences of meeting or not meeting those goals. In order to more fully understand the connections between self-regulation and stress and coping, we next review the literature on stress and coping in adolescence from a developmental-contextual perspective.

THE DEVELOPMENTAL CONTEXT
FOR AN INTEGRATIVE MODEL

Developmental Shifts in Magnitude, Type, and Gender Specificity of Life Stress

One commonality among previous reviews and models of adolescent depression is the inclusion of stress as a factor in the development of depression. Within the contexts of family, peers, and school, adolescents experience shifts in social roles and increasing responsibility (Graber & Brooks-Gunn,

1996). From a self-regulation perspective, those shifts reflect changes in goals or standards for adolescents and their behavior. While the shifts provide opportunities for growth and success, they also increase opportunities for stress. Indeed, typically teens report stress in all three of the contexts of family, peers and school (Rudolph & Hammen, 1999). Adolescents also experience stress regarding their futures (Nurmi, Poole, & Kalakoski, 1994; Nurmi, Poole, & Seginer, 1995), which can take the form of preoccupation about their education and career-related issues as well as a sense of aimlessness and insecurity (Frydenberg & Lewis, 1999; Matheney, Aycock, & McCarthy, 1993). The increase in stress during the transition to and across adolescence parallels, and is argued by many investigators to at least partially account for, the increase in depression during this period (Ge et al., 1994). In sum, adolescence is a time of changes in sources of stress and increases in stress levels, and these normative developmental changes may be partially due to changes in goals and standards that adolescents hold themselves and that their social worlds also hold for them.

In general, stress is associated with increased risk for depression and other forms of psychological maladjustment (Compas, Connor-Smith, Saltzman, Thomsen, & Wadsworth, 2001; Fields & Prinz, 1997; Seiffge-Krenke, 2000). However, gender appears to moderate the association between stressful life events and depressive symptoms. Stressful life events have a greater impact on girls' reports of depressive symptoms than boys' reports of depressive symptoms; that is, girls appear to be more reactive, at least with regard to internalizing symptoms, to environmental stressors than boys (Compas & Wagner, 1991; Dornbusch, Mont-Reynaud, Ritter, Chen, & Steinberg, 1991; Ge et al., 1994; Hankin, Mermelstein, & Roesch, 2007; Rudolph & Hammen, 1999; Siddique & D'Arcy, 1984). One possible explanation for the disproportionate effect of stress on depression for girls versus boys is that girls may hold their goals more strongly and have more difficulty disengaging from them (e. g., Van Hook & Higgins, 1988). Therefore, when stress arises due to the inability to meet a goal, a girl may have trouble reducing the discrepancy by changing the goal or decreasing the goal importance (e. g., by focusing on other salient goals).

It also appears that adolescent girls experience more stress than boys (e. g., Allgood-Merten et al., 1990; Davies & Windle, 1997; Graber et al., 1995; Hankin et al., 2007; Schwartz & Koenig, 1996). However, this finding is not always consistent (e. g., Rudolph & Hammen, 1999), and the inconsistency may result from differences in the type of stressors considered. Although stress appears to increase in adolescence for both boys and girls, there may be more nuanced patterns of gender-specific changes for different kinds of stressors. Indeed, a longitudinal analysis of gender-linked changes in stress suggests that while boys have more uncontrollable stressful life events before age 12, the pattern shifts at age 13, with girls reporting more uncontrollable stressful life events than boys (Ge et al., 1994). Also, for girls, interpersonal stress increases from preadolescence to adolescence; in contrast, for boys, *non*interpersonal stress increases from preadolescence to adolescence (Rudolph & Hammen, 1999). Interestingly, adolescent girls experience more self-generated interpersonal stress with parents and peers than do adolescent boys or preadolescents (Rudolph & Hammen, 1999). In contrast, adolescent boys experience more self-generated noninterpersonal stress than do adolescent girls or preadolescents (Rudolph & Hammen, 1999). Therefore, whereas some shifts in pressures during adolescence are common across boys and girls (e. g., to seek a career path, to gain more independence), other shifts seem to differ for girls and boys. It may also be the case that girls' orientation toward certain goals (e. g., interpersonal and relationship goals), that are not shared as strongly by boys, increases girls' risk for certain stressors. Adolescence also seems to bring on certain stressors that are specific to, or more common among, girls, in part because of the way that pubertal morphological changes alter adolescents' self-views and because of the way that others in the social environment interact with girls after those morphological changes.

Morphological Changes, Sexual Harassment, and Sexual Abuse

Pubertal changes in body shape typically lead girls to perceive themselves as differing in appearance from thin cultural ideals (Stice, 2003), which girls internalize, to a great degree, as goals for themselves. The perceived differences between their own body shape and the culturally established ideal body lead girls to have more negative body esteem than boys (Mendelson, Mendelson, & White, 2001; Polce-Lynch, Myers, Kliewer, & Kilmartin, 2001). This may occur because changes in body weight and weight distribution associated with puberty cause girls, but not boys, to feel that they are overweight (Ge, Elder, Regenerus, & Cox, 2001c). Indeed, body image and self-esteem may at least partially mediate the association between gender and depression in adolescence (Allgood-Merten et al., 1990). Further, longitudinal research suggests that body dissatisfaction is associated with increases in depressive symptoms, but the reverse is not true (Stice & Bearman, 2001; Stice & Whitenton, 2002). Within a self-regulatory perspective, these findings can be understood as girls having an increased vulnerability to not meeting internalized standards or goals related to body shape, compared to boys and preadolescent girls. That is, the content of their goals can lead to an increase in their perceived discrepancy from their goals and therefore increased stress and, consequently, depression.

In addition to the effects of morphological changes on their own self-views and depressive symptoms, changes in young girls' and boys' bodies during adolescence serve as a social stimulus for peers and adults to view and treat adolescents as maturing young women and men (Brooks-Gunn, 1991; Galambos et al., 1990; Lindberg, Grabe, & Hyde, 2007). With puberty, girls' bodies become a social stimulus for others to treat them in a more sexualized manner (Fredrickson & Roberts, 1997). Additionally, we suggest that girls' bodily changes serve as a stimulus for changes in their own understanding of themselves and their goals for themselves. When others begin to treat them as sexual beings and when they begin to see themselves more in that light, the issues and expectations in the sexual arena for adult women become more relevant and salient for adolescent girls. The new domain contains new goals and creates new opportunities for positive emotions and adjustment to the degree that girls are able to meet those goals. However, the conflicting goals and expectations for girls and women (e. g., to be both demure and yet also sexy) may make it complicated, or impossible, for them to meet all of their internalized goals and standards. Such inabilities to meet self-goals increase the risk for depression (Strauman, 2002).

Another unfortunate potential consequence of physical maturity for girls is that they face increased sexual harassment and abuse (Costello, Erkanli, Fairbank, & Angold, 2002; Hyde et al., 2008; Tolin & Foa, 2006). The increases in stress due to sexual harassment and abuse have been proposed as a partial explanation for the emergence of gender differences in depression (Hyde et al., 2008; Cutler & Nolen-Hoeksema, 1991). Further, sexual abuse victimization is a particularly deleterious form of stress that differentially affects girls compared to boys and has many long term effects, including depression (Kendler, Kuhn, & Prescott, 2004). Although the impact of sexual abuse on self-regulation has yet to be explored systematically, it is likely that such abuse at any point in development creates significant and lasting problems both for self-concept, as well as for the goals that girls pursue and the strategies they use to pursue them.

The issues that result from morphological changes may be particularly relevant for early-maturing girls. Although early puberty is stressful and a risk factor for maladjustment for both boys and girls, the effect of early maturity on depression is greater for girls than boys (Ge, Conger, & Elder, 2001a, 2001b). The stresses of the pubertal transition may be greater for early-maturing girls because they have to confront new environmental stressors, social norms, and behavioral expectations before they are psychologically prepared (Ge et al., 2001a). From a self-regulation perspective, early puberty creates particular challenges for preteens but especially for girls. In particular, changes in appearance have the effect of altering the expectations (implicit as well as explicit) that others in the girl's social environment have for her, which can lead to more conflicts among personal goals and therefore more in perceived failure, identity confusion, and distress.

Interpersonal Stress

Another type of stress that is important in adolescence is interpersonal stress. Between 46 and 82% of the stressful everyday events experienced by adolescents are interpersonal or relational in nature (Compas & Phares, 1991; Ebata & Moos, 1994; Seiffge-Krenke, 2006). These stressors occur within relationships with parents (Seiffge-Krenke, Weidemann, Fentner, Aegenheister, & Poeblau, 2001; Thornton, Orbuch, & Axinn, 1995), friends (Bowker, Bukowski, Hymel, & Sippola, 2000), and romantic partners (Nieder & Seiffge-Krenke, 2001; Pollina & Snell, 1999). There are also age- and gender-linked shifts in stressors in interpersonal stress. During adolescence, there is a shift in the social environment as the salience of the family decreases and the salience of peers increases (Larson & Asmussen, 1991; Laursen, 1996; Steinberg & Silverberg, 1986). Adolescents may experience more interpersonal stress than children because they are more focused on peer interactions and because they are more engaged in actively selecting their friends and companions and in creating their social worlds (Boyce, Frank, Jensen, & MacArthur Foundation Research Network on Psychopathology and Development, 1998; Rudolph & Asher, 2000; Scarr, 1992). Other social–environmental changes that compound interpersonal stress during adolescence are the increased importance of being in a popular clique and increased conformity pressures (Gavin & Furman, 1989). Such pressures and social jockeying may explain why there are more antagonistic interactions with peers during early and middle adolescence, compared to childhood or even late adolescence (Gavin & Furman, 1989).

Whereas adolescent boys experience more achievement-related stress, girls experience more interpersonal stress with peers, romantic partners, and family members (Gore, Aseltine, & Cohen, 1993; Larson & Ham, 1993; Leadbeater, Blatt, & Quinlan, 1995; Rudolph & Hammen, 1999; Rudolph, 2002; Towbes, Cohen, & Glyshaw, 1989; Wagner & Compas, 1990; Windle, 1992). However, some have argued that girls' characteristic interpersonal orientation during adolescence involves tradeoffs and may not be inherently more or less adaptive than boys' orientations (Rose & Rudolph, 2006). On one hand, girls experience more positive social interactions (Gavin & Furman, 1989) and the protective effects of social support (Burton, Stice, & Seeley, 2004). However, as interpersonal and friendship roles and expectations change in adolescence (see Greene & Larson, 1991; Fenzel & Blyth, 1986), girls may seek more emotional support from their friendships, and this increased need may place them at risk for greater interpersonal stress—which, in turn, may be more salient and a larger threat to their well-being to them than for boys (Rudolph & Hammen, 1999). Girls' greater interpersonal focus may also lead them to experience and be more sensitive to stressful life events among members of their social networks than boys; this effect appears to intensify from childhood through adolescence (Gore et al., 1993; Wagner & Compas, 1990). Girls' increases in interpersonal stress may also be due to changes in relationships during adolescence. Whereas boys' friendships typically are based on companionship and affiliation, girls' friendships are more focused on intimacy and disclosure (Berndt, 1982; Cooper & Ayers-Lopez, 1985; Youniss & Smollar, 1985), and adolescence brings on more intimacy, loyalty, and closeness in friendships (for a review, see Laursen, 1996). That increased intimacy may set the stage for increased possibilities for interpersonal stress, particularly among adolescent girls. Girls may have more stringent standards for themselves and their friends, which may set the stage for more trespasses within their friendships—and increased interpersonal stress.

In general, interpersonal stress is associated with distress and depression (Gore et al., 1993; Larson & Ham, 1993; Rudolph, 2002; Wagner & Compas, 1990). However, girls seem to be more affected than boys by interpersonal stressors (Goodyer & Altham, 1991; Hankin et al., 2007; Leadbeater et al., 1995; Moran & Eckenrode, 1991). Indeed, gender moderates the association between interpersonal stress, in general, and peer stress in particular, on emotional difficulties, with girls being more affected by stress than boys (Goodyer & Altham, 1991; Rudolph, 2002; Rudolph & Hammen, 1999). For example, girls report being more bothered by negative peer behaviors (Gavin & Furman, 1989), and peer social aggression has a greater negative impact on girls than boys (Crick, Bigbee, & Howes, 1996; Galen & Underwood, 1997; Paquette & Underwood, 1999). In contrast, boys may be more affected than girls by school stressors (Sund, Larsson, & Wichstrom, 2003). Whereas boys' negative moods tend to be associated with activities (e. g., competitive games), girls' negative moods tend to be associated with interpersonal encounters and events (Larson & Asmussen, 1991). These findings suggest that the effect of interpersonal stress on depression may be moderated by gender, but there is also evidence that the gender difference in depression is partially mediated by interpersonal stress involving peers (Hankin et al., 2007; Liu & Kaplan, 1999; Rudolph & Hammen, 1999; Rudolph, 2002) and family (Davies & Windle, 1997). These findings make sense when seen through the lens of the self-regulation framework. Gender may both moderate and mediate the effect of interpersonal stress on depression because interpersonal goals are particularly important and salient to girls. Therefore, when girls perceive that they are unable to meet interpersonal goals, it is likely to have a larger effect on their well-being and on symptoms of depression than for boys (a moderation effect). And, further, because they are more likely to have interpersonal goals, girls are more likely than boys to experience interpersonal stress—which increases their vulnerability to depression.

Not only does exposure to stress lead to increased depression in adolescents, but depressed adolescents may interact with their social environments in such a way that they increase their own stress levels (Hammen, 1991). Stress that is partially generated by the individual is referred to as dependent stress. In two longitudinal studies (Cole, Nolen-Hoeksema, Girgus, & Paul, 2006), Cole and colleagues found support for an association between depression and dependent stress. They found that not only does stress lead to higher levels of depression over time, but also, trait and state dysphoric symptoms predict subsequent stressful life events, even after controlling for prior stressful life events. And, it appears that there is a reciprocal association between depression and dependent stress, because dependent stress predicts depression (e. g., Rudolph & Hammen, 1999). However, to date, relatively few studies have examined potential gender-linked patterns of stress generation either during the transition to adolescence or during adolescence itself.

Responses to Stress—Coping

Although stress exposure and its effects on mood help to explain adolescent depression, it is also important to consider how individuals respond to stress (Lazarus & Folkman, 1984). We also suggest that there may be two ways that self-regulatory goal content and processes may be associated with coping. First, there is evidence in college students that goal failure may prompt coping; in particular, goal failure appears to be a stressor that is associated with more rumination and catastrophizing (Schroevers et al., 2007). Second, individuals' specific goals for themselves may influence the types of coping strategies that they will use in response to stress (Jones, Papadakis, Hogan, & Strauman, 2009).

In their broad model of responses to stress, Compas and colleagues suggest that responses vary along multiple dimensions (Compas et al., 2001; Connor-Smith, Compas, Wadsworth, Thomsen, & Saltzman, 2000). The broadest distinction is between voluntary and involuntary responses. Voluntary responses are purposeful, controlled reactions to stress and encompass what is generally referred to as coping. Coping can be defined as "conscious volitional efforts to regulate emotion, cognition, behavior, physiology, and the environment in response to stressful events or circumstances" (Compas et al., 2001, p. 89). Voluntary responses include those directed toward changing the stressor or one's reaction to it (engagement) as well as responses directed away from the stressor or one's reaction to it (disengagement; Connor-Smith et al., 2000). Voluntary disengagement strategies include responses such as acceptance and distraction (Connor-Smith et al., 2000). Involuntary responses to stress include reactions that "may or may not be within conscious awareness and are not under volitional control" (Compas et al., 2001, p. 977), and include engagement responses such as rumination and intrusive thoughts as well as disengagement responses such as involuntary avoidance and emotional numbing (Connor-Smith et al., 2000).

In addition to the gender-linked patterns in stress noted above, there are some gender-linked patterns in responses to stress. With regard to the emergence of a gender difference in depression, the most well studied gender-linked coping pattern involves rumination, which is a form of involuntary engagement and can be defined as a repetitive focus on negative mood and its causes and consequences (Nolen-Hoeksema, 1991). There are mixed findings about whether girls ruminate more than boys in childhood (Broderick, 1998; Broderick & Korteland, 2002; Broderick & Korteland, 2004). However, there are fairly consistent findings that adolescent girls ruminate more than boys (Compas, Malcarne, & Fondacaro, 1988; Jose & Brown, 2008; Li, DiGiuseppe, & Froh, 2006; Schwartz & Koenig, 1996), with one notable exception (Burwell & Shirk, 2007). In a careful analysis, Jose and Brown (2008) found that the gender difference in rumination begins at about age 12, which was 1 year prior to the emergence of gender differences in stress and depression in their sample. The relative timing of the increase in rumination and the increases in stress and depression suggest that rumination may be a causal factor in the development of gender differences in depression.

Studies also suggest that rumination is associated with the development and maintenance of depressed mood in adolescents, because it is predictive of depression in adolescence concurrently and prospectively (Burwell & Shirk, 2007; Jose & Brown, 2008; Kraaij et al., 2003; Schwartz & Koenig, 1996), as well as in adulthood (e. g., Treynor, Gonzalez, & Nolen-Hoeksema, 2003). In addition, gender differences in rumination may partially explain the gender difference in depression, because rumination partially mediates the gender difference in depression (Grant et al., 2004; Jose & Brown, 2008) and also partially mediates increases in depression over time for girls but not for boys (Burwell & Shirk, 2007). In addition, rumination mediates the association between stress and depression in preadolescent and adolescent girls and adolescent (though not preadolescent) boys (Jose & Brown, 2008). Although rumination appears to be part of the process by which stress levels lead to more depression, gender appears to moderate the association between rumination and depression, with rumination leading to more depression for girls than boys (Jose & Brown, 2008). In addition, there is some evidence that rumination intensifies the effect of stress on depression (Kraaij et al., 2003), although this is not a consistent finding (Jose & Brown, 2008).

Although girls tend to engage in more rumination, which is an isolative activity, they also seek more emotional and instrumental support than boys do. This is true in relation to stress in general and interpersonal stress in particular, and the gender difference in support seeking increases with age (for a review, see Rose & Rudolph, 2006). This gender difference is consistent with girls' more interpersonally oriented goals. However, girls' interpersonal orientation may also prompt their tendency to co-ruminate (Rose, 2002; Rose, Carlson, & Waller, 2007). Like rumination, co-rumination is a repetitive process focused on problems and distress; however, co-rumination occurs when individuals, usually friends, talk together repetitively about their problems and negative feelings (Rose, 2002). Co-rumination has been proposed as a possible explanation for the emergence of gender differences in depression. Indeed, girls report co-ruminating more than boys do, and co-rumination predicts depression prospectively (Rose et al., 2007) and partially explains gender differences in depression (Rose, 2002). However, co-rumination also partially mediates the gender difference in friendship quality (Rose, 2002). That is, co-rumination partially explains why girls have higher friendship quality than boys, but it also leads to more depression for girls versus boys.

From a self-regulation perspective, girls' tendencies to ruminate and co-ruminate are understandable. That is, they represent coping strategies that are consistent with girls' goals not to cause interpersonal difficulties and to have strong friendships. Rumination is an alternative to confrontational strategies, and co-rumination may simply be a manifestation of the interpersonal orientation and social support seeking gone awry. Rumination and co-rumination may also have particular importance in the self-regulatory process by keeping failures to meet self-goals salient. Indeed, rumination intensifies the negative effects of self-discrepancies on depression in adolescent girls (Papadakis et al., 2006) and college students (Jones et al., 2009). Therefore, rumination appears to intensify the effects of self-regulatory processes on depression.

In addition to rumination, co-rumination, and support seeking, there are other coping strategies that follow gender-linked patterns. Specifically, girls also use more passive avoidance (Hampel & Petermann, 2005), resignation (Donaldson, Prinstein, Donovsky, & Spirito, 2000), problem solving, and emotional expression (Connor-Smith et al., 2000; de Anda et al., 2000). At the same time, boys use more distraction (Broderick, 1998; Connor-Smith et al., 2000; Copeland & Hess, 1995; Hampel & Petermann, 2005; Kurdek, 1987), humor (e. g., Chapman & Mullis, 1999; Kurdek, 1987; Copeland & Hess, 1995) and positive self-instructions that are part of problem solving (Hampel & Petermann, 2005), as well as more cognitive restructuring, emotional regulation, acceptance, emotional numbing, and escape (Connor-Smith et al., 2000). It also appears that boys use more behavioral avoidance and withdrawal (Causey & Dubow, 1992; Chapman & Mullis, 1999; Copeland & Hess, 1995; Rose & Asher, 2004), but that finding is not consistent (e. g., Connor-Smith et al., 2000; Ebata & Moos, 1994; Kliewer, Fearnow, & Miller, 1996; Phelps & Jarvis, 1994).

In general, it is challenging to map the literature on gender differences in coping strategies onto the literature regarding the impact of coping strategies on depression, as there is little consistency in the coping strategies studied. However, research on the effects of coping strategies on depression suggest that voluntary engagement primary control strategies—that is, voluntary strategies aimed at changing the stressor, such as active coping and problem solving—are associated with fewer internalizing symptoms (Clarke, 2006; Compas et al., 1988). Similarly, secondary control strategies—that is, voluntary engagement strategies aimed at adjusting one's response to a stressor, such as positive reappraisal and positive thinking and distraction—are associated with less depression (Compas, Langrock, Keller, Merchant, & Copeland, 2002; Kraaij et al., 2003). In contrast, some disengagement strategies such as avoidance and some negative engagement strategies such as self-blame, rumination, and castrophizing are associated with more depression (Garnefski & Kraaij, 2006; Garnefski, Kraaij, & van Etten, 2005; Herman-Stahl, Stemmler, & Peterson, 1995; Seiffge-Krenke & Klessinger, 2000; Seiffge-Krenke & Stemmler, 2002).

Based on these findings (taken together with the literature on gender differences in coping), we suggest that adolescent girls are more likely to engage in and rely on coping strategies that increase their vulnerability to depression. This is not itself a novel insight from the perspective of the stress and coping literature, but we believe that a self-regulation perspective both reinforces that impression and helps to explain its origins and functions. It appears that girls' higher levels of passive avoidance and emotional expression and lower levels of distraction, cognitive restructuring, emotional numbing, and escape may represent clusters of coping strategies that are associated with more depression, in part because of their consequences for goal pursuit in social contexts. We also suggest that those coping strategies are also generally consistent with girls' goals, representing an additional source of vulnerability (e. g., the combination of an interpersonally oriented goal and certain types of coping styles that inadvertently exacerbate stress in social interactions).

While research suggests that coping has a main effect on depression, aside from studies on rumination, there are few reports that examine how coping may moderate the effect of stress on depression, and there are several that report null results. One possible reason for the inconsistent findings is that few studies have examined particular coping strategies within specific domains or types of stress. For example, ruminative coping may be more likely to moderate the effects of uncontrollable versus controllable stress, peer versus parental stress, dependent versus independent life events, or life events versus daily hassles. By characterizing coping and stress at a high level of abstraction and generality, we may inadvertently obscure subtler patterns within the data. A few studies have begun to disentangle the effects of particular coping strategies in particular domains. For example, in a study of college women, Mezulis, Abramson, and Hyde (2002) found that women ruminated more than men within the three domains of achievement, interpersonal relationships, and body image, but the gender differences in the achievement domain are small compared to differences in the interpersonal and body image domains. Although these findings do not directly test the moderation effect and were conducted with an older population, they suggest that a more nuanced analysis may yield clearer patterns. We suggest that it would be useful to consider a self-regulatory perspective when selecting which domain and coping strategy pairings to examine in future research. For example, following the Mezulis et al. (2002) finding, one might hypothesize that rumination will intensify the negative effects of problems with interpersonal relationships and body image for girls more so than for boys. And this also follows from the self-regulatory perspective, as interpersonal relationships and body image are more central and salient goals for girls versus boys.

Developmental Origins of Gender Differences in Stress and Coping

Certainly there are many sources for sex differences in stress, coping, and adjustment. Others have reviewed sexual and social challenges (Nolen-Hoeksema & Girgus, 1994), parent socialization (Keenan & Shaw, 1997; Zahn-Waxler, Cole, & Barrett, 1991), school contexts (Eccles et al., 1993), and hormonal and body image changes (Brooks-Gunn, Graber, & Paikoff, 1994; Susman, Dorn, & Chrousos, 1991). We will focus our discussion on parental and peer socialization influences, particularly as they pertain to a self-regulation perspective on emotional vulnerability.

Adults act as strong socialization agents for gender-linked characteristics (e.g., Ruble & Martin, 1998). For example, parents socialize their daughters to be more empathic and self-disclosing and their sons to be more independent and physically competent (Ruble & Martin, 1998; Zahn-Wexler, 2000; Zahn-Wexler et al., 1991). Those differences may interact with biological factors such as sex-linked hormonal reactions to stress, which are associated with oxytocin-related affiliative responses in girls and testosterone-related aggressive responses in boys (Geary & Flinn, 2002; Taylor et al., 2000). Indeed, the developmental postulates of self-discrepancy theory (Higgins, 1989) emphasize how the nature and sources of goals and standards vary predictably across childhood and how they are likely to differ as a function of gender, both during childhood and as children move into adolescence. Our comments in the previous section illustrate some of the vicissitudes of self-guides during the teen years, and both this chapter and others in the volume discuss how girls and boys are likely to self-regulate toward different goals and in different ways.

The gender differences in goals and characteristics may also be further reinforced and socialized by peers (Rose & Rudolph, 2006). The peer group is an important socializing context during adolescence (Larson & Asmussen, 1991; Laursen, 1996; Steinberg & Silverberg, 1986). The influence of peers begins early, and exposure to same-sexed peers in childhood leads to more sex-typed behavior (Martin & Fabes, 2001). Those socialization processes continue in adolescence; adolescents positively reinforce one another for displaying sex-typed behavior (Hibbard & Buhrmester, 1998). Even children of parents who are intent on treating their children in gender-neutral ways have children who live and interact in a highly sex-typed peer culture (Harris, 1995), which can lead to gender-linked patterns in their children. All of these sex-typed behaviors can be understood within a goals perspective. Girls and boys are socialized by parents and peers to have gender-typed internalized goals and standards and then to strive to meet them. In addition, from a self-regulation perspective, the shift toward peers as a primary source of self-evaluative standards and personal goals increases the salience of social interactions in general and peers in particular.

It has been shown repeatedly that gender socialization, particularly in terms of socialized gender characteristics, is relevant to vulnerability to depression because individuals with fewer masculine characteristics and more negative feminine characteristics have higher risk for depression (Allgood-Merten et al., 1990; Bassoff & Glass, 1982; Craighead & Green, 1989; Li et al., 2006; Roos & Cohen, 1987). Further, it appears that the negative association between masculine attributes and depression is mediated by coping (Li et al., 2006; Nezu & Nezu, 1987). Specifically, individuals with more masculine attributes engage in more active behavioral coping, more distractive coping, less avoidant coping reactions, more problem-focused coping, and less emotion-focused coping—coping styles that are, in turn, related to decreased levels of depression. These findings are consistent with a model that individuals' goals influence their actual characteristics, which in turn influence their behavior (specifically their coping responses to stress), and then depression.

Parent and peer socialization of gender-linked characteristics can also have profound implications for personal goals, standards, and the process of self-regulation, which can, in turn, affect depression. Socialization can be viewed as the process by which external (in this case, parent or peer) goals for an individual become the individual's own goals. According to theories of self-regulation (Carver & Scheier, 1998), when particular goals or standards become central to identity (both as one actually is and as one strives to be), those goals and standards become relevant to emotional well-being. The goals and standards can be a potential locus for perceived failure and lead to emotional vulnerabilities, or they may be a potential locus for perceived success and lead to emotional stability. When the goals and standards are associated with success, they likely reinforce the importance of such standards to make perceived progress toward being a particular kind of person. In this way, consistent with the principles of self-regulation, socialized goals and standards can influence self-regulatory *processes* and have emotional consequences. However, adolescent girls may also be more vulnerable to difficulties with self-regulation than adolescent boys because of the difficult and often contradictory standards that important adults and peers apply to them, and which they internalize themselves. That is, there are gender differences in the *content* of goals and standards.

As noted previously, girls are socialized into having more of an interpersonal focus and more goals regarding relationships. Although they do not differ from boys in their desire for overall peer popularity, adolescent girls care more about having dyadic friendships than boys do (Benenson & Benarroch, 1998). Further, girls have more specific kinds of goals that involve interpersonal relationships. Girls' goals include more social goals (e. g., having friends, helping others) versus nonsocial goals (e. g., getting good grades, making money) compared to boys (Ford, 1982). Also, adolescent girls have more goals regarding intimacy and nurturance (Jarvinen & Nicholls, 1996), relationship maintenance (Chung & Asher, 1996; Rose & Asher, 1999), supportiveness (Rose & Asher, 2004), and resolution of peer problems (Rose & Asher, 2004). Girls also have more worries about social approval, abandonment, and the status of their friendships, as well as more empathy or sensitivity to distress in others than do boys (for a review, see Rose & Rudolph, 2006). Girls' interpersonal orientation and their goals for relationships may place them at risk for developing emotional problems, such as low self-esteem, anxiety, and depression (Rose & Rudolph, 2006), and this risk may be due in part to their increased vulnerability to interpersonal stressors that results from their interpersonal orientation.

In contrast, boys have more agentic and status-oriented goals, such as goals of control (Chung & Asher, 1996; Rose & Asher, 1999; Strough & Berg, 2000), presenting themselves in a socially desirable manner (Rose & Asher, 2004), maintaining their privacy (Rose & Asher, 2004), controlling social situations (Chung & Asher, 1996), dominance (Jarvinen & Nicholls, 1996), and revenge seeking (Rose & Asher, 1999). All of these agentic and status-oriented goals are likely internalized to a greater extent in boys as a result of a gender-specific socialization process. We propose that failure to meet the types of goals that girls possess are more likely to induce stress and depression, compared to those goals espoused by boys.

Finally, this socialization toward an interpersonal focus may also affect how girls cope in response to stress. They may avoid using strategies that are overly assertive or involve conflict. And, although the reliance on friends is not a bad thing, in and of itself, it may be that an overreliance on friends and perhaps co-rumination increases girls' risk for depression, in part through the self-regulatory content and process factors noted above. The interpersonal focus also means that girls may have a more challenging time when faced with interpersonal stress because they cannot necessarily rely on their primary support (including friends) when faced with interpersonal stressors. In the next section we propose a conceptual framework for integrating existing models of vulnerability with a self-regulation model.

In summary, there are a number of ways in which socialization is likely to influence the emerging differential vulnerability to depression between girls and boys, particularly when viewed from a self-regulation perspective. First, the content of individuals' goals influences the type and level of stressors that they encounter. Second, the content of individuals' goals influences how they respond to stress. Third, people have problems with the process of self-regulation when they experience the inability to achieve a salient goal, and previous research suggests that failure to meet salient goals increases vulnerability to depression. We also posit that the consequences of self-regulatory failure (a process issue) are more potent during adolescence than childhood due to developmental changes. In addition to the vulnerabilities conferred by self-regulatory *processes*, we propose that a self-regulatory perspective and focus on the *content* of adolescents' goals can be helpful in understanding the emergence of gender differences in depression.

A Shift in Self-Regulation in Adolescence

As children become teenagers, the kinds of personal goals that they pursue undergo profound changes. From a self-discrepancy theory perspective, changes in the representational capacities of the child over the course of development lead to a major shift in self-regulation content and processes with the arrival of adolescence (Higgins, 1989). For instance, young adolescents are able to represent abstract, generalized personal characteristics and goals, and to represent the relation (congruent vs. discrepant) between such attributes or goals and their actual behavior. As for other self-regulatory processes, this increasing ability to represent desired and undesired end states brings both costs and benefits. In particular, as long as there is perceived congruency between a goal or standard and the individual's behavior, he or she is likely to feel a sense of well-being and to be motivated to continue such behavior. However, when the adolescent perceives discrepancy between a goal or standard (and, in particular, an expectation from a peer or friend) and his or her actual behavior, the emotional consequences will be more substantial and generalized than had been the case during childhood.

Given the substantial literature indicating that negative self-evaluation in general and self-discrepancy in particular are associated with distress as well as clinical disorders, is there evidence that these self-regulatory processes are relevant to emotional vulnerability during adolescence? And, can such processes help to account for the emergence of gender differences in vulnerability to depression during that critical period? Adolescence is a time when one's sense of identity, as well as one's goals, reach a level of abstraction and sophistication that allows teenagers to see themselves as distinctive and consistent individuals. While in middle childhood, the ability to cope through cognitive means (e. g., distraction, delay, problem solving) solidifies, in adolescence the emergence of metacognition allows for the regulation to be based on future concerns that include long-term goals (Skinner & Zimmer-Gembeck, 2007). As Higgins (1989) noted, the ability to evaluate oneself in terms of progress toward an abstract personal goal—for instance, being a particular kind of person—is itself a developmental achievement. Further, classic theories of cognitive development have long predicted that before adolescence, self-evaluation is more concrete and attribute-specific, whereas self-evaluation becomes more abstract and generalized in adolescence (Case, 1985). It is only when children develop the representational and executive-functioning capacity to perceive themselves in terms of abstract qualities (e. g., attractive, popular, shy, intelligent) that true self-regulatory cognition becomes part of their ongoing interactions with the social world (Harter, 1983).

Thus, a developmental perspective on self-regulation would predict that self-discrepancy takes on a significantly greater emotional potency during adolescence, when individuals are cognitively capable of representing their personal characteristics as stable attributes and also capable of identifying mismatches or inconsistencies between the kind of person they are and the kind of person they would like to be (Harter, 1983). In a landmark study, Moretti and Wiebe (1999) predicted that the same patterns of associations between different types of self-discrepancy and different types of distress observed among adults would be found for adolescents, and that because girls were more likely in general to develop strong self–other contingency beliefs than boys (Cross & Madson, 1997) due to differences in socialization, self-discrepancies would have greater emotional impact on adolescent girls versus boys. Moretti and Wiebe found evidence in support of both hypotheses, particularly that girls were more strongly influenced (in terms of experienced distress) than boys by discrepancies involving ideal and ought self-guides that were identified as coming from parents.

CONCLUSION: TOWARD AN INTEGRATIVE MODEL

The purpose of this chapter has been to explore the existing literature on the emergence of gender differences in depression during adolescence and to investigate how a perspective on self-regulation—the process of evaluating one's behavior in reference to motivationally significant goals and standards—might help to expand our understanding of why adolescent girls are at greater risk for depression than their male counterparts. Others (Hankin & Abramson, 1999; Hankin et al., 2007; Rudolph, 2002) have suggested two distinct conceptual models for how stressors may explain the gender difference in depression. One is a meditational stress exposure model, which postulates that girls are exposed to more stress, which in turn predicts higher levels of depression. The second is a moderational stress reactivity model, which postulates that gender moderates the association between stress and depression such that girls react to, or are affected by, stress more than boys are. Hankin et al. (2007) have noted that the models are not mutually exclusive; indeed, they are complementary. As reviewed above and elaborated in greater detail within the other chapters in this volume, there is solid evidence for both models. For the meditational stress exposure model, girls report more stress (e. g., Allgood-Merten et al., 1990; Davies & Windle, 1997; Graber et al., 1995; Hankin et al., 2007; Schwartz & Koenig, 1996), and stress is associated with more depression concurrently and prospectively, with interpersonal, dependent, family, and peer stressors explaining most of the association between gender and the trajectories of depressive symptoms (Hankin et al., 2007). For the moderational stress reactivity model, there is evidence that stress has a greater impact on depressive symptoms in girls versus boys, although this effect was found only for interpersonal, achievement, independent, peer, and overall level of stressors, and not for family, romantic, school, or athletic stressors, and only marginally for interpersonal and dependent stressors (Hankin et al., 2007).

Similarly, other researchers have argued that the gender difference in depression may be explained by girls' use of fewer adaptive, and more maladaptive, coping strategies; that is, they hypothesize that coping mediates the effect of gender on depression (e. g., Grant et al., 2004; Jose & Brown, 2008). There also is some evidence consistent with this prediction. It is a fundamental component of stress and coping models that how individuals cope with stress will alter the impact of stress on depression; that is, that coping moderates the effect of stress on depression. However, this postulate has not yet received extensive empirical testing within the adolescent stress and coping literature, particularly as it relates to the gender difference in depression.

What has also been lacking in the literature is a larger, integrative model that includes all of the moderation and mediation hypotheses for stress and coping. We propose that these complementary perspectives can be integrated by combining them with a self-regulation perspective that emphasizes both content (e. g., via the addition of socialization and internalized goals to the models) and process (e. g., by acknowledging how self-evaluation in reference to goals and standards, particularly those related to parent and peers, becomes a primary psychological task of adolescence that can lead to feelings of well-being or of failure). Indeed, the ongoing process of self-regulation represents a proximal locus for the distal contributory impact of genetic, biological, cognitive, interpersonal, and societal factors already associated with vulnerability to depression (Strauman, 2002). Our hope is that this chapter is a small step in the direction of integration by identifying points of overlap between existing models and a self-regulation perspective on emotional vulnerability.

What would be the implications of such an expanded model for intervention and prevention? We close with some initial observations and suggestions. In concordance with Abaied and Rudolph's (2010) suggestion, we propose that a comprehensive coping repertoire may be important for adolescents. Parents should consider socializing their children with multiple forms of coping, which may require an expansion and elaboration of the goals that parents typically socialize their children into acquiring. In addition to having a large repertoire, it is likely important for individuals to be flexible in response to stressors. It may be that certain forms of coping that are generally considered to be maladaptive (such as disengagement strategies, e. g., distraction) may in fact be helpful under certain conditions, when other forms of coping that are general considered to be adaptive (such as engagement strategies, e. g., problem solving) may not be effective. For example, consider the following situation. If an adolescent is faced with a relatively mild uncontrollable stressor, it might be better for him or her to use distraction and to ignore the stressor rather than attempt to engage and problem-solve. In addition to being flexible in selecting coping responses for particular stressors, flexibility in response to problems with achieving goals may also be important. For example, it is an important skill to recognize when to continue to try to achieve a goal or standard and when it is better to abandon or revise unattainable goals (Wrosch, Scheier, Miller, Schulz, & Carver, 2003), and not get caught in a cycle of catastrophizing, rumination, and self-blame in response to goal failure, as those coping responses are associated with depression (Schroevers et al., 2007). Parents can assist their children with developing the skills to recognize unattainable goals and to redirect their efforts toward more attainable goals.

We recognize that this integrative work is only in its infancy. Nonetheless, along with the other investigators contributing to this volume, we also recognize the need for research that is prospective, developmentally sound, and focuses on hypotheses across traditional models and levels of analysis. Self-regulation as a construct offers opportunities for such transtheoretical conceptual and empirical work, and we look forward to interactions with our colleagues to develop these ideas and to investigate their potential for expanding our understanding of the etiology, treatment, and prevention of depression in adolescent girls.

REFERENCES

Abaied, J. L., & Rudolph, K. D. (2010). Mothers as a resource in times of stress: Interactive contributions of socialization of coping and stress to youth psychopathology. *Journal of Abnormal Child Psychology, 38*(2), 273–289.

Abramson, L. Y, Alloy, L. B., Hankin, B. L., Haeffel, G. J., MacCoon, D, G., & Gibb, B. E. (2002). Cognitive vulnerability–stress models of depression in a self-regulatory and psychobiological context. In I. H. Gotlib & C. L. Hammen (Eds.), *Handbook of depression* (pp. 268–294). New York: Guilford Press.

Allgood-Merten, B., Lewinsohn, P. M., & Hops, H. (1990). Sex differences and adolescent depression. *Journal of Abnormal Psychology, 99*, 55–63.

Anderson, J. C., Williams, S., McGee, R., & Silva, P. A. (1987). DSM-III disorders in preadolescent children. *Archives of General Psychiatry, 44*, 69–76.

Angold, A. (1990). Childhood and adolescent depression: II. Research in clinical populations. In S. Chess & M. E. Hertzig (Eds.), *Annual progress in child psychiatry and child development, 1989* (pp. 355–384). Philadelphia: Brunner/Mazel.

Angold, A., Costello, E. J., & Worthman, C. M. (1998). Puberty and depression: The roles of age, pubertal status, and pubertal timing. *Psychological Medicine, 28*, 51–61.

Aubé, J., Fichman, L., Saltaris, C., & Koestner, R. (2000). Gender differences in adolescent depressive symptomatology: Toward an integrated social–developmental model. *Journal of Social and Clinical Psychology, 19*, 297–313.

Barefoot, J. C., Mortensen, E. L., Helms, M. J., Avlund, K., & Schroll, M. (2001). A longitudinal study of gender differences in depressive symptoms from age 50 to 80. *Psychology and Aging, 16*(2), 342–350.

Barry, L. C., Allore, H. G., Guo, Z., Bruce, M. L., & Gill, T. M. (2008). Higher burden of depression among older women: The effect of onset, persistence, and mortality over time. *Archives of General Psychiatry, 65*(2), 172–178.

Bassoff, E. S., & Glass, G. V. (1982). The relationship between sex roles and mental health: A meta-analysis of twenty-six studies. *Counseling Psychologist, 10*, 105–112.

Benenson, J. F., & Benarroch, D. (1998). Gender differences in responses to friends' hypothetical greater success. *Journal of Early Adolescence, 18*, 192–208.

Berndt, T. (1982). The features and effects of friendship in early adolescence. *Child Development, 53*(6), 1447–1460.

Bornstein, M. H. (1995). Parenting infants. In M. H. Bornstein (Ed.), *Handbook of parenting: Vol. 1. Children and parenting* (pp. 3–39). Mahwah, NJ: Erlbaum.

Bowker, A., Bukowski, W. M., Hymel, S., & Sippola, L. K. (2000). Coping with daily hassles in the peer group in early adolescence: Variations as a function of peer experience. *Journal of Research on Adolescence, 10,* 211–243.

Bowlby, J. (1973). *Separation: Anxiety and anger: Vol. 2. Attachment and loss.* New York: Basic Books.

Boyce, W. T., Frank, E., Jensen, P. S., & the MacArthur Foundation Research Network on Psychopathology and Development. (1998). Social context in developmental psychopathology: Recommendations for future research from the MacArthur network on psychopathology and development. *Development and Psychopathology, 10,* 143–164.

Broderick, P. C. (1998). Early adolescent gender differences in the use of ruminative and distracting coping strategies. *Journal of Early Adolescence, 18,* 173–191.

Broderick, P. C., & Korteland, C. (2002). Coping style and depression in early adolescence: Relationships to gender, gender role, and implicit beliefs. *Sex Roles, 46,* 201–213.

Broderick, P. C., & Korteland, C. (2004). A prospective study of rumination and depression in early adolescence. *Clinical Child Psychology and Psychiatry, 9,* 383–394.

Brooks-Gunn, J. (1991). How stressful is the transition to adolescence for girls? In M. E. Colten & S. Gore (Eds.), *Adolescent stress: Causes and consequences* (pp. 131–149). New York: Aldine de Gruyter.

Brooks-Gunn, J., Graber, J. A., & Paikoff, R. L. (1994). Studying links between hormones and negative affect: Models and measures. *Journal of Research on Adolescence, 4*(4), 469–486.

Burton, E., Stice, E., & Seeley, J. R. (2004). A prospective test of the stress-buffering model of depression in adolescent girls: No support once again. *Journal of Consulting and Clinical Psychology, 72,* 689–697.

Burwell, R. A., & Shirk, S. R. (2007). Subtypes of rumination in adolescence: Associations between brooding, reflection, depressive symptoms, and coping. *Journal of Clinical Child and Adolescent Psychology, 36,* 56–65.

Carver, C. S., & Scheier, M. F. (1990). Origins and functions of positive and negative affect: A control-process view. *Psychological Review, 97,* 19–35.

Carver, C. S., & Scheier, M. F. (1998). *On the self-regulation of behavior.* New York: Cambridge University Press.

Case, R. (1985). *Intellectual development: Birth to adulthood.* New York: Academic Press.

Causey, D. L., & Dubow, E. F. (1992). Development of a self-report coping measure for elementary school children. *Journal of Clinical Child Psychology, 21,* 47–59.

Chamberlain, P., & Patterson, G. R. (1995). Discipline and child compliance in parenting. In M. H. Bornstein (Ed.), *Handbook of parenting: Vol. 4. Applied and practical parenting* (pp. 205–229). Mahwah, NJ: Erlbaum.

Chapman, P. L., & Mullis, R. L. (1999). Adolescent coping strategies and self-esteem. *Child Study Journal, 29,* 69–77.

Chung, T., & Asher, S. R. (1996). Children's goals and strategies in peer conflict situations. *Merrill–Palmer Quarterly, 42,* 125–147.

Clarke, A. T. (2006). Coping with interpersonal stress and psychosocial health among children and adolescents: A meta-analysis. *Journal of Youth and Adolescence, 35*(1), 11–24.

Cole, D. A., Nolen-Hoeksema, S., Girgus, J., & Paul, G. (2006). Stress exposure and stress generation in child and adolescent depression: A latent trait-state-error approach to longitudinal analyses. *Journal of Abnormal Psychology, 115,* 40–51.

Compas, B. E., Connor-Smith, J. K., Saltzman, H., Thomsen, A. H., & Wadsworth, M. E. (2001). Coping with stress during childhood and adolescence: Problems, progress, and potential in theory and research. *Psychological Bulletin, 127*: 87–127.

Compas, B. E., Langrock, A. M., Keller, G., Merchant, M. J., & Copeland, M. E. (2002). Children coping with parental depression: Processes of adaptation to family stress. In S. H. Goodman & I. H. Gotlib (Eds.), *Children of depressed parents: Mechanisms of risk and implications for treatment* (pp. 227–252). Washington, DC: American Psychological Association.

Compas, B. E., Malcarne, V. L., & Fondacaro, K. M. (1988). Coping with stressful events in older children and young adolescents. *Journal of Consulting and Clinical Psychology, 56*(3), 405–411.

Compas, B. E., & Phares, V. (1991). Stress during childhood and adolescence: Sources of risk and vulnerability. In E. M. Cummings, A. L. Greene, & K. H. Karraker (Eds.), *Lifespan developmental psychology* (pp. 111–130). Hillsdale, NJ: Erlbaum.

Compas, B. E., & Wagner, B. M. (1991). Psychosocial stress during adolescence: Intrapersonal and interpersonal processes. In M. E. Colten & S. Gore (Eds.), *Adolescent stress: Causes and consequences* (pp. 67–85). New York: Aldine de Gruyter.

Connor-Smith, J. K., Compas, B. E., Wadsworth, M. E., Thomsen, A. H., & Saltzman, H. (2000). Responses to stress in adolescence: Measurement of coping and involuntary stress responses. *Journal of Consulting and Clinical Psychology, 68*(6), 976–992.

Cooley, C. H. (1964). *Human nature and the social order.* New York: Schocken Books.

Cooper, C. R., & Ayers-Lopez, S. (1985). Family and peer systems in early adolescence: New models of the role of relationships in development. *Journal of Early Adolescence, 5*(1), 9–21.

Copeland, E. P., & Hess, R. S. (1995). Differences in young adolescents' coping strategies based on gender and ethnicity. *Journal of Early Adolescence, 15,* 203–219.

Costello, E. J., Erkanli, A., Fairbank, J., & Angold, A. (2002). The prevalence of potentially traumatic events in childhood and adolescence. *Journal of Traumatic Stress, 15,* 99–112.

Costello, E. J., Mustillo, S., Erkanli, A., Keeler, G., & Angold, A. (2003). Prevalence and development of psychiatric disorders in childhood and adolescence. *Archives of General Psychiatry, 60,* 837–844.

Craighead, L. W., & Green, B. J. (1989). The relationship between depressed mood and sex-typed personality characteristics in adolescents. *Journal of Youth and Adolescence, 18,* 467–474.

Crick, N. R., Bigbee, M. A., & Howes, C. (1996). Gender differences in children's normative beliefs about aggression: How do I hurt thee? Let me count the ways. *Child Development, 67,* 1003–1014.

Cross, S. E., & Madson, L. (1997). Models of the self: Self-construal and gender. *Psychological Bulletin, 122*(1), 5–37.

Cutler, S. E., & Nolen-Hoeksema, S. (1991). Accounting for sex differences in depression through female victimization: Childhood sexual abuse. *Sex Roles, 24,* 425–438.

Cyranowski, J. M., Frank, E., Young, E., & Shear, M. K. (2000). Adolescent onset of the gender difference in lifetime rates of major depression. *Archives of General Psychiatry, 57*(1), 21–27.

Davies, P. T., & Windle, M. (1997). Gender-specific pathways between maternal depressive symptoms, family discord, and adolescent adjustment. *Developmental Psychology, 33*(4), 657–668.

de Anda, D., Baroni, S., Boskin, L., Buchwald, L., Morgan, J., Ow, J., et al. (2000). Stress, stressors, and coping strategies among high school students. *Child and Youth Services Review, 22*(6), 441–463.

Donaldson, D., Prinstein, M. J., Donovsky, M., & Spirito, A. (2000). Patterns of children's coping with life stress: Implications for clinicians. *American Journal of Orthopsychiatry, 70*(3), 351–359.

Dornbusch, S. M., Mont-Reynaud, R., Ritter, P. L., Chen, Z., & Steinberg, L. (1991). Stressful events and their correlates among adolescents of diverse backgrounds. In M. E. Colton & S. Gore (Eds.), *Adolescent stress: Causes and consequences* (pp. 21–41). New York: Aldine De Gruyter.

Duval, S., & Wicklund, R. A. (1972). *A theory of objective self-awareness.* New York: Academic Press.

Ebata, A. T., & Moos, R. H. (1994). Personal, situational, and contextual correlates of coping in adolescence. *Journal of Research on Adolescence, 4,* 99–125.

Eccles, J. S., Midgley, C., Wigfield, A., Buchanan, C. M., Reuman, D., Flanagan, C., et al. (1993). Development during adolescence: The impact of stage–environment fit on young adolescents' experiences in schools and in families. *American Psychologist, 48*(2), 90–101.

Fenzel, L. M., & Blyth, D. A. (1986). Individual adjustment to school transitions: An exploration of the role of supportive peer relations. *Journal of Early Adolescence, 6*(4), 315–329.

Fields, L., & Prinz, R. J. (1997). Coping and adjustment during childhood and adolescence. *Clinical Psychology Review, 17*(8), 937–976.

Ford, M. E. (1982). Social cognition and social competence in adolescence. *Developmental Psychology, 18,* 323–340.

Fredrickson, B. L., & Roberts, T. (1997). Objectification theory: Toward understanding women's lived experience and mental health risks. *Psychology of Women Quarterly, 21,* 173–206.

Frydenberg, E., & Lewis, R. (1999). Adolescent coping: The role of schools in facilitating reflection. *British Journal of Educational Psychology, 69,* 83–96.

Galambos, N. L., Almeida, D. M., & Petersen, A. C. (1990). Masculinity, femininity, and sex role attitudes in early adolescence: Exploring gender intensification. *Child Development, 61,* 1905–1914.

Galen, B. R., & Underwood, M. K. (1997). A developmental investigation of social aggression among children. *Developmental Psychology, 33,* 589–600.

Garnefski, N., & Kraaij, V. (2006). Relationships between cognitive emotion regulation strategies and depressive symptoms: A comparative study of five specific samples. *Personality and Individual Differences, 40,* 1659–1669.

Garnefski, N., Kraaij, V., & van Etten, M. (2005). Specificity of relations between adolescents' cognitive emotion regulation strategies and internalizing and externalizing psychopathology, *Journal of Adolescence, 28,* 619–631.

Gavin, L. A., & Furman, W. (1989). Age differences in adolescents' perceptions of their peer groups. *Developmental Psychology, 25*(5), 827–834.

Ge, X., Conger, R. D., & Elder, G. H. (2001a). Pubertal transition, stressful life events, and the emergence of gender differences in adolescent depressive symptoms. *Developmental Psychology, 37,* 404–417.

Ge, X., Conger, R. D., & Elder, G. H. (2001b). The relation between puberty and psychological distress in adolescent boys. *Journal of Research on Adolescence, 11,* 49–70.

Ge., X., Elder, G. H., Regenerus, M., & Cox, C. (2001c). Pubertal transitions, perceptions of being overweight, and adolescents' psychological maladjustment: Gender and ethnic differences. *Social Psychology Quarterly, 64*(4), 363–375.

Ge, X., Lorenz, F. O., Conger, R. D., Elder, G. H., & Simons, R. L. (1994). Trajectories of stressful life events and depressive symptoms during adolescence. *Developmental Psychology, 30,* 467–483.

Geary, D. C., & Flinn, M. V. (2002). Sex differences in behavioral and hormonal response to social threat: Commentary on Taylor et al. (2000). *Psychological Review, 109,* 745–750.

Goodyer, I. M., & Altham, P. M. (1991). Lifetime exit events and recent social and family adversities in anxious and depressed school-aged children. *Journal of Affective Disorders, 21,* 219–228.

Goodyer, I. M., Herbert, J., Tamplin, A., & Altham, P. M. (2000). Recent life events, cortisol, dehydroepiandrosterone, and the onset of major depression in high-risk adolescents. *British Journal of Psychiatry, 177,* 499–504.

Gore, S., Aseltine, R. H., & Cohen, M. E. (1993). Gender, social-relational involvement, and depression. *Journal of Research on Adolescence, 3,* 101–125.

Gotlib, I. H., & Hammen, C. L. (1992). *Psychological aspects of depression: Toward a cognitive–interpersonal integration.* Chichester, UK: Wiley.

Graber, J. A., & Brooks-Gunn, J. (1996). Transitions and turning points: Navigating the passage from childhood through adolescence. *Developmental Psychology, 32,* 768–776.

Graber, J. A., Brooks-Gunn, J., & Warren, M. P. (1995). The antecedents of menarcheal age: Heredity, family, and stressful life events. *Child Development, 66*(2), 346–359.

Grant, K. E., Lyons, A. L., Finkelstein, J. S., Conway, K. M., Reynolds, L. K., O'Koon, J. H., et al. (2004). Gender differences in rates of depressive symptoms among low-income, urban, African-American youth: A test of two meditational hypotheses. *Journal of Youth and Adolescence, 33*, 523–533.

Greene, A. L., & Larson, R. W. (1991). Variation in stress reactivity during adolescence. In E. M. Cummings, A. L. Greene, & K. H. Karraker (Eds.), *Life-span developmental psychology: Perspectives on stress and coping* (pp. 195–209). Hillsdale, NJ: Erlbaum.

Halbreich, U., & Kahn, L. (2001). Role of estrogen in the aetiology and treatment of mood disorders. *CNS Drugs, 15*, 797–817.

Hall, G. S. (1904). *Adolescence: Its psychology and its relations to physiology, anthropology, sociology, sex, crime, religion, and education.* New York: Appleton.

Hammen, C. (1991). Generation of stress in the course of unipolar depression. *Journal of Abnormal Psychology, 100*, 555–561.

Hampel, P., & Petermann, F. (2005). Age and gender effects on coping in children and adolescents. *Journal of Youth and Adolescence, 34*(2), 73–83.

Hankin, B. L. (2010). Personality and depressive symptoms: Stress generation and cognitive vulnerabilities to depression in a prospective daily diary study. *Journal of Social and Clinical Psychology, 29*(4), 369–401.

Hankin, B. L., & Abramson, L. Y. (1999). Development of gender differences in depression: Description and possible explanations. *Annals of Medicine, 31*, 372–379.

Hankin, B. L., & Abramson, L. Y. (2001). Development of gender differences in depression: An elaborated cognitive vulnerability–transactional stress theory. *Psychological Bulletin, 127*, 773–796.

Hankin, B. L., Abramson, L. Y., Miller, N., & Haeffel, G. J. (2004). Cognitive vulnerability–stress theories of depression: Examining affective specificity in the prediction of depression versus anxiety in three prospective studies. *Cognitive Therapy and Research, 28*, 309–345.

Hankin, B. L., Abramson, L. Y., Moffit, T. E., Silva, P., McGee, R., & Angell, K. E. (1998). Development of depression from preadolescence to young adulthood: Emerging gender differences in a 10-year longitudinal study. *Journal of Abnormal Psychology, 107*, 128–140.

Hankin, B. L., Mermelstein, R., & Roesch, L. (2007). Sex differences in adolescent depression: Stress exposure and reactivity models. *Child Development, 78*, 279–295.

Hankin, B. L., Roberts, J., & Gotlib, I. H. (1997). Elevated self-standards and emotional distress during adolescence: Emotional specificity and gender differences. *Cognitive Therapy and Research, 21*, 663–679.

Harris, J. R. (1995). Where is the child's environment?: A group socialization theory of development. *Psychological Review, 102*, 458–489.

Harter, S. (1983). Developmental perspectives on the self-system. In P. H. Mussen (Ed.), *Handbook of child psychology: IV. Socialization, personality, and social development* (pp. 275–385). New York: Wiley.

Herman-Stahl, M. A., Stemmler, M., & Petersen, A. C. (1995). Approach and avoidant coping: Implications for adolescent mental health. *Journal of Youth and Adolescence, 34*(6), 649–665.

Hibbard, D. R., & Buhrmester, D. (1998). The role of peers in the socialization of gender-related social interaction styles. *Sex Roles, 39,* 185–202.

Higgins, E. T. (1987). Self-discrepancy: A theory relating self and affect. *Psychological Review, 94,* 319–340.

Higgins, E. T. (1989). Continuities and discontinuities in self-regulatory and self-evaluative processes: A developmental theory relating self and affect. *Journal of Personality, 57,* 407–444.

Higgins, E. T. (1997). Beyond pleasure and pain. *American Psychologist, 52,* 1280–1300.

Higgins, E. T., Bond, R. N., Klein, R., & Strauman, T. (1986). Self-discrepancies and emotional vulnerability: How magnitude, accessibility, and type of discrepancy influence affect. *Journal of Personality and Social Psychology, 51,* 5–15.

Hyde, J. S., Mezulis, A. H., & Abramson, L. Y. (2008). The ABCs of depression: Integrating affective, biological, and cognitive models to explain the emergence of the gender difference in depression. *Psychological Review, 115*(2), 291–313.

Ingram, R. E., Miranda, J., & Segal, Z. V. (1998). *Cognitive vulnerability to depression.* New York: Guilford Press.

James, W. (1948). *Psychology.* New York: World Publishing.

Jarvinen, D. W., & Nicholls, J. G. (1996). Adolescents' social goals, beliefs about the causes of social success, and satisfaction in peer relations. *Developmental Psychology, 32,* 435–441.

Jones, N. P., Papadakis, A. A., Hogan, C. M., & Strauman, T. J. (2009). Over and over again: Rumination, reflection, and promotion goal failure and their interactive effects on depressive symptoms. *Behaviour Research and Therapy, 47,* 254–259.

Jose, P. E., & Brown, I. (2008). (2008). When does the gender difference in rumination begin?: Gender and age differences in the use of rumination by adolescents. *Journal of Youth and Adolescence, 37,* 180–192.

Kandel, D. B., & Davies, M. (1982). Epidemiology of depressive mood in adolescents. *Archives of General Psychiatry, 39,* 1205–1212.

Kandel, D. B., & Davies, M. (1986). Adult sequelae of adolescent depressive symptoms. *Archives of General Psychiatry, 43,* 255–262.

Karoly, P. (1999). A goal systems/self-regulatory perspective on personality, psychopathology, and change. *Review of General Psychology, 3,* 264–291.

Keenan, K., & Shaw, D. (1997). Developmental and social influences on young girls' early problem behavior. *Psychological Bulletin, 121*(1), 9–113.

Kendler, K. S. (2005). Toward a philosophical structure for psychiatry. *American Journal of Psychiatry, 162,* 433–440.

Kendler, K. S., Gardner, C. O., Neale, M. C., & Prescott, C. A. (2001). Genetic risk factors for major depression in men and women: Similar or different heritabilities and same or partly distinct genes? *Psychological Medicine, 31*(4), 605–616.

Kendler, K. S., Gardner, C. O., & Prescott, C. A. (2002). Toward a comprehensive developmental model for major depression in women. *American Journal of Psychiatry, 159,* 1133–1145.

Kendler, K. S., Kessler, R., Neale, M., Heath, A., & Eaves, L. (1993). The prediction of major depression in women: Toward an integrated etiologic model. *American Journal of Psychiatry, 150,* 1139–1148.

Kendler, K. S., Kuhn, J., & Prescott, C. A. (2004). Childhood sexual abuse, stressful life events and risk for major depression in women. *Psychological Medicine, 34,* 1475–1482.

Kessler, R. C., McGonagle, K. A., Swartz, M., & Blazer, D. G. (1993). Sex and depression in the National Comorbidity Survey: I. Lifetime prevalence, chronicity, and recurrence. *Journal of Affective Disorders, 29*(2–3), 85–96.

Kliewer, W., Fearnow, M. D., & Miller, P. A. (1996). Coping socialization in middle childhood: Tests of maternal and parental influences. *Child Development, 67* 2339–2357.

Kochanska, G., Clark, L. A., & Goldman, M. S. (1997). Implications of mothers' personality for their parenting and their young children's developmental outcomes. *Journal of Personality, 65*(2), 387–420.

Kochanska, G., Murray, K. T., & Harlan, E. T. (2000). Effortful control in early childhood: Continuity and change, antecedents, and implications for social development. *Developmental Psychology, 36*(2), 220–232.

Kovacs, M. (1996). The course of childhood-onset depressive disorders. *Psychiatric Annals, 26,* 326–330.

Kovacs, M. (1997). Depressive disorders in childhood: An impressionistic landscape. *Journal of Child Psychology and Psychiatry, 38,* 287–298.

Kraaij, V., Garnefski, N., de Wilde, E., Dijkstra, A., Gebhardt, W., Maes, S., et al. (2003). Negative life events and depressive symptoms in late adolescence: Bonding and cognitive coping as vulnerability factors? *Journal of Youth and Adolescence, 32,* 185–193.

Kurdek, L. A. (1987). Gender differences in the psychological symptomatology and coping strategies of young adolescents. *Journal of Early Adolescence, 7,* 395–410.

Larson, R., & Asmussen, L. (1991). Anger, worry, and hurt in early adolescence: An enlarging world of negative emotions. In M. E. Colton & S. Gore (Eds.), *Adolescent stress: Causes and consequences* (pp. 21–41). New York: Aldine De Gruyter.

Larson, R., & Ham, M. (1993). Stress and "storm and stress" in early adolescence: The relationship of negative events with dysphoric affect. *Developmental Psychology, 29,* 130–140.

Laursen, B. (1996). Closeness and conflict in adolescent peer relationships: Interdependence with friends and romantic partners. In W. M. Bukowski, A. F. Newcomb, & W. W. Hartup (Eds.), *The company they keep: Friendship in childhood and adolescence* (pp. 186–210). New York: Cambridge University Press.

Lazarus, R. S., & Folkman, S. (1984). *Stress, appraisal, and coping*. New York: Springer.

Lewinsohn, P. M., Hops, H., Roberts, R. E., Seeley, J. R., & Andrews, J. A. (1993). Adolescent psychopathology: I. Prevalence and incidence of depression and other DSM-III-R disorders in high school students. *Journal of Abnormal Psychology, 102*(1), 133–144.

Leadbeater, B. J., Blatt, S. J., & Quinlan, D. M. (1995). Gender-linked vulnerabilities to depressive symptoms, stress, and problem behaviors in adolescents. *Journal of Research on Adolescence, 5*, 1–29.

Li, C. E., DiGiuseppe, R., & Froh, J. (2006). The roles of sex, gender, and coping in adolescent depression. *Adolescence, 41*(163), 409–415.

Lindberg, S. M., Grabe, S., & Hyde, J. S. (2007). Gender, pubertal development, and peer sexual harassment predict objectified body consciousness in early adolescence. *Journal of Research on Adolescence, 17*(4), 723–742.

Liu, X., & Kaplan, H. B. (1999). Explaining gender differences in symptoms of subjective distress in young adolescents. *Stress Medicine, 15*(1), 41–51.

Lopez, C. M., Driscoll, K. A., & Kistner, J. A. (2009). Sex differences and response styles: Subtypes of rumination and associations with depressive symptoms. *Journal of Clinical Child and Adolescent Psychology, 38*(1), 27–35.

Maccoby, E. E., & Martin, J. A. (1983). Socialization in the context of the family: Parent–child interaction. In P. H. Mussen (Ed.), *Handbook of child psychology: Vol. 4. Socialization, personality and social development* (pp. 643–691). New York: Wiley.

Maes, S., Leventhal, H., & De Ridder, D. T. D. (1996). Coping with chronic diseases. In M. Zeidner & D. Endler (Eds.), *Handbook of coping* (pp. 221–251). New York: Wiley.

Manian, N., Papadakis, A. A., Strauman, T. J., & Essex, M. J. (2006). The development of children's ideal and ought self-guides: Parenting, temperament, and individual differences in guide strength. *Journal of Personality, 74*, 1619–1645.

Markus, H., & Nurius, P. (1986). Possible selves. *American Psychologist, 41*, 954–969.

Martin, C. L., & Fabes, R. A. (2001). The stability and consequences of young children's same-sex peer interactions. *Developmental Psychology, 37*, 431–446.

Matheney, K., Aycock, D., & McCarthy, C. (1993). Stress in school-aged children and youth. *Educational Psychological Review, 5*, 109–134.

Mendelson, B. K., Mendelson, M. J., & White, D. R. (2001). Body-Esteem Scale for Adolescents and Adults. *Journal of Personality Assessment, 76*(1), 90–106.

Mezulis, A. H., Abramson, L. Y., & Hyde, J. S. (2002). Domain specificity of gender differences in rumination. *Journal of Cognitive Psychotherapy, 16*, 421–434.

Moran, P. B., & Eckenrode, J. (1991). Gender differences in the costs and benefits of peer relationships during adolescence. *Journal of Adolescent Research, 6*, 396–409.

Moretti, M. M., & Wiebe, V. J. (1999). Self-discrepancy in adolescence: Own and parental standpoints on the self. *Merrill–Palmer Quarterly, 45*(4), 624–649.

Nezu, A. M., & Nezu, C. M. (1987). Psychological distress, problem solving, and coping reactions: Sex role differences. *Sex Roles, 16,* 205–214.

Nieder, T., & Seiffge-Krenke, I. (2001). Coping with stress in different phases of romantic development. *Journal of Adolescence, 24,* 297–311.

Nolen-Hoeksema, S. (1991). Responses to depression and their effects on the duration of depressive episodes. *Journal of Abnormal Psychology, 100,* 569–582.

Nolen-Hoeksema, S. (1994). An interaction model of emergence of gender differences in depression in adolescence. *Journal of Research on Adolescence, 4,* 519–534.

Nolen-Hoeksema, S. (2001). Gender differences in depression. *Current Directions in Psychological Science, 10*(5), 173–176.

Nolen-Hoeksema, S., & Girgus, J. S. (1994). The emergence of gender differences in depression during adolescence. *Psychological Bulletin, 115,* 424–443.

Nolen-Hoeksema, S., Girgus, J. S., & Seligman, M. E. P. (1991). Sex differences in depression and explanatory style in children. *Journal of Youth and Adolescence, 20,* 233–246.

Nurmi, J. E., Poole, M. E., & Kalakoski, V. (1994). Age differences in adolescent future-oriented goals, concerns, and related temporal extension in different sociocultural contexts. *Journal of Youth and Adolescence, 23,* 471–487.

Nurmi, J. E., Poole, M. E., & Seginer, R. (1995). Tracks and transition: A comparison of adolescent future-oriented goals, explorations, and commitment in Australia, Israel, and Finland. *International Journal of Psychology, 30,* 355–375.

Papadakis, A. A., Prince, R. P., Jones, N. P., & Strauman, T. J. (2006). Self-regulation, rumination, and vulnerability to depression in adolescent girls. *Development and Psychopathology, 18,* 815–829.

Paquette, J. A., & Underwood, M. K. (1999). Gender differences in young adolescents' experiences of peer victimization: Social and physical aggression. *Merrill–Palmer Quarterly, 45,* 242–266.

Petersen, A. C. (1988). Adolescent development. In M. R. Rosenzweig (Ed.), *Annual review of psychology* (pp. 583–607). Palo Alto, CA: Annual Reviews.

Petersen, A. C., Compas, B. E., Brooks-Gunn, J., Stemmler, M., Ey, S., & Grant, K. E. (1993). Depression in adolescence. *American Psychologist, 48*(2), 155–168.

Petersen, A. C., Sarigiani, P. A., & Kennedy, R. E. (1991). Adolescent depression: Why more girls? *Journal of Youth and Adolescence, 20*(2), 247–271.

Phelps, S. B., & Jarvis, P. A. (1996). Coping in adolescencelence: Empirical evidence for a theoretically based approach to assessing coping. *Journal of Youth and Adolescence, 23,* 359–371.

Piccinelli, M., & Wilkinson, G. (2000). Gender differences in depression. *British Journal of Psychiatry, 177,* 486–492.

Polce-Lynch, M., Myers, B. J., Kliewer, W., & Kilmartin, C. (2001). Adolescent self-esteem and gender: Exploring relations to sexual harassment, body image, media influence, and emotional expression. *Journal of Youth and Adolescence, 30*(2), 225–244.

Pollina, L. K., & Snell, W. E., Jr. (1999). Coping in intimate relationships: Development of the Multidimensional Intimate Coping Questionnaire. *Journal of Social and Personal Relationships, 16,* 133–144.

Rogers, C. R. (1961). *On becoming a person.* Boston: Houghton Miffin.

Roos, P. E., & Cohen, L. H. (1987). Sex roles and social support as moderators of life stress adjustment. *Journal of Social Psychology, 52,* 576–585.

Rose, A. J. (2002). Co-rumination in the friendships of girls and boys. *Child Development, 67,* 449–470.

Rose, A. J., & Asher, S. R. (1999). Children's goals and strategies in response to conflicts within a friendship. *Developmental Psychology, 35,* 69–79.

Rose, A. J., & Asher, S. R. (2004). Children's strategies and goals in response to help-giving and help-seeking tasks within a friendship. *Child Development, 75,* 749–763.

Rose, A. J., Carlson, W., & Waller, E. M. (2007). Prospective associations of co-rumination with friendship and emotional adjustment: Considering the socio-emotional trade-offs of co-rumination. *Developmental Psychology, 43,* 1019–1031.

Rose, A. J., & Rudolph, K. D. (2006). A review of sex differences in peer relationship processes: Potential tradeoffs for the emotional and behavioral development of girls and boys. *Psychological Bulletin, 132,* 98–131.

Ruble, D. N., & Martin, C. L. (1998). Gender development. In W. Damon (Series Ed.) & N. Eisenberg (Vol. Ed.), *Handbook of child psychology: Vol. 3. Social, emotional, and personality development* (pp. 933–1016). New York: Wiley.

Rudolph, K. D. (2002). Gender differences in emotional responses to interpersonal stress during adolescence. *Journal of Adolescent Health, 30,* 3–13.

Rudolph, K. D., & Asher, S. R. (2000). Adaptation and maladaptation in the peer system: Developmental processes and outcomes. In A. J. Sameroff & M. Lewis (Eds.), *Handbook of developmental psychopathology* (2nd ed., pp. 157—175). Dordrecht, The Netherlands: Kluwer Academic.

Rudolph, K. D., & Hammen, C. (1999). Age and gender as determinants of stress exposure, generation, and reactions in youngsters: A transactional perspective. *Child Development, 70,* 660–677.

Scarr, S. (1992). Developmental theory for the 1990's: Development and individual differences. *Child Development, 63,* 1–19.

Schroevers, M., Kraaij, V., & Garnefski, N. (2007). Goal disturbance, cognitive coping strategies, and psychological adjustment to different types of stressful life event. *Personality and Individual Differences, 43,* 413–423.

Schwartz, J. A. J., & Koenig, L. J. (1996). Response styles and negative affect among adolescents. *Cognitive Therapy and Research, 20,* 13–36.

Scott, L., & O'Hara, M. (1993). Self-discrepancies in clinically anxious and depressed university students. *Journal of Abnormal Psychology, 102,* 282–287.

Seiffge-Krenke, I. (2000). Causal links between stressful events, coping style, and adolescent symptomatology. *Journal of Adolescence, 23*(6), 675–691.

Seiffge-Krenke, I. (2006). Coping with relationship stressors: The impact of different working models of attachment and links to adaptation. *Journal of Youth and Adolescence, 35,* 25–39.

Seiffge-Krenke, I., & Klessinger, N. (2000). Long-term effects of avoidant coping on adolescents' depressive symptoms. *Journal of Youth and Adolescence, 29*(6), 617–630.

Seiffge-Krenke, I., & Stemmler, M. (2002). Factors contributing to gender differences in depressive symptoms: A test of three developmental models. *Journal of Youth and Adolescence, 31*(6), 405–417.

Seiffge-Krenke, I., Weidemann, S., Fentner, S., Aegenheister, N., & Poeblau, M. (2001). Coping with school-related stress and family stress in healthy and clinically referred adolescents. *European Psychologist, 6*, 123–132.

Shah, J. Y., & Higgins, E. T. (2001). Regulatory concerns and appraisal efficiency: The general impact of promotion and prevention. *Journal of Personality and Social Psychology, 80*, 693–705.

Siddique, C. M., & D'Arcy, C. (1984). Adolescence, stress, and psychological well-being. *Journal of Youth and Adolescence, 13*(6), 459–473.

Silberg, J., Pickles, A., Rutter, M., Hewitt, J., Simonoff, E., Maes, H., et al. (1999). The influence of genetic factors and life stress on depression among adolescent girls. *Archives of General Psychiatry, 56*, 225–232.

Skinner, E. A., & Zimmer-Gembeck, M. J. (2007). The development of coping. *Annual Review of Psychology, 58*, 119–144.

Sonnenberg, C. M., Beekman, A. T. F., Deeg, D. J. H., & van Tilburg, W. (2000). Sex differences in late-life depression. *Acta Psychiatrica Scandinavica, 101*(4), 286–292.

Steinberg, L. (2010). A dual-systems model of adolescent risk-taking. *Developmental Psychobiology, 52*, 216–224.

Steinberg, L., & Silverberg, S. B. (1986). The vicissitudes of autonomy in early adolescence. *Child Development, 57*(4), 841–851.

Steiner, M., Dunn, E., & Born, L. (2003). Hormones and mood: From menarche to menopause and beyond. *Journal of Affective Disorders, 74*, 67–83.

Stice, E. (2003). Puberty and body image. In C. Hayward (Ed.), *Gender differences at puberty* (pp. 129–135). New York: Cambridge University Press.

Stice, E., & Bearman, S. K. (2001). Body-image and eating disturbances prospectively predict increases in depressive symptoms in adolescent girls: A growth curve analysis *Developmental Psychology, 37*(5), 597–607.

Stice, E., & Whitenton, K. (2002). Risk factors for body dissatisfaction in adolescent girls: A longitudinal investigation. *Developmental Psychology, 38*(5), 669–678.

Strauman, T. J. (1989). Self-discrepancies in clinical depression and social phobia: Cognitive structures that underlie affective disorders? *Journal of Abnormal Psychology, 98*, 14–22.

Strauman, T. J. (1992). Self-guides, autobiographical memory, and anxiety and dysphoria: Toward a cognitive model of vulnerability to emotional distress. *Journal of Abnormal Psychology, 101*, 87–95.

Strauman, T. J. (1996). Self-beliefs, self-evaluation and depression: A perspective on emotional vulnerability. In L. L. Martin & A. Tesser (Eds.), *Striving and feeling: Interactions among goals, affect and self-regulation* (pp. 175–201). Mahwah, NJ: Erlbaum.

Strauman, T. J. (2002). Self-regulation and depression. *Self and Identity, 1*, 151–157.

Strough, J., & Berg, C. A. (2000). Goals as a mediator of gender differences in high-affiliation dyadic conversations. *Developmental Psychology, 36,* 117–125.

Sund, A. M., Larsson, B., & Wichstrom, L. (2003). Psychosocial correlates of depressive symptoms among 12–14-year-old Norwegian adolescents. *Journal of Child Psychology and Psychiatry, 44*(4), 588–597.

Susman, E. J., Dorn, L. D., & Chrousos, G. P. (1991). Negative affect and hormone levels in young adolescents: Concurrent and predictive perspectives. *Journal of Youth and Adolescence, 20*(2), 167–190.

Taylor, S. E., Klein, L. C., Lewis, B. P., Gruenewald, T. L., Gurung, R. A. R., & Updegraff, J. A. (2000). Biobehavioral responses to stress in females: Tend-and-befriend, not fight-or-flight. *Psychological Review, 107,* 411–429.

Thornton, A., Orbuch, T. L., & Axinn, W. G. (1995). Parent child relationships during the transition to adulthood. *Journal of Family Issues, 16,* 538–564.

Tolin, D. F., & Foa, E. B. (2006). Sex differences in trauma and posttraumatic stress disorder: A quantitative review of 25 years of research. *Psychological Bulletin, 132,* 959–992.

Towbes, L. C., Cohen, L. H., & Glyshaw, K. (1989). Instrumentality as a life-stress moderator for early versus middle adolescents. *Journal of Personality and Social Psychology, 57,* 109–119.

Treynor, W., Gonzalez, R., & Nolen-Hoeksema, S. (2003). Rumination reconsidered: A psychometric analysis. *Cognitive Therapy and Research, 27,* 247–259.

Twenge, J., & Nolen-Hoeksema, S. (2002). Age, gender, race, socioeconomic status, and birth cohort differences in the Children's Depression Inventory: A meta-analysis. *Journal of Abnormal Psychology, 111,* 578–588.

Van Hook, E., & Higgins, E. T. (1988). Self-related problems beyond the self-concept: Motivational consequences of discrepant self-guides. *Journal of Personality and Social Psychology, 55,* 625–633.

Wade, R. J., Cairney, J., & Pevalin, D. (2002). Emergence of gender differences in depression during adolescence: National panel results from three countries. *Journal of the American Academy of Child and Adolescent Psychiatry, 41,* 190–198.

Wagner, B. M., & Compas, B. E. (1990). Gender, instrumentality, and expressivity: Moderators of the relation between stress and psychological symptoms during adolescence. *American Journal of Community Psychology, 18,* 383–406.

Weissman, M. M., Bland, R. C., Canino, G. J., Faravelli, C., Greenwald, S., Hwu, H.-G., et al. (1996). Cross-national epidemiology of major depression and bipolar disorder. *Journal of the American Medical Association, 276*(4), 293–299.

Wichstrom, L. (1999). The emergence of gender difference in depressed mood during adolescence: The role of intensified gender socialization. *Developmental Psychology, 35,* 232–245.

Windle, M. (1992). A longitudinal study of stress buffering for adolescent problem behaviors. *Developmental Psychology,28,* 522–530.

Wrosch, C., Scheier, M. F., Miller, G. E., Schulz, R., & Carver, C. S. (2003). Adaptive self-regulation of unattainable goals: Goal disengagement, goal reengagement, and subjective well-being. *Personality and Social Psychology Bulletin, 29*, 1494–1508.

Youniss, J., & Smollar, J. (1985). *Adolescent relations with mothers, fathers, and friends.* Chicago: University of Chicago Press.

Zahn-Waxler, C. (2000). The development of empathy, guilt, and internalization of distress: Implications for gender differences in internalizing and externalizing problems. In R. J. Davidson (Ed.), *Anxiety, depression, and emotion* (pp. 222–265). New York: Oxford University Press.

Zahn-Waxler, C., Cole, P. M., & Barrett, K. C. (1991). Guilt and empathy: Sex differences and implications for the development of depression. In J. Garber & K. A. Dodge (Eds.), *The development of emotion regulation and dysregulation* (pp. 243–272). New York: Cambridge University Press.

Zubenko, G. S., Hughes, H., Maher, B., Stiffler, J., Zubenko, W., & Marazita, M. (2002). Genetic linkage of region containing the *CREB1* gene to depressive disorders in women from families with recurrent, early-onset, major depression. *American Journal of Medical Genetics, 114,* 980–987.

PART III

PREVENTION SCIENCE PERSPECTIVES

CHAPTER 9

Prevention of Depression in Youth

Sex Differences in Effects

Judy Garber *and* Lindsay E. Downs

The present chapter examines the evidence regarding sex differences in the effects of depression prevention programs in youth. Several facts provide the context for this review: (1) the rates of depression increase from childhood to adolescence (Costello & Angold, Chapter 2, this volume; Costello, Foley, & Angold, 2006); (2) sex differences emerge during this time, with girls showing higher levels of depressive symptoms and disorders than boys by early to mid-adolescence (Costello, Mustillo, Erkanli, Keeler, & Angold, 2003; Hankin et al., 1998); and (3) efforts to prevent depressive symptoms and disorders in youth have yielded small to moderate effects (Horowitz & Garber, 2006; Merry, McDowell, Hetrick, Bir, & Muller, 2005). The purpose of this chapter is to address several questions that follow logically from these three facts:

1. Are depression prevention programs differentially efficacious for girls versus boys?
2. If so, what is the nature and direction of these sex differences?
3. What might account for these differences?

DEPRESSION IN ADOLESCENTS

The prevalence rates of mood disorders rise sharply from childhood to adolescence (Costello et al., 2003). A meta-analysis (Costello et al., 2006) showed that the overall prevalence estimate of depression in children is

2.8%, although the rates vary by age, informant, and type of depression (i.e., major depressive disorder [MDD], dysthymia). For example, the rates of diagnosed depressive disorders in preadolescents are relatively low, although the rates are higher when based on children's as compared to parents' reports (Rubio-Stipec, Fitzmaurice, Murphy & Walker, 2003).

In adolescents, the point prevalence rates are estimated to be between 3 and 8%; lifetime prevalence rates of MDD in adolescents have ranged from 9 to 24% (Lewinsohn & Essau, 2002; Merikangas & Knight, 2009). The National Comorbidity Study, an epidemiological survey in the United States, reported a lifetime prevalence rate of 15% for MDD in adolescents (Kessler & Walters, 1998). Similar rates have been found in other community samples of adolescents (Lewinsohn, Rohde, Seeley, Klein, & Gotlib, 2003; Rao, Hammen, & Daley, 1999). Overall, an estimated 20% of youth will have a depressive episode by age 18 (Lewinsohn, Rohde, & Seeley, 1998). Depression during adolescence is associated with impairment in interpersonal relationships and academic functioning, and increased risk of cigarette smoking, substance use problems, high-risk sexual behaviors, physical health problems, and suicide, accounting for a substantial proportion of the health care costs incurred by this age group (Birmaher et al., 1996; Brent et al., 1993; Le, Munoz, Ippen, & Stoddard, 2003; Lewinsohn et al., 2003; Pickles et al., 2001; Stolberg, Clark, & Bongar, 2002).

The average depressive episode in youth lasts between 6 and 8 months (Kaminski & Garber, 2002; Kovacs, 1996; Lewinsohn, Clarke, Seeley, & Rohde, 1994). Longer episodes are associated with worse functioning over time (Rao et al., 1999) and are more difficult to treat (Brent & Birmaher, 2006). Early-onset depressions are associated with recurrent episodes during adolescence (Emslie et al., 1997; McCauley et al., 1993) and adulthood (Rao et al., 1999; Weissman et al., 2006). Many cases of recurrent adult depression had their initial onsets during adolescence (Kessler, Wai, Demler, & Walters, 2005; Pine, Cohen, Gurley, Brook, & Ma, 1998). Thus, adolescence is a particularly opportune developmental window during which to intervene to prevent the onset and recurrence of depressive disorders and associated impairment.

SEX DIFFERENCES

The increasing rate of depressive disorders is especially evident in female adolescents (Angold, Erkanli, Silberg, Eaves, & Costello, 2002). In preadolescents, the rate of MDD has been found to be about equal in girls and boys (Angold & Rutter, 1992; Fleming, Offord, & Boyle, 1989), although some studies have reported higher rates among preadolescent boys than girls (e.g., Angold, Costello, & Worthman, 1998; Steinhausen & Metzke,

2003). Angold and colleagues (1998) showed that girls had higher rates of depressive disorders after Tanner Stage III of pubertal development, whereas boys had higher rates before this stage. Girls begin to show higher levels of depressive symptoms and disorders by early to midadolescence (i.e., about 12–14 years old; Hankin et al., 1998). This sex difference persists throughout adolescence, reaching the 2:1 female-to-male ratio found in adults across cultures (Weissman & Olfson, 1995). Moreover, MDD tends to be more recurrent and insidious in adolescent females than males (Lewinsohn & Essau, 2002).

Findings of sex differences in minor depression or depressive symptoms have been less clear (e.g., Gónzalez-Tejera et al., 2005). A meta-analysis of 310 studies that assessed depressive symptoms with the Children's Depression Inventory found no significant sex differences in children ages 8–12, although boys reported slightly higher scores than girls; girls' depressive symptoms started to increase around age 13, whereas boys' levels of depressive symptoms remained more stable over adolescence (Twenge & Nolen-Hoeksema, 2002).

Theoretical models proposed to explain the increasing rates of depression in females during adolescence emphasize the contributions of biological, psychological, interpersonal, and contextual factors and their interactions during the transition to adolescence (e.g., Cyranowski, Frank, Young, & Shear, 2000; Hankin & Abramson, 2001; Hyde, Mezulis, & Abramson, 2008; Keenan & Hipwell, 2005; Nolen-Hoeksema & Girgus, 1994). Sex differences have been found with regard to various correlates of depression, including hormones, genetic liability, interpersonal stressors, affiliative tendencies, rejection sensitivity, rumination and co-rumination, cognitive vulnerability, and body image (Hankin, Cheely, & Wetter, 2008).

Hormonal changes during puberty have been proposed as one possible explanation of emerging sex differences in depression during adolescence (Angold, Costello, Erkanli, & Worthman, 1999; Susman, Trickett, Ianotti, Hollenbeck, & Zahn-Waxler, 1985). Angold, Worthman, and Costello (2003) reported that higher levels of androgen and estradiol were associated with depression in girls at puberty; when sex steroid levels (combined testosterone and estradiol) reached the upper 30th percentile, girls were five times more likely to be depressed than were girls with lower levels; reaching the upper 10% further quadrupled the rates of depression.

With regard to genes, major depression has been found to be moderately heritable, with estimates ranging from 30 to 50% (Rice, Harold, & Thapar, 2002). In a twin study, significant heritability of depression was found for pubertal girls, but not pubertal boys or prepubertal children (Silberg et al., 1999). Silberg and colleagues also suggested that genetic liability to life events may partially account for the higher rates of depression in girls after puberty. Additionally, a test of the diathesis–stress model in adolescents showed that a functional polymorphism in the promoter region of the serotonin transporter (5-HTT) predicted heightened depression in the face of life stress for adolescent girls but not boys (Eley et al., 2004). Thus, a genetic liability to depression may be activated during adolescence and trigger or interact with biological, psychological, and social changes around the pubertal transition, particularly in girls.

Girls report and experience more stressful life events than boys. Interpersonal stressors (e.g., peer rejection, conflicts with romantic partners, family discord) are especially linked to depression in young adolescent females (e.g., Hankin, Mermelstein, & Roesch, 2007; Rudolph, 2002; Sheeber, Davis, & Hops, 2002). During the transition to adolescence, interpersonal relationships become increasingly salient and undergo many changes, including the formation of new social networks and the emergence of romantic relationships. Girls generally show more negative reactions to relationship problems such as romantic breakups or covert aggression than boys (Hankin et al., 2007; Rudolph, 2002; Rudolph & Hammen, 1999; Shih, Eberhart, Hammen, & Brennan, 2006). Girls also experience more dependent stressors, which they play a role in generating, such as interpersonal problems (Hankin et al., 2007; Rudolph & Hammen, 1999). Thus, the greater exposure and reactivity to interpersonal difficulties in females are especially likely to contribute to the emerging sex difference in depression during adolescence.

Sex differences also have been found with regard to several psychological variables, including cognitive vulnerability, rumination, social evaluative concerns, and interpersonal dependency (e.g., Little & Garber, 2005; Mezulis, Abramson, Hyde, & Hankin, 2004; Rudolph & Conley, 2005; Ziegert & Kistner, 2002). Moreover, females might be more vulnerable to depression due to greater negative affectivity (e.g., Chorpita, Plummer, & Moffitt, 2000), excessive empathy (e.g., Zahn-Waxler, 2000), overcompliance (e.g., Kochanska, Coy, & Murray, 2001), and difficulties with emotion regulation (e.g., Zeman, Shipman, & Suveg, 2002). The extent to which these various cognitive and emotional vulnerabilities mediate or moderate the relation between sex and depression, as well as interact with stress, needs further study, particularly in regard to prevention.

An important distinction relevant to the present discussion is between sex differences in risk versus sex differences in response to an intervention. Although female adolescents are at greater risk for depression compared to their male peers, this does not necessarily mean sex differences will be found in treatment response. In general, males are less likely to become depressed, but those who do may respond similarly to treatment as do females. For example, antidepressant medications may effectively reduce depression in both males and females, even if the causes of their depressions were quite different. The link between risk and prevention, however, likely is stronger than between risk and treatment. Therefore, identifying what factors increase the probability of depression in girls versus boys is particularly important for constructing gender-relevant preventive interventions.

PREVENTION OF DEPRESSION

Several qualitative (Garber & McCauley, 2002; Gillham, Shatté, & Freres, 2000; Merry & Spence, 2007; Munoz, Le, Clarke, & Jaycox, 2002; Sutton, 2007) and quantitative (Brunwasser, Gillham, & Kim, 2009; Horowitz & Garber, 2006; Jané-Llopis, Hosman, Jenkins, & Anderson, 2003; Merry et al., 2005; Stice, Shaw, Bohon, Marti, & Rohde, 2009) reviews of studies testing interventions to prevent depression in children and adolescence have been conducted in the last decade. Whereas qualitative reviews generally summarize and synthesize findings across multiple studies, meta-analyses amalgamate effect sizes from different studies with various numbers of participants, and allow for an examination of other study characteristics that can influence effect sizes, such as the age and sex of the participants, type of intervention, and baseline symptom levels. The present chapter reports the results of a meta-analysis of the effects of depression prevention programs specifically as a function of sex.

Since the report by the Institute of Medicine in 1994 (Mrazek & Haggerty, 1994) prevention programs have been classified into three categories (universal, selective, and indicated) based on the population groups to whom the interventions are directed. Universal preventive intervention is administered to all members of a population and does not select participants based on risk. Selective prevention is given to a subgroup of a population whose risk is deemed to be above average (e.g., offspring of depressed parents). Indicated prevention is provided to individuals who have detectable, subclinical levels of signs or symptoms of the disorder, but who do not currently meet diagnostic criteria for the disorder. Selective and indicated samples sometimes are lumped together into a category called "targeted." The type of sample used in each study included in the current review is designated in the first column of Table 9.1.

Sex × Intervention Interactions

When a randomized control trial testing the efficacy of a depression prevention program finds a significant Sex × Intervention interaction, several different patterns of results are possible. This interaction could reflect within-sex effects of the intervention (Figure 9.1), within-intervention effects for sex (Figure 9.2), both (Figure 9.3), or various other outcome configurations. In Figure 9.1, the effect of the preventive intervention was significant

TABLE 9.1. Effect Sizes of Depression Prevention Programs

Program	Age M (SD)	Total N (% female)	Girls N Boys N	Overall effect sizes	Girls' effect sizes	Boys' effect sizes	Dep. measure	Comments
Penn Prevention Program: cognitive-behavioral, social problem solving								
U Cardemil et al. (2002, 2007)[a, c]								
Study 1	M = 11.3 yr	53 (45%)	G = 24 B = 29	0.58 (post) 0.68 (6 mo)	Girls 0.23 (post) 0.14 (6 mo)	Boys 0.31 (post) 0.37 (6 mo)	CDI	Significant effects for Latino, but not African American, youth
Study 2	M = 10.9 yr	115 (55%)	G = 63 B = 52	0.12 (post) −0.06 (6 mo)				
Chaplin et al. (2006)[a]	11–14 yr M = 12.16 (0.89)	208 (50%)	G = 103 B = 105	0.29 (post) 0.08 (12 mo)	Girls-only vs. cntrl 0.33 (post)	Coed vs. cntrl 0.47 (post)	CDI	Girls-only > coed girls in hopelessness, attendance; girls-only = coed groups in dep sxs
Pattison & Lynd-Stevenson (2001)[a]	9–12 yr M = 10.44 (0.69)	66 (52%)	G = 34 B = 32	0.08 (post) 0.48 (6 mo)	No sex difference		CDI	Cognitive then social component vs. social then cognitive component
Quayle et al. (2001)[a, b] (Australia)	11–12 yr	N = 47 (100%)	G = 47 B = 0	−0.42 (post) 0.82 (6 mo)		No boys in the sample	CDI	
Gillham et al. (2007)[a]	9–15 yr M = 12.13 (1.03)	N = 697 (46%)	G = 321 B = 377	(PRP vs. cntrl) 0.05 (post) 0.06 (6 mo) 0.21 (12 mo)	No sex difference		CDI CDRS-R	PRP vs. cntrl vs. PEP: PRP better in schools A & B; PEP better in

198

	Study	Population	N		Effect size (PEP vs. cntrl)	Sex difference	Boys	Measure	Notes
S	Seligman et al. (1999)[a]	College freshmen	231 (52%)	G = 120 B = 111	(PEP vs. cntrl) 0.13 (post) 0.06 (6 mo)	No sex difference		BDI	school C
	Seligman et al. (2007)[a] (replication and extension of Seligman et al. [1999])	College freshmen	N = 240 (65%)	G = 156 B = 84	0.16 (post) 0.16 (6 mo) 0.25 (36 mo)	NR		BDI	CBT web-based program Lower dep sxs at posttest, but not at 6-mo f-up
I	Jaycox et al. (1994) (reported in Gillham et al. [1995])	10–13 yr $M = 11.4$ (0.67)	N = 143 (46%)	G = 66 B = 77	0.47 (post) 0.23 (6 mo)	No sex difference		CDI	First test of PPP
	Gillham et al. (1995)[a,b,c] (2-yr follow-up of Jaycox et al.)	$M = 11.37$	N = 118 (47%)	G = 55 B = 63	0.18 (post) 0.32 (6 mo) 0.65 (12 mo)	Girls 0.18 (post) −0.24 (6 mo) −0.11 (12 mo)	Boys 0.64 (post) 0.62 (6 mo) 0.92 (12 mo)	CDI	More effective for males; cntrl boys had highest sxs at each time point
	Gillham & Reivich (1999) (follow-up of Gillham et al. [1995])	$M = 11.37$	N = 118 (46%)	G = 55 B = 63	0.16 (30 mo) 0.20 (36 mo)	NR		CDI	No significant effect of condition at 30 or 36 mo

(cont.)

TABLE 9.1. (cont.)

Program	Age M (SD)	Total N (% female)	Girls N Boys N	Overall effect sizes	Girls' effect sizes	Boys' effect sizes	Dep. measure	Comments
Gillham, Hamilton, et al. (2006)[a,b,c]	11–12 yr	N = 271 (53%)	G = 144 B = 127	−0.02 (post) 0.22 (6 mo)	Girls 0.21 (post) 0.27 (6 mo)	Boys −0.33 (post) 0.16 (6 mo)	CDI	Girls > boys; primary care, moderated by sex and intervention fidelity
Gillham, Reivich, et al. (2006)[a]	Grades 6 & 7	N = 44 (30%)	G = 13 B = 31	0.08 (post) 0.57 (6 mo)	NR		CDI	Pilot of parent intervention component; small N
I Gillham, Reivich, & Seligman (2007)[a]	10–15 yr M = 11.98	N = 427 (48%)	G = 204 B = 223	0.14 (post) 0.12 (6 mo) 0.15 (12 mo)	NR		CDI, RADS	Adolescent-only PRP, adolescent and parent PRP, or no-intervention cntrl
Roberts et al. (2003, 2004)[a,b,c] (Australia)	11–13 yr M = 11.92 (0.32)	N = 189 (50%)	G = 94 B = 95	0.05 (post) 0.07 (6 mo) 0.13 (30 mo)	Girls 0.09 (30 mo)	Boys 0.27 (30 mo)	CDI	Effects on anxiety but not on dep (30-mo f-up)
Yu & Seligman (2002)[a] (Chinese children)	8–15 yr M = 11.8 (1.69)	N = 220 (45%)	G = 98 B = 122	0.23 (post) 0.39 (6 mo)	No sex difference		CDI, CASQ	Penn Optimism Program; changes in explanatory style mediated intervention effect

Coping with Depression: cognitive-behavioral

	Study	Age	N	G/B		Girls	Boys		Measure	Comparison/Outcome
U	Clarke et al. (1993)									
	Study 1	Grades 9 & 10 M = 15.4	N = 513 (42.4%)	G = 216 B = 297	0.06 (post) 0.03 (3 mo)	No sex difference at 12 mo	Boys Improved in dep sxs at post and 3 mo		CDI	
	Study 2	Grades 9 & 10 M = 15.1	N = 300 (46%)	G = 138 B = 162	0.09 (post) 0.14 (3 mo)					
U	Horowitz et al. (2007)[a,c]	M = 14.43 (0.70)	N = 380 (54%)	G = 205 B = 175	(post) CBT = 0.37 IPT-AST = 0.24 (6 mo) CBT = 0.22 IPT-AST = 0.05	Girls (CBT) 0.32 (post) 0.35 (6 mo) Girls (IPT-AST) 0.32 (post) −0.04 (6 mo)	Boys (CBT) 0.44 (post) 0.01 (6 mo) Boys (IPT-AST) 0.14 (post) 0.13 (6 mo)		CDI, CES-D	Group CBT vs. group IPT-AST vs. no intervention
I	Clarke et al. (1995)[a]	Grades 9 & 10 M = 15.3 (0.70)	N = 150 (70%)	G = 105 B = 45	0.31 (post) −0.07 (6 mo) −0.01 (12 mo)	No sex differences			CES-D	
I S	Clarke et al. (2001)[a,b,c]	13–18 yr M = 14.6	N = 94 (60%)	G = 56 B = 38	0.42 (post) 0.47 (12 mo) 0.04 (24 mo)	Girls 0.63 (post) 0.30 (12 mo) −0.14 (24 mo)	Boys −0.003 (post) 0.77 (12 mo) 0.24 (24 mo)		CES-D	Significantly reduced depressive disorders

(cont.)

TABLE 9.1. *(cont.)*

Program	Age M (SD)	Total N (% female)	Girls N Boys N	Overall effect sizes	Girls' effect sizes	Boys' effect sizes	Dep. measure	Comments
Garber et al. (2009)[a,b,c]	13–17 yr	N = 316 (59%)	G = 185 B = 131	0.30 (post) 0.31 (9 mo)	Girls 0.21 (post) 0.13 (9 mo)	Boys 0.39 (post) 0.57 (9 mo)	CES-D	Replicated Clarke et al. (2001); significantly fewer dep episodes in CBT vs. usual care
I Burton et al. (2007)[a,b,c]	14–23 yr M = 18.6	N = 145 (100%)	G = 145 B = 0	0.52 (post) 0.05 (6 mo)		No boys in sample	BDI	Change in dep sxs mediated the effect on change in bulimic sxs; four sessions

Resourceful Adolescent Program: cognitive-behavioral and interpersonal

Program	Age M (SD)	Total N (% female)	Girls N Boys N	Overall effect sizes	Girls' effect sizes	Boys' effect sizes	Dep. measure	Comments
U Harnett & Dadds (2004)[a,c]	12–16 yr M = 13.58 (0.61)	N = 212 (100%)	G = 212 B = 0	0.28 (post) 0.21 (6 mo) 0.16 (3 yr)		No boys in sample	RADS	No significant effect overall
Merry et al. (2004)[a] (New Zealand)	13–15 yr M = 14.2 (0.6)	N = 364 (52%)	G = 188 B = 176	0.04 (post) −0.25 (6 mo) −0.25 (18 mo)	No sex difference		RADS, BDI-II	
Shochet et al. (2001)[a,c] (Australia)	Year 9 12–15 yr M = 13.5 (.54)	N = 228 (53.5%)	G = 121 B = 107	0.39 (post) 0.25 (10 mo)	Girls 0.46 (post) 0.28 (10 mo)	Boys 0.31 (post) 0.23 (10 mo)	RADS, CDI	RAP-A (adolescents only) RAP-F (+ parent groups); results for RAP programs combined

Problem-Solving for Life

						Girls	Boys		
U	Spence et al. (2003, 2005)[a,c]	12–14 yr M = 12.9	N = 1500 (52%)	G = 780 B = 720	0.24 (post) −0.03 (1 yr)	Girls 0.09 (post) −0.10 (1 yr) −0.04 (4 yr)	Boys 0.40 (post) 0.06 (1 yr) 0.15 (4 yr)	BDI	More effective for boys at postintervention, but not at f-up
U I	Sheffield et al. (2006)[a,b,c]	13–15 M = 14.3	N = 521 (69%)	G = 358 B = 163	U = 0.08 (post) I = 0.15 (post) + = −0.02 (post) Follow-up U = −0.02 (12 mo) I = −0.08 (12 mo) + = −0.15 (12 mo)	Girls (indicated) −0.04 (post) −0.16 (6 mo)	Boys (indicated) 0.03 (post) 0.16 (6 mo)	CDI, CES-D	+ = U + I No significant sex difference reported

LARS and LISA: cognitive-behavioral and social skills

						Girls	Boys		
U	Pössel et al. (2004, 2005)[a,c]	8th grade M = 13.82 (0.71)	N = 347 (48%)	G = 166 B = 181	0.42 (post) 0.20 (3 mo) 0.44 (6 mo)	Girls 0.18 (post) 0.41 (6 mo)	Boys 0.07 (post) 0.53 (6 mo)	CES-D	Single-sex groups; effects stronger for those with high dep scores at baseline
U	Pössel et al. (2008)[a,c]	8th grade M = 13.73 (0.64)	N = 301	G = 140 B = 161	0.01 (post) 0.02 (6 mo)	Girls −0.01 (post) 0.06 (6 mo)	Boys 0.02 (post) 0.003 (6 mo)	SBB-DES	Single-sex groups

(cont.)

203

TABLE 9.1. (cont.)

Program	Age M (SD)	Total N (% female)	Girls N Boys N	Overall effect sizes	Girls' effect sizes	Boys' effect sizes	Dep. measure	Comments
Family Psychoeducation: education and communication								
S Beardslee et al. (1997)[a]	8–15 yr M = 11.5 (2.03)	N = 52 (38.5%)	G = 21 B = 31	0.20 (post) 0.41 (18 mo)	No sex difference		CDI YSR	Two intervention conditions; no group differences on dep sxs
Beardslee et al. (2003)	8–15 yr M = 11.6 (1.9)	N = 121 (43%)	G = 59 B = 62		Girls −0.43 (post)	Boys 0.05 (post)	YSR	Internalizing sxs decreased, but no group differences
Beardslee et al. (2007)[b,c] (follow-up to Beardslee et al. [2003])	8–15 yr M = 12	N = 105 (42%)	G = 44 B = 61		Girls 0.05 (18 mo)	Boys −0.25 (18 mo)	YSR, YASR	Better communication and understanding of parent's illness
Family Bereavement Program: parenting, coping								
S Sandler et al. (2003)[a,b,c]	8–16 yr M = 11.4 (2.43)	N = 244 (49%)	G = 120 B = 124	0.06 (post) 0.11 (11 mo)	Girls 0.12 (post) 0.26 (11 mo)	Boys 0.004 (post) −0.09 (11 mo)	CDI	Significant group × sex effect (11 mo); girls and those with high baseline scores improved more
New Beginnings: divorce								
S Wolchik et al. (2002)[a,b,c]	15–19 yr M = 10.7	N = 218 (50%)	G = 109 B = 109	MP 0.01 (post) −0.04 (6 mo)	Girls MPCP 0.17 (post) 0.14 (6 mo)	Boys MPCP −0.06 (post) 0.01 (6 mo)	CDI	Overall, no significant reduction in internalizing sxs;

Study	Age	N (%)	G / B	Effect size	Girls	Boys	Measure	Notes
				MPCP 0.06 (post) 0.06 (6 mo) −0.04 (72 mo)				stronger effects for those with higher baseline symptoms
Parenting, Child Coping								
S Compas et al. (2009)[a]	M = 11.4 (2.00)	N = 155 (45%)	G = 70 B = 85	0.04 (post) 0.18 (6 mo) 0.42 (12 mo)	NR		CES-D	Significant effects at 12-mo f-up
Education Support Group								
S Gwynn & Brantley (1987)	9–11 yr	N = 60 (50%)	G = 30 B = 30	1.37 (post)	No sex difference		CDI	Social support; children of divorce
Interpersonal Therapy–Adolescent Skills Training								
I Young et al. (2006)[a]	11–16 yr M = 13.4	N = 41 (85%)	G = 35 B = 6	1.03 (post) 0.79 (6 mo)		Few boys in sample	CES-D	Teach communication skills; mostly Hispanic females
I Young et al. (2010)[b,c]	M = 14.51 (0.76)	N = 57 (59%)	G = 34 B = 23	NR	Girls 0.67 (post) 0.18 (6 mo)	Boys 0.63 (post) 0.80 (6 mo)	CDI	
Interpersonal Therapy								
I Forsyth (2001) (dissertation)	18–25 yr M = 19.4	N = 59 (97%)	G = 57 B = 3	1.51 (post) 1.95 (12 mo)	Very few boys in sample			Female college students; teach interpersonal skills

(cont.)

TABLE 9.1. *(cont.)*

Program	Age M (SD)	Total N (% female)	Girls N Boys N	Overall effect sizes	Girls' effect sizes	Boys' effect sizes	Dep. measure	Comments
Brief Cognitive-Behavioral								
I Stice et al. (2007)[a,b,c]	15–22 yr M = 18.4	N = 225 (70%)	G = 158 B = 67	0.68 (post) 0.13 (6 mo)	Girls CBT vs. WL 0.76 (post) –0.02 (6 mo)	Boys CBT vs. WL 1.44 (post) 0.46 (6 mo)	BDI	CBT > WL, supportive-expressive, bibliotherapy, expressive writing, journaling
Stice et al. (2008)[a,b,c]	M = 15.6 (1.20)	N = 341 (56%)	G = 191 B = 150	CB vs. cntrl 0.63 (post) 0.49 (6 mo)	Girls CB vs. cntrl 0.55 (post) 0.56 (6 mo)	Boys CBT vs. cntrl 0.62 (post) 0.43 (6 mo)	BDI	Brief CB > waitlist, supportive-expressive, bibliotherapy, expressive writing, journaling
Cognitve-Behavioral								
I Peden et al. (2001)[a,b,c]	18–24 yr M = 19.3	N = 92 (100%)	G = 92 B = 0	0.73 (post) 0.82 (6 mo) 0.31 (18 mo)		No boys in the sample	CES-D, BDI	Young adult females
S Hyun et al. (2005)[a,b,c] (Korea)	M = 15.6 (2.10)	N = 27 (0%)	G = 0 B = 27	0.60 (post)	No girls in sample		BDI	Homeless, runaway youth in a shelter

206

						Girls	Boys		
Penn State Adolescent Study: coping									
U	Petersen et al. (1997)	Grades 6 & 9	N = 335	NR	−0.12 (post)	Girls sxs decreased	Boys sxs increased	CDI	Improved coping; significant effect for dep sxs at posttest; no sex difference at 6 mo
Coping Skills									
I	Lamb et al. (1998)	14–19 yr M = 15.8	N = 41 (56%)	G = 23 B = 18	0.70 (post)	Girls Significant decrease in sxs	Boys No significant effect	RADS	Rural sample
Friends Program: reduce anxiety to prevent depression									
U	Lock & Barrett (2003)	Grade 6 9–10 yr Grade 9 14–16 yr	N = 733 (51%)	G = 371 B = 362	NR	Girls 0.14 (post) 0.43 (12 mo) 0.12 (post) −0.21 (12 mo)	Boys 0.22 (post) 0.35 (12 mo) 0.02 (post) 0.07 (12 mo)	CDI	Significant effects only at 12 mo for sixth-grade boys and girls and ninth-grade girls
U	Barrett et al. (2006) (follow-up of Lock & Barrett [2003])	Grade 7 10–11 yr Grade 10 15–17 yr	N = 669 (51.3%)	G = 344 B = 325	NR	Girls 0.21 (24 mo) 0.55 (36 mo) 0.01 (24 mo) 0.20 (36 mo)	Boys 0.38 (24 mo) 0.31 (36 mo) 0.21 (24 mo) 0.30 (36 mo)	CDI	No change in CDI at 24 or 36 mo; lower dep scores for children in intervention vs. cntrls in sixth grade, but not in ninth-grade cohort *(cont.)*

TABLE 9.1. (cont.)

Program	Age M (SD)	Total N (% female)	Girls N Boys N	Overall effect sizes	Girls' effect sizes	Boys' effect sizes	Dep. measure	Comments
U Lowry-Webster et al. (2003)[a] (Australia)	Grades 5–7 10–13 yr	N = 594 (53%)	G = 314 B = 280	0.17 (post) 0.30 (12 mo)	No sex difference		CDI	
Stress Inoculation								
U Hains & Ellman (1994)	Grades 9–12	N = 21 (76%)	G = 16 B = 5	0.36 (post) −0.04 (2 mo)		Few boys in the sample		Stress management
Cognitive-Behavioral + Interpersonal								
U Cecchini (1997); Johnson (2000) (dissertations)	Grade 5	N = 100	NR	0.11 (post) −0.15 (12 mo)	NR			Increased social skills; no effect on dep
Mastery Learning Program								
U Kellam et al. (1994)[a, c]	Grade 1 M = 6.3 4.7–9.4	N = 575 (49%)	G = 282 B = 293	−0.01 (post)	Girls 0.15 (post)	Boys −0.11 (post)	CDI	School-based; improved reading achievement, not dep sxs

208

Family–School Partnership

	Study	Grade/Age	N	G/B	Effect size	Sex difference	Measure	Notes
U	Ialongo et al. (1999, 2001)	Grade 1 M = 6.2 yr (0.34)	N = 678 (46%)	G = 312 B = 366	Not reported	No change in "shy/withdrawn" sxs post or f-up	More effective for boys than girls at post	TOCA-R, POCA-R	School-based; improved reading achievement, not dxs
I	Bearman et al. (2003)[a,b,c]	M = 18.9 (0.75)	N = 74 (100%)	G = 74 B = 0	0.25 (post) −0.06 (6 mo)	No boys in the sample	BDI	Girls with body dissatisfaction; significant at post, not at 6 mo
U	Sawyer et al. (2008)[a]	M = 13.1 (0.50)	N = 5,634 (53%)	G = 2,986 B = 2,648	−0.05 (post) −0.06 (24 mo)	No sex difference	CES-D	School-based; no significant effects at posttest for dxs

Note. Unbiased effect sizes reported; effect sizes calculated using the standard deviation of the control group. U, universal; S, selective; I, indicated; dep, depression; sxs, symptoms; yr, years; mo, months; f-up, follow-up; BDI, Beck Depression Inventory; CBT, cognitive-behavioral therapy; CASQ, Children's Attributional Style Questionnaire; CDI, Children's Depression Inventory; CDRS, Children's Depression Rating Scale; CES-D, Center for Epidemiologic Studies Depression Scale; MP, Mother Program; MPCP, Mother Plus Child Program; PEP, Penn Enhancement Program; PPP, Penn Prevention Program; POCA-R, Parent Observation of Child Adaptation—Revised; PRP, Penn Resilience Program; RADS, Reynolds Adolescent Depression Scale; SBB-DES, Self-Report Questionnaire; TOCA-R; Teacher Observation of Classroom Adaptation—Revised; YASR, Young Adult Self-Report; YSR, Youth Self-Report; cntrl, controls; NR, not reported, indicates that analyses of sex differences either were not conducted or were not reported by the authors; "No sex difference" indicates that the authors reported that they tested and found no sex differences, but the means and standard deviations were not provided separately for girls and boys; WL, waitlist.

[a]Data included in analyses for Table 9.2a.
[b]Data included in analyses for Table 9.2b.
[c]Data included in analyses for Table 9.2c.

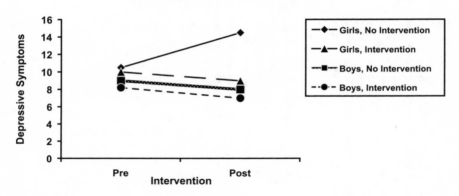

FIGURE 9.1. Within-sex effects of the intervention: No significant difference between boys and girls in the intervention group, but girls in the no-intervention condition had significantly higher postintervention depression scores compared to girls in the intervention condition, indicating prevention in girls.

for females but not males; that is, depressive symptoms increased significantly for girls in the no-intervention control condition, but not for girls in the preventive intervention; no significant intervention effect was found for boys. Such a finding would be consistent with epidemiological data showing that depression increases during adolescence for females (Hankin et al., 1998). Thus, the effects for depression prevention programs might be expected to appear larger for girls than boys because of the typically higher levels of depression in adolescent girls as compared to boys. Therefore, a

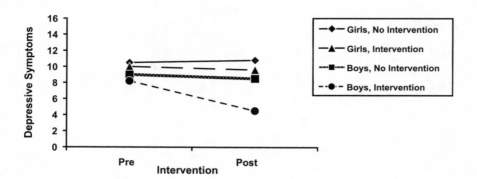

FIGURE 9.2. Within-intervention effects for sex: At postintervention for youth in the intervention group, boys had significantly lower depression scores than girls; no significant differences were found for girls in the intervention versus no intervention conditions, indicating a treatment effect.

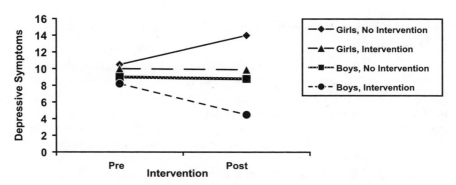

FIGURE 9.3. Girls in the no-intervention group increased in depression compared to girls in the intervention condition (within-sex effects of the intervention), and boys in the intervention group significantly decreased in depression compared to girls in the intervention group (within-intervention effects of sex).

prevention effect may be easier to demonstrate for girls even if the efficacy of the intervention is not significantly different for girls and boys.

Alternatively, one of the sexes could respond better than the other to the intervention, and there could be no difference within sex as a function of condition, as displayed in Figure 9.2. Here the sex × intervention interaction was due to a significant difference between girls and boys in the intervention condition. Another possibility is that both of these outcomes could occur (Figure 9.3); that is, a significant sex × intervention interaction could indicate both that girls in the no-intervention group increased in depression and boys in the intervention group decreased in depression. These are only examples of possible patterns of results when a significant interaction is found between sex and the intervention. The important point is that both within-intervention and within-sex effects should be explored when unpacking this interaction.

These figures highlight another issue relevant to the prevention literature. The outcome displayed in Figure 9.1 would be considered "prevention" because the expected trajectory for girls receiving no intervention would be to increase in depressive symptoms over time. In this case, girls receiving the intervention presumably were prevented from manifesting this rise in depression. In contrast, the results depicted in Figure 9.2 may be characterized as "treatment" because those receiving the intervention showed a decrease in symptoms, whereas those receiving no intervention showed no change. Although the difference between what is referred to as *prevention* versus *treatment* may be mostly semantic, the distinction is useful when describing the nature of the effects observed (Horowitz & Garber, 2006).

Evidence of Sex Differences in the Prevention of Depression

In most meta-analyses of the depression prevention literature (Horowitz & Garber, 2006; Stice et al., 2009), sex has been defined as percent of females in the sample and then tested as a moderator. Separate effect sizes for females versus males, however, are not reported consistently in this literature. We present here the effect sizes for girls and boys separately when those data were available (see Table 1), and compare the overall effect sizes for girls versus boys (see Table 9.2).

Among studies of depression prevention programs that have examined sex differences, some have found that girls responded better than boys (e.g., Gillham, Hamilton, Freres, Patton, & Gallop, 2006; Petersen, Leffert, Graham, Alwin, & Ding, 1997; Schmiege, Khoo, Sandler, Ayers, & Wolchik, 2006; Seligman, Schulman, DeRubeis, & Hollon, 1999); others have found that boys responded better than girls (e.g., Clarke, Hawkins, Murphy, & Sheeber, 1993; Ialongo et al., 1999; Kellam, Rebok, Mayer, Ialongo, & Kalodner, 1994); and still others have found no sex differences (e.g., Horowitz, Garber, Ciesla, Young, & Mufson, 2007; Jaycox, Reivich, Gilham, & Seligman, 1994; Merry, McDowell, Wild, Bir, & Cunliffe, 2004; Pattison & Lynd-Stevenson, 2001). It is noteworthy that universal programs have tended to show no sex differences or better effects for males than females, whereas some targeted programs have found stronger effects for females.

A meta-analysis of studies that specifically tested the Penn Resiliency Programs (PRP) found evidence of the program's effectiveness for both boys and girls, although the range of the effect sizes was large and varied across studies and length of follow-ups (Brunwasser et al., 2009). In one of the earlier trials, Reivich (1996) found moderate effect sizes for boys (0.35–0.61), whereas the effects for girls were quite poor (–0.39–0.06). In contrast, a more recent study (Gillham, Hamilton, et al., 2006) found consistently positive effects for girls (0.21–0.34) and worse effects for boys (–0.33–0.16).

There is some evidence that girls may respond better to more interpersonally focused programs. For example, the Penn Enhancement Program (PEP), which is a more social–emotional intervention, was found to be more effective for girls than boys. In contrast, the Penn Optimism Program (POP), which is a cognitive-behavioral (CB) skills training approach, was effective for boys but not girls (Reivich, 1996; Shatté, 1996).

In a study testing an interpersonally oriented prevention program with a predominantly female sample, Forsyth (2001) found one of the largest effect sizes of any program tested to date. Without a male sample for comparison, however, we do not know whether this program would have

TABLE 9.2. Mean Effect Sizes by Sample Type and by Sex

a. Mean effect sizes for targeted and universal samples, combined across sex

	Targeted (k = 22) [95% CI]	Universal (k = 17) [95% CI]	Between-Ggroups ANOVA (fixed effects)
Posttest	0.30*** [0.23–0.37]	0.06** [0.02–0.10]	Q_B = 32.7*** (df = 1, 37)
Follow-up (6 mo)	0.23*** [0.16–0.30]	0.02 [−0.03–0.06]	Q_B = 24.0*** (df = 1, 35)

b. Mean effect sizes for females and males across (targeted and universal) samples

	Females (k = 23) [95% CI]	Males (k = 19) [95% CI]	Between-groups ANOVA (fixed effects)
Posttest	0.18*** [0.11–0.24]	0.19*** [0.11–0.27]	Q_B = 0.064 (df = 1, 40)
Follow-up (6 mo)	0.09* [0.02–0.16]	0.18*** [0.10–0.27]	Q_B = 2.85~ (df = 1, 39)

c. Mean effect sizes for females and males in targeted samples only

	Females (k = 14) [95% CI]	Males (k = 12) [95% CI]	Between-groups ANOVA (fixed effects)
Posttest	0.20*** [0.11–0.30]	0.13* [0.01–0.24]	Q_B = 1.00 (df = 1, 24)
Follow-up (6 mo)	0.07 [−0.02–0.16]	0.21** [0.10–0.33]	Q_B = 3.61~ (df = 1, 25)

~p < .10; *p < .05; **p < .01; ***p < .001. For mean effect sizes, asterisks indicate that they were significantly different from zero. k = number of studies in the analyses.

worked for males as well. Nevertheless, the Forsyth study is consistent with the idea that an interpersonal approach may be particularly effective for females.

Young and colleagues (Young, Mufson, & Davies, 2006; Young, Mufson, & Gallop, 2010) developed interpersonal psychotherapy–adolescent skills training (IPT-AST), a depression prevention program for adolescents that explicitly focuses on social relationships. Their first study used a predominantly female sample and found positive results (Young et al., 2006). Their next trial included both sexes and showed positive effects for both boys and girls (Young et al., 2010).

Horowitz et al. (2007) directly compared Young's IPT-AST to a CB intervention and found that both programs were more effective than a no-intervention control group in reducing depressive symptoms; no significant group × sex interaction effects were found, however. A closer analysis of these data indicated that the CB intervention yielded small to modest effects for both girls (0.32) and boys (0.44) immediately postintervention, whereas at the 6-month follow-up the effect sizes remained about the same for girls (0.35), but diminished for boys (0.01). Interestingly, the effect of IPT-AST was not significantly different for girls (0.32 at postintervention; −0.04 at 6 months) versus boys (0.14 at postintervention; 0.13 at 6 months).

Meta-analyses of the depression prevention literature have reported a significant effect for sex, that is, a higher percent of females in the sample was associated with a bigger effect size (Horowitz & Garber, 2006; Stice et al., 2009). However, when studies comprised of only college students were excluded from the meta-analysis, the impact of sex on effect sizes became nonsignificant (Horowitz & Garber, 2006). Stice and colleagues (2009) suggested that this pattern of findings may result from age × sex interactions. Testing this hypothesis, they found that at postintervention the largest effects were associated with studies involving older, predominantly female samples. These analyses may be somewhat misleading, however, because some of the older samples were all or mostly female, and hence the effects of the programs for males could not be tested.

Given the inconsistencies in this literature, the question of sex differences in the effects of depression prevention programs remains unresolved. The aim of the current review and meta-analysis is to provide a more in-depth examination of sex differences by providing effects sizes separately for males and females, when available, and by using different operational definitions of sex differences in the analyses.

META-ANALYSIS OF DEPRESSION PREVENTION PROGRAMS: EXAMINATION OF SEX DIFFERENCES

For the present meta-analysis, we identified relevant studies through a computer search of the PsycINFO database using the keywords *depression* and *prevention*. In addition, we examined references of all obtained studies to identify any additional relevant articles, and we reviewed the reference lists of other recent meta-analyses (Brunwasser et al., 2009; Stice et al., 2009). We also conducted a manual search of all journals within which an obtained study was published, from 1971 through December, 2009, including *Archives of General Psychiatry, Journal of the American Academy of Child and Adolescent Psychiatry, Prevention and Treatment, Psychological Science, Psychology in the Schools, School Psychology Quarterly,* the

International Journal of Mental Health Promotion, American Journal of Community Psychology, Behavior Research and Therapy, Family Relations, Journal of Abnormal Child Psychology, Journal of Consulting and Clinical Psychology, Journal of American College Health, Journal of the American Medical Association, and *International Journal of Eating Disorders.*

To be included in the current meta-analysis, studies had to meet the following criteria: (1) one of the goals involved preventing depressive symptoms in children or adolescents; (2) participants were randomly assigned to condition; (3) the study compared a specific preventive intervention with a control condition; (4) depressive symptoms were assessed using a generally accepted measure; and (5) data broken down for girls and boys separately were available in the published article or were provided by the authors. If the necessary data were not provided, we used the procedures suggested by Smith, Glass, and Miller (1980) to derive effect sizes using alternative statistical data (e.g., t or F values).

Effect sizes for each study were calculated by dividing the postintervention difference between the control group and intervention group depression scores by the standard deviation of the control group. Interventions may produce greater variability in the treatment group than in the control group. Therefore, we calculated effect sizes using the standard deviation of the control group because it is presumed to be a more accurate estimate of the population variance (Weiss & Weisz, 1990; Weisz, Weiss, Han, Granger, & Morton, 1995), rather than using the pooled standard deviation of the groups (Cohen, 1977; Lipsey & Wilson, 2001). Effect sizes (Cohen's d) of 0.2 are considered small, 0.5 is moderate, and 0.8 is large (Cohen, 1977). Effect sizes were standardized so that a positive effect size indicated that the intervention group had lower depressive symptoms than the control group.

To preserve independence of effect size estimates, we used only one effect size from each subject sample in the analyses (Weiss & Weisz, 1990; Wilson, Lipsey, & Derzon, 2003). In the few studies (e.g., Reivich, 1996; Wolchik et al., 2002) that included two variations of an intervention and a control group, we pooled results for both intervention groups and compared them to the one control group. One study (Stice, Burton, Bearman, & Rohde, 2006) compared a CB intervention to a waiting-list control condition and four alternative interventions. Given the significant differences among the alternative conditions, and for the sake of consistency, in this meta-analysis we used the comparison of the CB intervention group to the waiting-list control condition.

All of the studies reviewed here used a self-report measure of depressive symptoms; far fewer also included diagnostic interviews. Therefore, we computed effect sizes for all studies using data from the self-report measures. The most common self-report depression measure was the Children's Depression Inventory (CDI). In all studies reviewed here, depressive symptoms were assessed at baseline and immediately postintervention; many studies also conducted follow-up assessments ranging from as short as 1 month to as long as 6 years; the most common follow-up period was 6 months. In the current meta-analysis, we computed effect sizes for immediately postintervention and at the follow-up closest to 6 months (range = 3–18 months).

Because effect sizes from small samples are known to be biased estimates of population parameters, an adjustment for small sample bias was applied to each effect size (Hedges & Olkin, 1985). In addition, to give more weight to effect sizes from studies with larger samples and with smaller standard errors, each effect size was weighted by the inverse of its variance (Hedges & Olkin, 1985).

Results

To test whether effect size values differed significantly from zero, we used SPSS macros created by Wilson (2005), which generate z tests. To examine whether the various effect sizes in the meta-analysis were estimating the same population mean, we conducted a homogeneity analysis based on Hedges and Olkin's (1985) Q statistic, which is designed to test whether the observed variability across effect sizes is greater than expected from subject-level sampling error. Potential moderators of effect size variability were examined using a meta-analytic analog to the analysis of variance (ANOVA) for categorical independent variables (e.g., type of intervention) and using a modified weighted regression for continuous variables (e.g., percent of females; Lipsey & Wilson, 2001). All analyses were conducted using inverse-variance-weighted, fixed-effects models (Hunter & Schmidt, 2000; Lipsey & Wilson, 2001). Standardized beta weights are reported in the moderator analyses.

Table 9.1 presents sample characteristics of each study, overall effect sizes, and when available, separate effect sizes for girls and boys. We identified 39 studies that met the inclusion criteria and were used in the analyses. Of these studies, 17 were universal samples and 22 were targeted (selective or indicated). Thirteen of the 54 studies listed in Table 9.1 were not included in the analyses or were included only in analyses by sex; 5 of these 13 reports were follow-up studies, so only the most recent publication was included in the analyses; two studies did not report the overall effect sizes, but rather reported only the effect sizes broken down by sex; and six studies did not provide sufficient information to enable calculating an unbiased effect size.

Positive effect sizes reflect lower levels of depressive symptoms in the intervention group relative to controls at that time point (i.e., postintervention or follow-up). In Table 9.1, effect sizes are presented separately for girls and boys, when available; that is, the sixth column, labeled "Girls' effect size," and the seventh column, labeled "Boys' effect size," present the effect of the intervention versus control for girls only or for boys only, respectively, in that sample. Across all sample types (i.e., universal and targeted), we were able to calculate 23 effect sizes for girls and 19 effect sizes for boys. The total number of studies differed by sex because some studies were male-only (e.g., Hyun, Cho Chung, & Lee, 2005) and some were female-only (e.g., Bearman, Stice, & Chase, 2003; Burton, Stice, Bearman, & Rohde, 2007; Harnett & Dadds, 2004). Within targeted (i.e., selective, indicated) samples only, we were able to calculate 14 effects sizes for girls and 12 for boys. The specific studies used in each of the analyses reported in Table 9.2 are shown in Table 1 with superscripts (a, b, c).

Overall Effects

At postintervention, weighted effect sizes across all studies ranged from −0.61 to 1.03. The weighted overall mean effect size was 0.12, which is considered small (Cohen, 1977). This effect was significantly different from 0 ($z = 6.55$, $p < .001$). At follow-up, weighted effect sizes ranged from −.25 to 0.81. The weighted overall mean effect size was 0.08, which was small but also significantly different from 0 ($z = 3.91$, $p < .001$). Effect size distributions were significantly heterogeneous at both postintervention ($Q = 143.83$, $p < .001$) and follow-up ($Q = 98.34$, $p < .001$), indicating that the various effect sizes may not be estimating a common population mean and that their variability was greater than expected from sampling error alone. Therefore, we next examined potential moderators of this variability.

Type of Intervention. At postintervention, the weighted mean effect size for the studies with targeted samples was 0.30 ($z = 8.25$, $p < .001$), and for universal samples was 0.06 ($z = 2.96$, $p < .003$). This difference in effect sizes was statistically significant [$Q (1, 37) = 32.70$, $p < .001$]. At follow-up, the weighted mean effect size for targeted sample studies was 0.23 ($z = 6.24$, $p < .001$), and for universal sample studies was 0.02 ($z = .70$, $p = .48$). This difference in effect sizes also was significant [$Q (1, 35) = 23.95$, $p < .001$]. Thus, consistent with what has been reported elsewhere (e.g., Horowitz & Garber, 2006; Merry et al., 2005; Stice et al., 2009), effects were stronger in studies using targeted as compared to universal samples. Results for these analyses are presented in Table 9.2a.

Sex: Percentage of Females in the Sample. For the moderator analysis of the overall sample, analyses were conducted using fixed-effects regressions with sex operationalized as the percentage of female participants in the sample. At postintervention, the effect of sex was significant ($z = 2.11$, $p = .04$, $B = 0.18$, $k = 36$ studies), indicating that studies with a percentage of females at or above the median had slightly larger effect sizes. This effect was not significant at follow-up ($z = .91$, $p = .37$, $B = 0.10$, $k = 34$ studies).

Interventions with a high and low percentage of females were then examined separately. At posttest, those studies with a lower percentage of females ($\leq 52\%$) yielded a weighted mean effect size of 0.15, which was significantly different from zero ($z = 3.72$, $p < .001$, $k = 16$ studies). The weighted mean effect size for interventions with a greater percentage of females (above 52%) was 0.11, which also was significantly different from zero ($z = 5.72$, $p < .001$, $k = 23$ studies). The effect size for interventions with a greater percentage of females was not significantly different from those with a lower percentage [$Q (1, 37) = .65$, $p = .42$].

A similar pattern was found at follow-up: Interventions with a lower percentage of females ($\leq 53\%$) had a weighted mean effect size of 0.07, which was significantly different from zero ($z = 2.08$, $p = .04$, $k = 17$ studies). The weighted mean effect size for interventions with a greater percentage of females was 0.07 ($z = 3.16$, $p = .002$, $k = 19$ studies). The effect size for interventions with a greater percentage of females was not significantly different from those with a lower percentage [$Q (1, 34) = .04$, $p = .85$].

Sex Differences by Treatment Type

Universal and Targeted Samples. Across all studies (i.e., universal and targeted samples) at posttest, the weighted mean effect size for females ($k = 23$ studies) was 0.18 (95% confidence interval [CI] = .11–.24), which was significantly different from zero ($z = 5.13$, $p < .001$). The weighted mean effect size for males ($k = 19$ studies) was .19 (95% CI = .11–.27), which also was significantly different from zero ($z = 4.73$, $p < .001$). At posttest, meta-ANOVAs revealed that these effect sizes for females versus males were not significantly different [$Q (1, 40) = .064$, $p = .80$].

At follow-up, the mean effect size for females ($k = 23$ studies) was 0.09 (95% CI = .02–.16), which was significantly different from zero ($z = 2.51$, $p = .01$), and the mean effect size for males ($k = 18$ studies) was 0.18 (95% CI = .10–.27), which also was significantly different from zero ($z = 4.28$, $p < .001$). At follow-up, meta-ANOVA revealed that these effect sizes for females versus males were not significantly different [$Q (1, 39) = 2.84$, $p = .09$], although there was a nonsignificant trend for the effect size to be larger for boys than girls (see Table 9.2b).

Targeted Samples Only. At posttest, within studies using targeted samples only, the weighted mean effect size for females (k = 14 studies) was 0.20 (95% CI = .11–.30), and significantly different from zero (z = 4.23, p < .001). For males (k = 12 studies), the weighted mean effect size was 0.13 (95% CI = .01–0.24), and also was significantly different from zero (z = 2.16, p = .03). At posttest among targeted samples, meta-ANOVA analyses revealed that there were no significant differences in these effect sizes by sex [Q (1, 24) = 1.00, p = .32].

At follow-up, the mean effect size for females in targeted samples was 0.07 (95% CI = –.02–.16), which was not significantly different from zero (z = 1.47, p = .14). For males, the mean effect size was 0.21 (95% CI = .10–.33), which was significantly different from zero (z = 3.6, p < .05). At follow-up among targeted samples, meta-ANOVAs revealed a nonsignificant trend for a larger effect size for males than females [Q (1, 25) = 3.61, p = .06] (see Table 9.2c).

Discussion

The primary aim of this meta-analysis was to examine sex differences in the effects of interventions for preventing depression in youth. To address this issue, sex differences were tested in three different ways, yielding some similar and some inconsistent findings. In one set of analyses, we tested sex as a potential moderator of the effect size variability in the overall set of 36 studies. Consistent with other meta-analyses of this literature (e.g., Horowitz & Garber, 2006; Stice et al., 2009), we operationalized *sex* as the percentage of participants in each study who were female. These analyses revealed a significant effect of sex at postintervention, indicating that studies with a higher percentage of females had slightly larger effect sizes. This effect was not significant at follow-up, however.

We next contrasted the effect sizes of samples with higher ($\geq$ 53%) versus lower percentages of females by conducting separate analyses of these two types of samples. At both postintervention and follow-up, we found significant weighted mean effect sizes for both high- and low-percentage female samples. That is, studies that had more females and those with more males both produced significant effect sizes; these effect sizes, however, were not significantly different from each other. Thus, analyzing the data this way yielded no sex differences in the size or significance of the effects.

In the third data-analytic approach, we (1) calculated separate effect sizes for girls and boys in each study, (2) obtained an overall weighted mean effect size for girls and boys separately, and (3) compared the effect sizes for girls versus boys statistically. This more demanding strategy was used in the meta-analyses of the larger depression prevention literature by Merry and colleagues (2005) and in the recent meta-analysis of studies specifically testing the Penn Prevention Program (Brunwasser et al., 2009). The current meta-analysis found that at postintervention, the mean effect sizes were low to moderate for both males and females, with a nonsignificant trend for a larger effect for males. At follow-up, the mean effect size also showed a nonsignificant trend to be larger for males than females, indicating that the effect of the intervention compared to the control condition tended to be greater for boys than girls. This pattern of results was stronger when analyses were conducted only on studies using targeted samples (see Table 9.2c).

Thus, we are left with three different conclusions based on the three analytic methods. Although each method has limitations, the third approach of calculating the actual effect sizes for girls and boys separately in each study likely is a more precise estimate of the actual effects as compared to using the percentage of females in the sample. One clear recommendation from these results is that *future randomized controlled trials aimed at preventing depression in youth should report the data (i.e., means, standard deviations, effect sizes) regarding the outcomes (i.e., depressive symptoms and disorders) separately for males and females, in addition to presenting the overall sample statistics.*

Moderators

As with any meta-analysis, the studies included here varied in the following ways: sample size, number of males and females in the samples, participants' ages, size and composition (single vs. mixed sex) of the groups, sex of the group leaders/therapists, training and skills of the group leaders/therapists, fidelity and quality of implementation of the interventions, content of the interventions (e.g., cognitive, interpersonal), measures of depression, baseline symptom levels, length of the interventions, and duration of the follow-ups. An advantage of meta-analysis is that it combines studies with different size samples in order to calculate an overall effect size. A disadvantage, however, is that lumping studies together in this way may ignore some potentially important study characteristics, particularly the quality of the study design and implementation (Moncrieff, Churchill, Drummond, & McGuire, 2001).

Other than adjusting for sample size, most meta-analyses of the depression prevention literature in youth have not taken into consideration many of the study features noted above. Some of these variables have been tested as potential moderators as a way of unpacking significant variability in effect sizes across studies. In general, the characteristics selected depend on the question(s) being asked and the number of studies with data available to be included in such analyses. The present meta-analysis tested sex and type of sample (i.e., universal, targeted) as moderators. Other meta-analyses of this literature have tested additional study features such as length of the program, level of baseline symptoms, characteristics of the group leaders/ therapists, and program content (Brunwasser et al., 2009; Merry et al., 2005; Stice et al., 2009). Few individual studies or meta-analyses of the depression prevention literature, however, have examined the interaction of sex with these other potential moderators, with the exception of the meta-analysis by Stice and colleagues (2009) that explicitly tested a sex × age interaction. Thus, we do not know yet, for example, whether the effect sizes for girls and boys differ for depression prevention programs involving mixed- versus single-sex groups, same- versus opposite-sex group leaders, or cognitive- versus interpersonally focused curriculum. Not enough studies have been conducted to allow for testing the interaction of sex with these as well as other study characteristics in a meta-analysis.

Studies using the PRP have been particularly attentive to the possibility that contextual factors (e.g., the intervention setting, group composition, or group leader characteristics) may affect boys and girls differently. For example, in an earlier study that found larger effect sizes for boys than girls, the clinicians observed that girls appeared more comfortable, engaged, and open when the group was mostly or completely female, whereas boys were more attentive and better behaved in groups with girls (Reivich, 1996). In a more recent study that explicitly tested differences as a function of the configuration of the groups, Chaplin and colleagues (2006) found that girls in single-sex groups attended more PRP sessions and had lower hopelessness scores than girls in co-ed groups; both all-girls and co-ed PRP groups, however, showed similar improvements in depressive symptoms as compared to a no-intervention control (Chaplin et al., 2006). Gillham and colleagues (Brunwasser et al., 2009; Chaplin et al., 2006 Gillham et al., 2000) have suggested that various contextual factors such as group leader characteristics or whether the group is single- versus mixed-sex may affect outcomes differently for girls versus boys. More such intervention studies that experimentally manipulate variables hypothesized to vary by sex are needed.

Implications of Sex Differences for Preventive Interventions

Prevalence. Sex differences in rates of depression have two important implications for prevention. First, given limited resources, should depression prevention programs target girls, in particular, because of their elevated risk? That is, because a greater number of girls than boys are likely to develop depressive symptoms and disorders, should depression prevention efforts concentrate on girls? One problem with this perspective, however, is that boys also get depressed. Given that depression is associated with other serious problems (e.g., academic difficulties, substance use, suicide) in boys as well as girls (Angold, Costello, & Erkanli, 1999), then boys, particularly those at risk, also should have access to preventive interventions. Thus, although adolescent females are at greater risk for depression than their male counterparts, results of this meta-analysis indicate that boys do benefit from some prevention programs, possibly even more so than girls.

A second implication of the greater prevalence of depression in females than males concerns the likelihood of finding a significant prevention effect. As noted earlier in reference to Figure 9.1, finding a significant intervention effect might be more likely for girls than boys, not because the intervention works better for girls than boys, but because without the intervention, girls will show a greater increase in depression than boys. Contrary to the assertion that "Given the gender differences in prevalence . . . it is likely that girls and boys will respond differently to interventions" (Merry et al., 2005; p. 2), we suggest that sex differences in prevalence do not necessarily mean that girls will *respond* better or even differently than boys to the same intervention. A head-to-head comparison of girls' and boys' responses to a prevention program might show no significant sex differences. The effect sizes for girls and boys, however, might differ because girls in the no-intervention condition may increase significantly in depression in contrast to girls who received the intervention, whereas boys in the no-intervention group might not show such an increase in symptoms. Thus, sex differences in prevalence and in response to an intervention do not readily map on to each other and may result from different processes.

Risk. Despite the various speculations about why females are at greater risk of depression than males (e.g., Nolen-Hoeksema & Hilt, 2009), depression prevention programs generally have not been designed to explicitly target the hypothesized mechanisms underlying these sex differences. Identifying specific risk factors associated with the increased likelihood of depression in either girls or boys is central to selecting *who* should be targeted for prevention. Understanding the specific risk processes underlying the relation between these risk factors and depression can inform the design of *what* actually to do (i.e., content) in the preventive program.

Discovering *who* is at risk for depression will help determine which individuals should be targeted for preventive. Such "selective" samples have included youth who were offspring of depressed parents (Beardslee et al., 1997; Clarke et al., 2001; Compas et al., 2009; Garber et al., 2009), exposed to specific stressors such as family conflict, parental divorce, death of a loved one (Gillham, Reivich, Jaycox, & Seligman, 1995; Sandler et al., 2003; Wolchik et al., 2002), high in anxiety (Lock & Barrett, 2003; Lowry-Webster, Barrett, & Lock, 2003), characterized by negative cognitive styles (Seligman et al., 1999), or had prior depressive episodes (Clarke et al., 2001; Garber et al., 2009). The content of the prevention programs with these samples, however, has varied regarding how much direct attention has been paid to the risk factor(s) for which the participants were selected. For example, some depression prevention studies using offspring of depressed parents as the index of risk have emphasized cognitive restructuring and problem solving, and only briefly addressed the parents' mood disorder in particular (Clarke et al., 2001; Garber et al., 2009). In contrast, other studies of at-risk offspring have explicitly attempted to alter the consequences of the parents' depression on their behaviors toward their children and to provide the children with skills for coping with their parents' depression (Compas et al., 2009). Both of these approaches have been shown to be efficacious; their relative efficacy has not been tested yet, however.

Even if an underlying cause of depression is not malleable (e.g., genes), the more proximal endophenotypes that link such a distal cause to subsequent depression (Roberts & Kendler, 1999) may be amenable to change. For example, the temperamental characteristic of "stress reactivity" may be the phenotypic expression of a genetic predisposition. Training stress-reactive individuals to reduce their initial response to stress and cope with the stress once it has occurred may be an effective strategy for preventing subsequent depression when such individuals are faced with negative life events. Identifying the specific mechanisms associated with a particular child's risk will allow us to better individualize the prevention program for him or her.

Thus, future research efforts should identify the risk processes that increase the likelihood of depression in females as well as males, recognizing that these etiological pathways may differ. Basic knowledge of what accounts for sex differences in depression then can be translated into the construction of gender-sensitive preventive interventions. A more comprehensive understanding of the mechanisms through which depression emerges in females and males is needed in order to design the most gender-appropriate interventions for preventing it.

ACKNOWLEDGMENTS

This work was supported in part from grants from the National Institute of Mental Health (R01 MH64735; RC1 MH088329) and the William T. Grant Foundation (173096).

REFERENCES

Asterisk (*) indicates studies for which means and standard deviations were available by gender, which were used in gender analyses.

Angold, A., Costello, E. J., & Erkanli, A. (1999). Comorbidity. *Journal of Child Psychology and Psychiatry, 40,* 57–87.

Angold, A., Costello, E. J., Erkanli, A., & Worthman, C. M. (1999). Pubertal changes in hormones of adolescent girls. *Psychological Medicine, 29,* 1043–1053.

Angold A., Costello E. J., & Worthman C. M. (1998). Puberty and depression: The roles of age, pubertal status, and pubertal timing. *Psychological Medicine, 28,* 51–61.

Angold, A., Erkanli, A., Silberg, J., Eaves, L., & Costello, E. J. (2002). Depression scale scores in 8–17-year-olds: Effects of age and gender. *Journal of Child Psychology and Psychiatry, 43,* 1052–1063.

Angold, A., Worthman, C., & Costello, E. J. (2003). Puberty and depression. In C. Hayward (Ed.), *Gender differences at puberty* (pp. 137-164). New York: Cambridge University Press.

Barrett, P. M., Farrell, L. J., Ollendick, T. H., & Dadds, M. (2006). Long-term outcomes of an Australian universal prevention trial of anxiety and depression symptoms in children and youth: An evaluation of the Friends Program. *Journal of Clinical Child and Adolescent Psychology, 35,* 403–411.

Beardslee, W. R., Gladstone, T. R. G., Wright, E. J., Cooper, A. (2003). A family-based approach to the prevention of depressive symptoms in children at risk: Evidence of parental and child change. *Pediatrics, 112,* 119–131.(*)

Beardslee, W. R., Wright, E. J., Gladstone, T. R. G., & Forbes, P. (2007). Long-term effects from a randomized trial of two public health preventive interventions for parental depression. *Journal of Family Psychology, 21,* 703–713.(*)

Beardslee, W. R., Wright, E. J., Salt, P., Drezner, K., Gladstone, T. R. G., Versage, E. M., et al. (1997). Examination of children's responses to two preventive intervention strategies over time. *Journal of the American Academy of Child and Adolescent Psychiatry, 36,* 196–204.

Bearman, S. K., Stice, E., & Chase, A. (2003). Evaluation of an intervention targeting both depressive and bulimic pathology: A randomized prevention trial. *Behavior Therapy, 34,* 277–293.(*)

Birmaher, B., Ryan, N., Williamson, D., Brent, D., Kaufman, J., Dahl, R., et al. (1996). Childhood and adolescent depression: A review of the past 10 years, Part I. *Journal of the American Academy of Child and Adolescent Psychiatry, 35,* 1427–1439.

Brent, D. A., & Birmaher, B. (2006). Treatment-resistant depression in adolescents: Recognition and management. *Child and Adolescent Psychiatric Clinics of North America, 15,* 1015–1034.

Brent, D. A., Perper, J. A., Moritz, G., Allman, C., Friend, A., Roth, C., et al. (1993). Psychiatric risk factors for adolescent suicide: A case-control study. *Journal of the American Academy of Child and Adolescent Psychiatry, 32,* 521–529.

Brunwasser, S. M., Gillham, J. E., & Kim, E. S. (2009). A meta-analytic review of the Penn Resiliency Program's effect on depressive symptoms. *Journal of Consulting and Clinical Psychology, 77,* 1042–1054.

Burton, E. M., Stice, E., Bearman, S. K., & Rohde, P. (2007). An experimental test of the affect-regulation theory of bulimic symptoms and substance use: A randomized trial. *International Journal of Eating Disorders, 40,* 27–36.(*)

Cardemil, E. V., Reivich, K. J., Beevers, C. G., Seligman, M. E. P., & James, J. (2007). The prevention of depressive symptoms in low-income minority children: Two-year follow-up. *Behaviour Research and Therapy, 45,* 313–327. (*)

Cardemil, E. V., Reivich, K. J., & Seligman, M. E. P. (2002). The prevention of depressive symptoms in low-income minority middle-school students. *Prevention and Treatment, 5,* Article 8. Available at *journals. apa.org/prevention/volume5/pre0050008a.html.*(*)

Cecchini, T. B. (1997). An interpersonal and cognitive-behavioral approach to childhood depression: A school-based primary prevention study (doctoral dissertation, Utah State University). *Dissertation Abstracts International, 58,* 12B. (UMI No. 9820698)

Chaplin, T. M., Gillham, J. E., Reivich, K., Elkon, A. G. L., Samuels, B., Freres, D. R., et al. (2006). Depression prevention for early adolescent girls: A pilot study of all-girls verses co-ed groups. *Journal of Early Adolescence, 26,* 110–126.

Chorpita, B. F., Plummer, C. P., & Moffitt, C. (2000). Relations of tripartite dimensions of emotion to childhood anxiety and mood disorders. *Journal of Abnormal Child Psychology, 28,* 299–310.

Clarke, G. N., Hawkins, W., Murphy, M., & Sheeber, L. B. (1993). School-based primary prevention of depressive symptomatology in adolescents: Findings from two studies. *Journal of Adolescent Research, 8,* 183–204.

Clarke, G. N., Hawkins, W., Murphy, M., & Sheeber, L. B., Lewinsohn, P. M., & Seeley, J. R. (1995). Targeted prevention of unipolar depressive disorder in an at-risk sample of high school adolescents: A randomized trial of a group cognitive intervention. *Journal of the American Academy of Child and Adolescent Psychiatry, 34,* 312–321.

Clarke, G. N., Hornbrook, M., Lynch, F., Polen, M., Gale, J., Beardslee, W., et al. (2001). A randomized trial of a group cognitive intervention for preventing depression in adolescent offspring of depressed parents. *Archives of General Psychiatry, 58,* 1127–1134.(*)

Cohen, J. (1977). *Statistical power analysis for the behavioral sciences* (rev. ed.). New York: Academic Press.

Compas, B. E., Forehand, R., Keller, G., Champion, J. E., Rakow, A., Reeslund, K. L., et al. (2009). Randomized controlled trial of a family cognitive-behavioral preventive intervention for children of depressed parents. *Journal of Consulting and Clinical Psychology, 77,* 1007–1020.

Costello, E. J., Foley, D. L., & Angold, A. (2006). 10-year research update review: The epidemiology of child and adolescent psychiatric disorders: II. Developmental epidemiology. *Journal of the American Academy of Child and Adolescent Psychiatry, 45,* 8–25.

Costello, E. J., Mustillo, S., Erkanli, A., Keeler, G., & Angold, A. (2003). Prevalence and development of psychiatric disorders in childhood and adolescence. *Archives of General Psychiatry, 60,* 837–844.

Cyranowski, J. M., Frank, E., Young, E., & Shear, K. (2000). Adolescent onset of the gender difference in lifetime rates of depression. *Archives of General Psychiatry, 57,* 21–27.

Eley, T. C., Sugden, K., Corsico, A., Gregory, A. M., Sham, P., McGuffin, P., et al. (2004). Gene–environment interaction analysis of serotonin system markers with adolescent depression. *Molecular Psychiatry, 9,* 908–915.

Emslie, G. J., Rush, A. J., Weinberg, W. A., Gullion, C. M., Rintelmann, J., & Hughes, C. W. (1997). Recurrence of major depressive disorder in hospitalized children and adolescents. *Journal of the American Academy of Child and Adolescent Psychiatry, 36,* 785–792.

Fleming, J. E., Offord, D. R., & Boyle, M. H. (1989). Ontario Child Health Study: Prevalence of childhood and adolescent depression in the community. *British Journal of Psychiatry, 155,* 647–654.

Forsyth, K. M. (2001). *The design and implementation of a depression prevention program* (doctoral dissertation, University of Rhode Island). *Dissertation Abstracts International, 61*(12), 6704B. (UMI No. 9999536)

Garber, J., Clarke, G. N., Weersing, V. R., Beardslee, W. R., Brent, D. A., Gladstone, T. R., et al. (2009). Prevention of depression in at-risk adolescents: A randomized controlled trial. *Journal of the American Medical Association, 21,* 2215–2224.(*)

Garber, J., & McCauley, E. (2002). Prevention of depression and suicide in children and adolescents. In M. Lewis (Ed.), *Child and adolescent psychiatry: A comprehensive text* (3rd ed., pp. 805–821). Baltimore: Williams & Wilkins.

Gillham, J. E., Hamilton, J., Freres, D. R., Patton, K., & Gallop, R. (2006). Preventing depression among early adolescents in the primary care setting: A randomized controlled study of the Penn Resiliency Program. *Journal of Abnormal Child Psychology, 34,* 203–219.(*)

Gillham, J. E., & Reivich, K. J. (1999). Prevention of depressive symptoms in school children: A research update. *Psychological Science, 10,* 461–462.

Gillham, J. E., Reivich, K. J., Freres, D. R., Chaplin, T. M., Shatte, A. J., Samuels, B., et al. (2007). School-based prevention of depressive symptoms: A randomized controlled study of the effectiveness and specificity of the Penn Resiliency Program. *Journal of Consulting and Clinical Psychology, 75,* 9–19.

Gillham, J. E., Reivich, K. J., Freres, D. R., Lascher, M., Litzinger, S., Shatté, A., et al. (2006). School-based prevention of depression and anxiety symptoms in early adolescence: A pilot of a parent intervention component. *School Psychology Quarterly, 21,* 323–348.

Gillham, J. E., Reivich, K. J., Jaycox, L. H., & Seligman, M. P. E. (1995). Prevention of depressive symptoms in schoolchildren: Two-year follow-up. *Psychological Science, 6,* 343–351.(*)

Gillham, J. E., Reivich, K. J., & Seligman, M. P. E. (2007, November). Prevention of depressive symptoms in children and parents. In J. Garber (Chair.), *Preventing depression in youths: Moderators of outcome.* Symposium conducted at the annual meeting of the Association for Behavioral and Cognitive Therapies, Philadelphia, PA.

Gillham, J. E., Shatté, A. J., & Freres, D. R. (2000). Preventing depression: A review of cognitive-behavioral and family interventions. *Applied & Preventive Psychology, 9,* 63–88.(*)

González-Tejera, G., Canino, G., Ramirez, R., Chï¿½vez, L., Shrout, P., Bird, H., et al. (2005). Examining minor and major depression in adolescents. *Journal of Child Psychology and Psychiatry, 46*, 888–899.

Gwynn, C. A., & Brantley, H. T. (1987). Effects of a divorce group intervention for elementary school children. *Psychology in the Schools, 24,* 161–164.

Hains, A. A., & Ellman, S. W. (1994). Stress inoculation training as a preventive intervention for high school youths. *Journal of Cognitive Psychotherapy: An International Quarterly, 8,* 219–232.

Hankin, B. L., & Abramson, L. Y. (2001). Development of gender differences in depression: An elaborated cognitive vulnerability–transactional stress theory. *Psychological Bulletin, 127,* 773–796.

Hankin, B. L., Abramson, L. Y., Moffitt, T. E., Silva, P. A., McGee, R., & Angell, K. A. (1998). Development of depression from preadolescence to young adulthood: Emerging gender differences in a 10-year longitudinal study. *Journal of Abnormal Psychology, 107,* 128–141.

Hankin, B. L., Cheely, C., & Wetter, E. (2008). Sex differences in child and adolescent depression: A developmental psychopathological approach. In J. R. Z. Abela & B. L. Hankin (Eds.), *Handbook of child and adolescent depression* (pp. 377–414). New York: Guilford Press.

Hankin, B. L., Mermelstein, R., & Roesch, L. (2007). Sex differences in adolescent depression: Stress exposure and reactivity models in interpersonal and achievement contextual domains. *Child Development, 78,* 279–295.

Harnett, P. H., & Dadds, M. R. (2004). Training school personnel to implement a universal school-based prevention of depression program under real world conditions. *Journal of School Psychology, 42,* 343–357.(*)

Hedges, L. V., & Olkin, I. (1985). *Statistical methods for meta-analysis.* Orlando, FL: Academic Press.

Horowitz, J. L., & Garber, J. (2006). The prevention of depressive symptoms in children and adolescents: A meta-analytic review. *Journal of Consulting and Clinical Psychology, 74,* 401–415.

Horowitz, J. L., Garber, J., Ciesla, J. A., Young, J., & Mufson, L. (2007). Prevention of depressive symptoms in adolescents: A randomized trial of cognitive-behavioral and interpersonal prevention programs. *Journal of Consulting and Clinical Psychology, 75,* 693–706.(*)

Hunter, J. E., & Schmidt, F. L. (2000). Fixed effects vs. random effects meta-analysis models: Implications for cumulative research knowledge. *International Journal of Selection and Assessment, 8,* 275–292.

Hyde, J. S., Mezulis, A., & Abramson, L. Y. (2008). The ABCs of depression: Integrating affective, biological, and cognitive models to explain the emergence of the gender difference in depression. *Psychological Review, 115,* 291–313.

Hyun, M.-S., Cho Chung, H.-I., & Lee, Y.-J. (2005). The effect of cognitive–behavioral group therapy on the self-esteem, depression, and self-efficacy of runaway adolescents in a shelter in South Korea. *Applied Nursing Research, 18,* 160–166.(*)

Ialongo, N. S., Poduska, J., Werthamer, L., & Kellam, S. (2001). The distal impact of two first grade preventive interventions on conduct problems and disorder and mental health service need and utilization in early adolescence. *Journal of Emotional and Behavioral Disorders, 9,* 146–160.(*)

Ialongo, N. S., Werthamer, L., Kellam, S. G., Brown, C. H., Wang, S., & Lin, Y. (1999). Proximal impact of two first-grade preventive interventions on the early risk behaviors for later substance abuse, depression, and antisocial behavior. *American Journal of Community Psychology, 27,* 599–641.

Jané-Llopis, E., Hosman, C., Jenkins, R., & Anderson, P. (2003). Predictors of efficacy in depression prevention programmes. *British Journal of Psychiatry, 183,* 384–397.

Jaycox, L. H., Reivich, K. J., Gillham, J., & Seligman, M. E. P. (1994). Prevention of depressive symptoms in school children. *Behaviour Research and Therapy, 32,* 801–816.

Johnson, N. C. (2000). A follow-up study of a primary prevention program targeting childhood depression (doctoral dissertation, Utah State University, 2000). (UMI No. 1402700)

Kaminski, K. M., & Garber, J. (2002). Depressive spectrum disorders in adolescents: Episode duration and predictors of time to recovery. *Journal of the American Academy of Child and Adolescent Psychiatry, 41,* 410–418.

Keenan, K., & Hipwell, A. E. (2005). Preadolescent clues to understanding depression in girls. *Clinical Child and Family Psychology Review, 8,* 89–105.

Kellam, S. G., Rebok, G. W., Mayer, L. S., Ialongo, N., & Kalodner, C. R. (1994). Depressive symptoms over first grade and their response to a developmental epidemiologically based preventive trial aimed at improving achievement. *Development and Psychopathology, 6,* 463–481.(*)

Kessler, R. C., Wai, T. C., Demler, O., & Walters, E. E. (2005). Prevalence, severity, and comorbidity of 12-month DSM-IV disorders in the National Comorbidity Survey replication. *Archives of General Psychiatry, 62,* 617–627.

Kessler, R. C., & Walters, E. E. (1998). Epidemiology of DSM-III-R major depression and minor depression among adolescents and young adults in the National Comorbidity Survey. *Depression and Anxiety, 7,* 3–14.

Kochanska, G., Coy, K. C., & Murray, K. T. (2001). The development of self-regulation in the first four years of life. *Child Development, 72,* 1091–1111.

Kovacs, M. (1996). The course of childhood-onset depressive disorders. *Psychiatric Annals, 26,* 326–330.

Lamb, J. M., Puskar, K. R., Sereika, M., & Corcoran, M. (1998). School-based intervention to promote coping in rural teens. *American Journal of Maternal and Child Nursing, 23,* 187–194.

Le, H., Munoz, R. F., Ippen, C. G., & Stoddard, J. L. (2003). Treatment is not enough: We must prevent major depression in women. *Prevention and Treatment, 6*(2). Retrieved from *journals.apa.org/prevention/volume6/pre0060010a.html.*

Lewinsohn, P. M., Clarke, G. N., Seeley, J. R., & Rohde, P. (1994). Major depression in community adolescents: Age at onset, episode duration, and time to recurrence. *Journal of the American Academy of Child and Adolescent Psychiatry, 33,* 809–818.

Lewinsohn, P. M., & Essau, C. A. (2002). Depression in adolescents. In I. H. Gotlib & C. L. Hammen (Eds.), *Handbook of depression* (pp. 541–559). New York: Guilford Press.

Lewinsohn, P. M., Rohde, P., & Seeley, J. R. (1998). Major depressive disorder in older adolescents: Prevalence, risk factors, and clinical implications. *Clinical Psychology Review, 18,* 765–794.

Lewinsohn, P. M., Rohde, P., Seeley, J. R., Klein, D. N., & Gotlib, I. H. (2003). Psychosocial characteristics of young adults who have experienced and recovered from major depressive disorder during adolescence. *Journal of Abnormal Psychology 112,* 353–363.

Lipsey, M. W., & Wilson, D. B. (2001). *Practical meta-analysis: Applied social research methods series* (Vol. 49). Thousand Oaks, CA: Sage.

Little, S. A., & Garber, J. (2005). The role of social stressors and interpersonal orientation in explaining the longitudinal relation between externalizing and depressive symptoms. *Journal of Abnormal Psychology, 114,* 432–443.

Lock, S., & Barrett, P. M. (2003). A longitudinal study of developmental differences in universal preventive intervention for child anxiety. *Behaviour Change, 20,* 183–199.

Lowry-Webster, H., Barrett, P. M., & Lock, S. (2003). A universal prevention trial of anxiety symptomatology during childhood: Results at one-year follow-up. *Behaviour Change, 20,* 25–43.

Mrazek, P. J., & Haggerty, R. J. (1994). *Reducing risks for mental disorders: Frontiers for preventive intervention research.* Washington, DC: National Academy Press.

McCauley, E., Myers, K., Mitchell, J. Calderon, R., Scholredt, K., & Treder, R. (1993). Depression in young people: Initial presentation and clinical course. *Journal of the American Academy of Child and Adolescent Psychiatry, 32,* 714–722.

Merikangas, K. R., & Knight, E. (2009). The epidemiology of depression in adolescents. In Nolen-Hoeksema, S. Hilt, L. M. (Eds.), *Handbook of depression in adolescents* (pp. 53–74). New York: Routledge/Taylor & Francis Group.

Merry, S. N., McDowell, H., Hetrick, S., Bir, J., & Muller, N. (2005). Psychological and/or educational interventions for the prevention of depression in children and adolescents (Review). *The Cochrane Collaboration.* New York: Wiley.

Merry, S. N., McDowell, H., Wild, C. J., Bir, J., & Cunliffe, R. (2004). A randomized placebo controlled trial of a school-based depression prevention program. *Journal of the American Academy of Child and Adolescent Psychiatry, 43,* 538–547.

Merry, S. N., & Spence, S. H. (2007). Attempting to prevent depression in youth: A systematic review of the evidence. *Early Intervention in Psychiatry, 1,* 128–137.

Mezulis, A. H., Abramson, L., & Hyde, J. S. (2002). Domain specificity of gender differences in rumination. *Journal of Cognitive Psychotherapy: An International Quarterly, 16,* 421–434.

Mezulis, A. H., Abramson, L., Hyde, J. S., & Hankin, B. L. (2004). Is there a universal positivity bias in attributions?: A meta-analytic review of individual, developmental, and cultural differences in the self-serving attributional bias. *Psychological Bulletin, 130,* 711–746.

Moncrieff, J., Churchill, R., Drummond, C., & McGuire, H. (2001). Development of a quality assessment instrument for trials of treatments for depression and neurosis. *International Journal of Methods in Psychiatric Research, 10,* 126–133.

Munoz, R. F., Le, H. N., Clarke, G., & Jaycox, L. (2002). Preventing the onset of major depression. In C. L. Hammen & I. H. Gotlib (Eds.), *Handbook of depression* (pp. 343–359). New York: Guilford Press.

Nolen-Hoeksema, S., & Girgus, J. S. (1994). The emergence of gender differences in depression in adolescence. *Psychological Bulletin, 115,* 424–443.

Nolen-Hoeksema, S., & Hilt, L. (2009). The emergence of gender differences in depression in adolescence. In S. Nolen-Hoeksema & L. Hilt (Eds.), *Handbook of depression in adolescents* (pp. 111–136). New York: Routledge.

Pattison, C., & Lynd-Stevenson, R. M. (2001). The prevention of depressive symptoms in children: Immediate and long-term outcomes of a school-based program. *Behavior Change, 18,* 92–102.

Peden, A. R., Rayens, M. K., Hall, L. A., & Beebe, L. H. (2001). Preventing depression in high-risk college women: A report of an 18-month follow-up. *Journal of American College Health, 49,* 299–306.(*)

Petersen, A. C., Leffert, N., Graham, B., Alwin, J., & Ding, S. (1997). Promoting mental health during the transition into adolescence. In J. Schulenberg, J. L. Muggs, & A. K. Hierrelmann (Eds.), *Health risks and developmental transitions during adolescence* (pp. 471–497). New York: Cambridge University Press.

Pickles, A., Rowe, R., Simonoff, E., Foley, D., Rutter, M., & Silberg, J. (2001). Child psychiatric symptoms and psychosocial impairment: Relationship and prognostic significance. *British Journal of Psychiatry, 179,* 230–235.

Pine, D. S., Cohen, E., Gurley, D., Brook, J., & Ma, Y. (1998). The risk for early-adulthood anxiety and depressive disorders in adolescents with anxiety and depressive disorders. *Archives of General Psychiatry, 55,* 56–64.

Pössel, P., Baldus, C., Horn, A. B., Groen, G., & Hautzinger, M. (2005). Influence of general self-efficacy on the effects of a school-based universal primary prevention program of depressive symptoms in adolescents: A randomized and controlled follow-up study. *Journal of Child Psychology and Psychiatry, 46,* 982–994.(*)

Pössel, P., Horn, A. B., Groen, G., & Hautzinger, M. (2004). School-based prevention of depressive symptoms in adolescents: A 6-month follow-up. *Journal of the American Academy of Child and Adolescent Psychiatry, 43,* 1003–1010. (*)

Pössel, P., Seemann, S., & Hautzinger, M. (2008). Impact of comorbidity in prevention of adolescent depressive symptoms. *Journal of Counseling Psychology, 55,* 106–117.(*)

Quayle, D., Dzuirawiec, S., Roberts, C., Kane, R., & Ebsworthy, G. (2001). The effect of an optimism and life skills program on depressive symptoms in preadolescence. *Behaviour Change, 18,* 194–203.(*)

Rao, U., Hammen, C., & Daley, S. E. (1999). Continuity of depression during the transition to adulthood: A 5-year longitudinal study of young women. *Journal of the American Academy of Child and Adolescent Psychiatry, 38,* 908–915.

Reivich, K. (1996). *The prevention of depressive symptoms in adolescents* (doctoral dissertation, University of Pennsylvania). (UMI No. 9627995)

Rice, F. J., Harold, G. T., & Thapar, A. (2002). Assessing the effects of age, sex and shared environment on the genetic aetiology of depression in childhood and adolescence. *Journal of Child Psychology and Psychiatry, 43,* 1039–1051.

Roberts, C., Kane, R., Bishop, B., Matthews, H., & Thomson, H. (2004). The prevention of depressive symptoms in rural school children: A follow-up study. *International Journal of Mental Health Promotions, 6,* 4–16.(*)

Roberts, C., Kane, R., Thomson, H., Bishop, B., & Hart, B. (2003). The prevention of depressive symptoms in rural school children: A randomized controlled trial. *Journal of Consulting and Clinical Psychology, 71,* 622–628.(*)

Roberts, S., & Kendler, K. (1999). Neuroticism and self-esteem as indices of the vulnerability to major depression in women. *Psychological Medicine, 29,* 1101–1109.

Rubio-Stipec, M., Fitzmaurice, G. M., Murphy, J. M., & Walker, A. (2003). The use of multiple informants in identifying the risk factors of depressive and disruptive disorders: Are they interchangeable? *Social Psychiatry and Psychiatric Epidemiology, 38,* 51–58.

Rudolph, K. D. (2002). Gender differences in emotional responses to interpersonal stress during adolescence. *Journal of Adolescent Health, 30,* 3–13.

Rudolph, K. D., & Conley, C. S. (2005). Socioemotional costs and benefits of social-evaluative concerns: Do girls care too much? *Journal of Personality, 73,* 115–137.

Rudolph, K. D., & Flynn, M. (2007). Childhood adversity and youth depression: The role of gender and pubertal status. *Development and Psychopathology, 19,* 497–521.

Rudolph, K. D., & Hammen, C. (1999). Age and gender determinants of stress exposure, generation, and reactions in youngsters: A transactional perspective. *Child Development, 70,* 660–677.

Sandler, I. N., Ayers, T. S., Wolchik, S. A., Tien, J., Kwok, O., Haine R. A., et al. (2003). The Family Bereavement Program: Efficacy evaluation of a theory-based prevention program for parentally bereaved children and adolescents. *Journal of Consulting and Clinical Psychology, 71,* 587–600.(*)

Sawyer, M., Pfeiffer, S., Spence, S., Bond, L., Graetz, B., Kay, D., et al. (2008). School-based prevention of depression: A randomized controlled study of the Beyond Blue School Research Initiative. *Journal of Consulting and Clinical Psychology, 76,* 595–606.

Schmiege, S. J., Khoo, S. T., Sandler, I. N., Ayers, T. S., & Wolchik, S. A. (2006). Symptoms of internalizing and externalizing problems: Modeling recovery curves following death of a parent. *American Journal of Preventive Medicine, 31*(Suppl. 5), 152–160.

Seligman, M. E. P., Schulman, P., DeRubeis, R. J., & Hollon, S. D. (1999). The prevention of depression and anxiety. *Prevention and Treatment, 2* (Electronic version, Retrieved October 19, 2007, from *journals.apa.org/prevention/volume2/pre0020008a.html*).

Seligman, M. E., Schulman, P., & Tryon, A. M. (2007). Group prevention of depression and anxiety symptoms. *Behavior Research and Therapy, 45,* 1111–1126.

Shatté, A. J. (1996). *Prevention of depressive symptoms in adolescents: Issues of dissemination and mechanisms of change* (doctoral dissertation, University of Pennsylvania). (UMI No. 9713001)

Sheeber, L., Davis, B., & Hops, H. (2002). Gender-specific vulnerability to depression in children of depressed mothers. In S. H. Goodman & I. H. Gotlib (Eds.), *Children of depressed parents: Mechanisms of risk and implications for treatment* (pp. 253-274). Washington, DC: American Psychological Association.

Sheffield, J. K., Spence, S. H., Rapee, R. M., Kowalenko, N., Wignall, A., Davis, A., et al. (2006). Evaluation of universal, indicated, and combined cognitive-behavioral approaches to the prevention of depression among adolescents. *Journal of Consulting and Clinical Psychology, 74,* 66–79.(*)

Shih, J. H., Eberhart, N. K., Hammen, C. L., & Brennan, P. A. (2006). Differential exposure and reactivity to interpersonal stress predict sex differences in adolescent depression. *Journal of Clinical Child and Adolescent Psychology, 35,* 103–115.

Shochet, I., Dadds, M., Holland, D., Whitefield, K., Harnett, P., & Osgarby, S. (2001). The efficacy of a universal school-based program to prevent adolescent depression. *Journal of Clinical Child Psychology, 30,* 303–315.(*)

Silberg, J. L., Pickles, A., Rutter, M., Hewitt, J., Simonoff, E., Maes, H., et al. (1999). The influence of genetic factors and life stress on depression among adolescent girls. *Archives of General Psychiatry, 56,* 225–232.

Smith, M. L., Glass, G. V., & Miller, T. I. (1980). *The benefits of psychotherapy.* Baltimore: Johns Hopkins University Press.

Spence, S. H., Sheffield, J. K., & Donovan, C. L. (2003). Preventing adolescent depression: An evaluation of the Problem Solving for Life Program. *Journal of Consulting and Clinical Psychology, 71,* 3–13.(*)

Spence, S. H., Sheffield, J. K., & Donovan, C. L. (2005). Long-term outcome of a school-based, universal approach to prevention of depression in adolescents. *Journal of Consulting and Clinical Psychology, 73,* 160–167.(*)

Steinhausen, H.-C., & Metzke, C. W. (2003). The validity of adolescent types of alcohol use. *Journal of Child Psychology and Psychiatry, 44,* 677–686.

Stice, E., Burton, E., Bearman, S. K., & Rohde, P. (2006). Randomized trial of a brief depression prevention program: An elusive search for a psychosocial placebo control condition. *Behavior Research and Therapy, 45,* 863–876.(*)

Stice, E., Rohde, P., Seeley, J., & Gau, J. (2008). Brief cognitive-behavioral depression prevention program for high-risk adolescents out-performs two alternative interventions: A randomized efficacy trial. *Journal of Consulting and Clinical Psychology, 76,* 595–606.(*)

Stice, E., Shaw, H., Bohon, C., Marti, C. N., & Rohde, P. (2009). A meta-analytic review of depression prevention programs for children and adolescents: Factors that predict magnitude of intervention effects. *Journal of Consulting and Clinical Psychology, 77,* 486-503.

Stolberg, R. A., Clark, D. C., & Bongar, B. (2002). Epidemiology, assessment, and management of suicide in depressed patients. In I. H. Gotlib & C. L. Hammen (Eds.), *Handbook of depression* (pp. 581–601). New York: Guilford Press.

Susman, E. J., Trickett, P. K., Iannotti, R. J., Hollenbeck, B. E., & Zahn-Waxler, C. (1985). Child-rearing patterns in depressed, abusive, and normal mothers. *American Journal of Orthopsychiatry, 59,* 410–419.

Sutton, J. M. (2007). Prevention of depression in youth: A qualitative review and future suggestions. *Clinical Psychology Review, 27,* 552–571.

Sutton, J. M. (2007). Prevention of depression in youth: A qualitative review and future suggestions. *Clinical Psychology Review, 27,* 552–571.

Twenge, J. M., & Nolen-Hoeksema, S. (2002). Age, gender, race, socioeconomic status, and birth cohort differences on the Children's Depression Inventory: A meta-analysis. *Journal of Abnormal Psychology, 111,* 578–588.

Weiss, B., & Weisz, J. R. (1990). The impact of methodological factors on child psychotherapy outcome research: A meta-analysis for researchers. *Journal of Abnormal Child Psychology, 18,* 639–670.

Weissman, M. M., & Olfson, M. (1995). Depression in women: Implication for health care research. *Science, 269,* 799–801.

Weissman, M. M., Pilowsky, D. J, Wickramaratne, P. J., Talati, A., Wisnieski, S. R., Fava, M., et al. (2006). Remission in Maternal Depression and Child Psychopathology. *Journal of the American Medical Association, 295,* 1389–1397.

Weisz, J. R., Weiss, B., Han, S. S., Granger, D., & Morton, T. (1995). Effects of psychotherapy with children and adolescents revisited: A meta-analysis of treatment outcome studies. *Psychological Bulletin, 117,* 450–468.

Wilson, D. B. (2005). *SPSS macros.* Retrieved March 3, 2007, from *mason.gmu. edu/~dwilsonb/ma.html.*

Wilson, S. J., Lipsey, M. W., & Derzon, J. H. (2003). The effects of school-based intervention programs on aggressive behavior: A meta-analysis. *Journal of Consulting and Clinical Psychology, 71,* 136–139.

Wolchik, S. A., Sandler, I. N., Milsap, R. E., Plummer, B. A., Greene, S. M., Anderson, E. R., et al. (2002). Six-year follow-up of preventive interventions for children of divorce: A randomized controlled trial. *Journal of the American Medical Association, 288,* 1874–1881.(*)

Young, J. F., Mufson, L., & Davies, M. (2006). Efficacy of interpersonal psychotherapy–adolescent skills training: An indicated preventive intervention for depression. *Journal of Child Psychology and Psychiatry 47,* 1254–1262.

Young, J. F., Mufson, L., & Gallop, R. (2010). Preventing depression: A randomized trial of Interpersonal Psychotherapy–Adolescent Skills Training. *Depression and Anxiety, 27,* 426-433.(*)

Yu, D. L., & Seligman, M. E. P. (2002). Preventing depressive symptoms in Chinese children. *Prevention and Treatment, 5,* Article 9. Retrieved from *journals. apa.org/prevention/volume5/pre0050009a.html*

Zahn-Waxler, C. (2000). The early development of empathy, guilt, and internalization of responsibility: Implications for gender differences in internalizing and externalizing problems. In R. Davidson (Ed.), *Wisconsin symposium on emotion: Vol. 1. Anxiety, depression, and emotion* (pp. 222–265). Oxford, UK: Oxford University Press.

Zeman, J., Shipman, K., & Suveg, C. (2002). Anger and sadness regulation: Predictions to internalizing and externalizing symptoms in children. *Journal of Clinical Child and Adolescent Psychology, 31,* 393–398.

Ziegert, D. I., & Kistner, J. A. (2002). Response styles theory: Downward extension to children. *Journal of Clinical Child and Adolescent Psychology, 31,* 325–334.

CHAPTER 10

Primary Prevention
of Secondary Depression

Indirect Prevention of Depression in Girls by Treating or Preventing Primary Obesity or Insomnia

Greg Clarke, Lynn DeBar, *and* Bobbi Jo Yarborough

Most interventions tested to date for preventing adolescent depression employ variants of psychotherapies originally employed as *treatments* for persons in active depression episodes. These include cognitive restructuring, behavioral activation, problem solving, and/or interpersonal approaches (Clarke, Hawkins, Murphy, & Sheeber, 1993; Clarke et al., 1995; Gillham, Reivich, Jaycox, & Seligman, 1995; Horowitz, Gerber, Ciesla, Young, & Mufson, 2007; Possel, Horn, Groen, & Hautzinger, 2004; Spence, Sheffield, & Donovan, 2003; Stice Burton, Bearman, & Rohde, 2007; Young, Mutson, & Davies, 2006). Reviews suggest that universal prevention programs targeting all youth regardless of risk status are generally not very successful (Spence & Shortt, 2007). However, targeted prevention programs aimed at youth with some elevated risk for depression and/or prodromal symptoms generally demonstrate good effects (Horowitz & Garber, 2006). The groups most often targeted include "indicated" youth demonstrating some prodromal signs of depression but not at a full diagnostic level (Clarke et al., 1995) or "selected" youth with risk factor(s) for future depression, most often the offspring of depressed parents (Clarke et al., 2001; Beardslee et al., 1997). These represent legitimate and productive approaches to depression prevention, but they may not be the only strategies worth pursuing.

It may also be possible to prevent depression by preventing or treating *other* disorders or conditions with onsets that may precede (are "primary"

235

to) subsequent depression, and which may play a causal or contributory role in the development of depression. This approach, often called "primary prevention of secondary disorders" (De Graaf, Bijl, Ten, Beekman, & Vollerbergh, 2004; Johnson, Roth, & Breslau, 2006a; Kendall & Kessler, 2002; Kessler & Price, 1993), has many positive benefits to recommend it. First, if successful, this approach avoids the onset of prodromal depressive symptoms (Clarke et al., 1995), which must occur first as a mark of risk in indicated prevention (Clarke et al., 1995, 2001). This is important because these subdiagnostic depressive states are themselves associated with significant morbidity and impairment and are to be avoided if possible (Judd, Paulus, Wells, & Rapaport, 1996; Sadek & Bona, 2000). This strategy is also an efficient approach to health promotion; the effort and cost required to prevent or treat the primary condition helps avoid the costs of treating the subsequent depression, potentially yielding an economic and health care "two for one" advantage. This approach also allows advocates of depression prevention to make common cause with advocacy groups promoting intervention for the primary conditions. The stronger, combined voice coming from this collaboration may be more likely to garner a greater share of social attention and health care funding to achieve an intervention that will benefit both conditions. Further, some of the primary conditions may have more societal appeal and less (or at least different) stigma associated with them, and thus may elicit more health resources than depression has to date.

Adequate epidemiological data are a necessary prerequisite for this approach, permitting the identification of candidate primary conditions. Fortunately, there are now several large, prospective epidemiological panel studies with initial assessments in childhood or early adolescence which permit us to examine the precursors to depression in adolescence, or early adulthood (Bittner et al., 2004; Breslau, Roth, Rosenthal, & Andreski, 1996; Chavira, Stein, Bailey, & Stein, 2004; Costello, Mustillo, Erkanli, Keeler, & Angold, 2003; De Graaf et al., 2004; Hasin & Grant, 2002; Johnson et al., 2006a; Kessler & Walters, 1998; Merikangas et al., 1996; Patton, Coffey, & Sawyer, 2003; Pine, Cohen, Gurley, Brook, & Ma, 1998; Rohde, Lewinsohn, & Seeley, 1991; Rohde, Lewinsohn, Kahler, Seeley, & Brown, 2001; Stein et al., 2001; Wittchen, Kessler, Pfister, & Lieb, 2000; Anderson, Cohen, Naumova, Jacques, & Must, 2007; Kimm et al., 2002). This literature identifies several possible contributing primary conditions, including social phobia, generalized anxiety disorder, obesity and subdiagnostic eating disorders, physical inactivity, substance abuse or dependence disorders, and insomnia and other sleep disturbances. We focus here on evidence suggesting that depression occurs *after* (secondary to) these other comorbid mental and physical health problems. This is a generally necessary pattern for this preventive approach to be feasible.

In the remainder of this chapter we describe two candidate primary conditions or disorders, selected to represent physical health and lifestyle risk factors; insomnia and other sleep disorders, and obesity and subdiagnostic eating disorders (weight/eating issues). We selected these exemplar conditions on the basis of their high and/or increasing prevalence during adolescence, particularly among adolescent girls. Although the case to be made for anxiety disorder or substance abuse is also particularly strong (Bittner et al., 2004; Costello et al., 2003; Lewinsohn, Gotlib, & Seeley, 1995; Wittchen et al., 2000), we selected insomnia and obesity in order to illustrate that primary conditions need not be limited to psychiatric or addiction comorbidities. Further, these primary conditions are important because, over the last decade, increasing social attention, policy discussions, and resources have been devoted to obesity, and to a lesser extent, insomnia (Metlaine, Leger, & Choudat, 2005; Leger, 2000; National Institutes of Health, 2005). Yoking depression prevention to the substantial societal resources being marshaled to address these somatic conditions may prove to be a significantly more fruitful strategy than remaining wholly within the mental health or addictions fields.

We review the literature supporting the possible contributing role of these conditions in depression onset. We also examine the time lines for the relative onset of these primary conditions to best identify windows of opportunity where prevention and/or treatment efforts may be most effective. Finally, we identify interventions that might successfully prevent or treat these initial conditions, with a particular focus on interventions that have established efficacy with, or which may be particularly suited for, adolescent females.

INSOMNIA AND OTHER SLEEP DISORDERS

Epidemiology

Researchers and policymakers have increasingly identified an epidemic of sleep deprivation in youth (Gibson et al., 2006; Hansen, Janssen, Schiff, Zee, & Dubocovich, 2005; Millman, 2005). An estimated 25% of adolescents have some form of sleep disturbance (Mindell et al., 1999; Roberts, Roberts, & Chen, 2002). This is a persistent problem for many, with 12.4% of adolescents reporting insomnia symptoms nearly every day of the past month, with higher rates for girls and lower socioeconomic status (SES) youth (Roberts, Lee, Hemandez, & Solari, 2004). The lifetime adolescent prevalence of DSM-IV insomnia through age 18 has been reported as 10.7% (Johnson et al., 2006b). Community rates of adolescent DSM-IV insomnia have been reported as 4.7% with 1-month prevalence (Roberts, Roberts, & Xing, 2006) and approximately 4% point prevalence (Ohayon,

Roberts, Zulley, Smirne, & Priest, 2000). Not surprisingly, rates of insomnia are even higher in depressed adolescents (Liu et al., 2007), our ultimate target population.

Gender Differences

Gender differences in sleep problems have been studied more frequently in adults. Compared to men, women report better sleep quality, more hours of sleep, and shorter time to sleep onset, and there appear to be no gender differences in objective markers of sleep such as sleep duration, sleep efficiency, arousal index, and slow wave or rapid eye movements (REM) sleep (Voderholzer, Al Shajlawi, Weske, Feige, & Riemann, 2003). However, women report more sleep-related complaints than men, and epidemiology studies indicate higher insomnia diagnosis rates among females (Krishnan & Collop, 2006). This discrepancy has led some to speculate that elevated insomnia diagnosis rates among women are actually a reflection of higher rates of anxiety or depression in females (Voderholzer et al., 2003).

Similar to depression, the insomnia gender difference appears to emerge at puberty. In a large adolescent community epidemiology sample Johnson Roth, Schultz, and Breslau (2006b) found no prepubertal gender differences in insomnia rates, but increased prevalence in girls after menses onset. In contrast, boys' insomnia prevalence was not related to their stage of maturational development. This finding suggests that insomnia may be a more common target in girls, and thus an important depression prevention target in girls.

Morbidity

Studies suggest a strong link between sleep disturbance and behavioral problems in youth (Dahl & Lewin, 2002). Adolescent insomnia and other sleep disturbances clearly contribute to school absenteeism and dropout (Carskadon, Wolfson, Acebo, Tzischinsky, & Seifer, 1998). Academic performance also declines (Wolfson & Carskadon, 1998, 2003), along with cognitive performance and attention (Fallone, Acebo, Arnedt, Seifer, & Canskadon, 2001).

Persons with insomnia also report more medical problems, have more physician office visits, are hospitalized more often, use more medication, have higher absenteeism, and have more problems at work or school, including more accidents (Leger, Guilleminault, Bader-Levy, & Paillard, 2002). Persons with insomnia have twice the normal rate of motor vehicle accidents (Aldrich, 1989; Carskadon, 2002). All of these affected areas incur direct and indirect costs for the patients, the health care delivery systems, and for society. The loss of productivity due to adult insomnia was estimated at nearly $42 billion in 1988 (Stoller, 1994), and the costs of sleep-related work and motor vehicle accidents was estimated at \$46–\$52 billion in 1988 (Balter & Uhlenhuth, 1992; Leger, 1994). Neither of these cost estimates includes the *direct costs* of medical services for sleep disorders, nor the costs of treating other disorders (e.g., depression) caused in part or whole by sleep disorders. Overall, the *total* annual cost of insomnia has been estimated at \$92.5–\$107.5 billion (Stoller, 1994). There may be even greater, as-yet unestimated costs associated with poor academic performance and reduced school attendance resulting from youth sleep disorder, which may in turn reduce high school and college graduation rates and lead to lower lifetime income.

Comorbidity with Depression

Sleep disturbances are frequently comorbid with depression and anxiety (Wolfson & Carskadon, 1998; Goetz et al., 1987; Brunello, et al., 2000). In the past it has been assumed that insomnia was a symptom, or epiphenomenon, of major depressive disorder (MDD). However, evidence has steadily accrued to indicate a bidirectional relationship between insomnia and MDD. Insomnia is both a symptom of depression and an independent risk factor (Dahl & Ryan, 1996; Dahl & Harvey, 2007; Harvey, 2001, 2006; Riemann, Berger, & Voderholzer, 2001; Ford & Kamerow, 1989; Riemann & Voderholzer, 2003; Ohayon & Roth, 2003). More specifically, a robust finding is that insomnia is a significant risk factor for both a first episode of MDD and for recurrent depressive episodes. A recent review of nine studies estimated that adults with persistent insomnia have a 3.5-fold increased risk for depression relative to individuals without insomnia (Perlis et al., 2006). The studies conducted to date suggest that this finding is relevant across the lifespan: in older adults (Livingston, Blizard, & Mann, 1993; Mallon, Broman, & Hetta, 2000), adults in the middle years (Ohayon & Roth, 2003; Eaton, Badawi, & Melton, 1995; Dryman & Eaton, 1991; Weissman, Warner, Wickramaratne, Moreau, & Olfson, 1997), and young adults (Breslau et al., 1996; Chang, Ford, Mead, Cooper-Patrick, & Klag, 1997). Insomnia may also be an independent predictor of suicidal behavior in depressed patients (Agargun Kara, & Solmaz, 1997; Pigeon & Perlis, 2006). Pigeon and Perlis (2006) similarly conclude that there is strong evidence that insomnia is a predisposing risk factor for depression, and that there is limited but intriguing evidence that insomnia may also play a precipitating or prodromal role in depression onset. Speaking to the possible preventive benefits, Eaton and colleagues (1995) calculated that 47% of the incidence of depression at a 1-year follow-up could be prevented, had sleep problems at baseline been eliminated.

Similar results are reported in adolescents. A community-based sample of 1,014 youth ages 13–16 found that primary insomnia significantly predicted future depression (hazard rate = 3.8) but that primary depression did not predict subsequent insomnia (Johnson et al., 2006a); interestingly, the reverse pattern was true for the association between anxiety and insomnia. Insomnia symptomatology also predicted subsequent depression in another large adolescent community panel (Roberts et al., 2002); elevated insomnia at wave 1 predicted greater depression severity at wave 2, even when controlling for wave 2 insomnia. Insomnia has also been found to predict adolescent hospitalization for suicide attempt (Gasquet & Choquet, 1994). In our own sample of adolescents at risk for depression and enrolled in a prevention trial (Clarke et al., 2001), we have found that insomnia symptomatology at baseline significantly predicted the onset of major depression episodes at subsequent follow-up points.

This high degree of association would be expected if insomnia were simply a symptom of depression. However, a recent review examined the epidemiological, sleep-EEG architecture, neuronimaging, neuroendocrine, and neuroimmune research and found distinct differences between depression and insomnia, suggesting that these are distinct but highly associated disorders with bidirectional impacts (Pigeon & Perlis, 2006).

Possible Mechanisms of Risk

How does insomnia contribute to depression risk? What mediational pathways are most important? One possible mechanism lies in the research demonstrating that sleep deprivation undermines emotion regulation the following day (Pilcher & Huffcutt, 1996; Van Dongen, Maislin, Mullington, & Dinges, 2003). If chronic insomnia leads to sustained emotional dysregulation, the resulting excess reactivity, irritability, and moodiness could, in turn, contribute to social rejection and other interpersonal problems that might precipitate depression in vulnerable persons. Another possible underlying mechanism is hyperactivity of the hypothalamic–pituitary–adrenal (HPA) axis, which is thought to play a causal role in primary sleep disorders and which may directly or indirectly (via insomnia) contribute to secondary problems such as insulin resistance, hypertension, and also depression (Buckley & Schatzberg, 2005).

One of the more paradoxical research findings in this field has been the short-acting antidepressant effects of induced sleep deprivation (Giedke & Schwarzler, 2002). That is, modest, elective sleep deprivation may lead to improved next-day mood in depressed persons. This phenomena is short-lived; chronic sleep deprivation is more strongly associated with increased depression. Based in part on this finding, it has been hypothesized (Adrien, 2002) that sleep loss in patients with insomnia at risk for depression might represent a unconscious adaptive mechanism in which sleep loss is endogenously initiated (without conscious intent) as an attempt to compensate for prodromal, subclinical depression. In this model insomnia is not so much a contributing factor for depression as it is an early attempt to moderate or compensate for emergent depression. In some cases the self-induced insomnia may be sufficient to counteract the underlying depressive mood for short periods of time, via moderation of the serotoninergic deficit believed to fuel depression development. However, in other cases the underlying serotoninergic deficit may be too profound for adaptive sleep loss to ameliorate. In these cases clinical depression may emerge and give rise to the observed epidemiological relationship between insomnia and depression.

Period of Greatest Prevention Opportunity

Ideally, we would intervene to prevent depression when the primary condition—in this case, insomnia—is present or developing but depression has not yet emerged. Epidemiological studies may shed light on those ages when these circumstances are most likely. In a random community sample of 1,014 adolescents ages 13–16 (Johnson et al., 2006a) the median age of onset for a first episode of insomnia was 11 years old. In this same sample, cases of MDD had a median onset of 12.5 years old, or an average of 1.5 years later. These limited data suggest that the ideal time for an insomnia intervention to reduce the risk of future depression would be around 11 or 12 years old. However, more research is needed to clearly identify the age span with the greatest opportunity for insomnia intervention to prevent depression.

Evidence-Based Interventions

There are several broad categories of established treatments for insomnia and other disordered sleep conditions. The "biological" or agent/device-based approaches include prescription medications such as hypnotics and sedatives (Glaze, 2004; Owens, Rosen, & Mindell, 2003; Younus & Labellarte, 2002), supplementation with exogenous melatonin (Coppola et al., 2004; Jan, Freeman, & Fast, 1999; Okawa, Uchiyama, Ozaki, Shibui, & Ichikawa, 1998; Paavonen et al., 2003; Weiss, Wasdell, Bomben, Rea, & Freeman, 2006; Smits, Nagtegaal, van der Heijden, Coenen, & Kerkhof, 2001), and phototherapy or light therapy (Yamadera, Takahashi, & Okawa, 1996; Papatheodorou & Kutcher, 1995; Okawa et al., 1998; Garcia, Rosen, & Mahowald, 2001). We do not review these biological therapies in this chapter. None of the pharmacological sleep agents has received Food and Drug Administration (FDA) approval for use with children and adolescents (Dahl & Harvey, 2007), and there have been no controlled trials of prescription sleep agents in youth. Further, patients with insomnia indicate clear preferences for psychological insomnia treatments over pharmacological interventions (Morin, Gaulier, Barry, & Kowatch, 1992; Vincent & Lionberg, 2001). Finally, although both psychotherapies and medications are effective short-term insomnia treatments, following discontinuation of active treatment the benefits of behavioral therapy endure whereas medication benefits are lost (Morin, Colecchi, Stone, Sood, & Brink, 1999; Sivertsen et al., 2006).

The main psychotherapeutic or behavioral interventions for insomnia include stimulus control therapy, sleep restriction, cognitive therapy, and sleep hygiene psychoeducation. Each of these approaches employs different tactics and skills, described in turn below. However, they are often used in combination and are collectively referred to as cognitive-behavioral therapy for insomnia (CBT-I). There are several existing, evidence-based CBT-I protocols for adult insomnia (Harvey, 2005; Morin & Espie, 2003; Perlis, Smith, Jungquist, & Posner, 2005).

The evidence base for CBT-I with adults has been summarized in three meta-analyses (Morin, Culbert, & Schwartz, 1994; Murtagh & Greenwood, 1995; Smith et al., 2002) and two practice parameters papers commissioned by the American Academy of Sleep Medicine (Chesson et al., 1999; Morin et al., 2006), encompassing the relevant randomized clinical trials. The clear conclusion to emerge is that CBT-I produces reliable and durable changes in adult sleep. However, little is known about its effect with adolescent insomnia and other sleep disorders.

Stimulus Control Therapy

Stimulus control therapy is one of the most established of all the behavioral interventions for insomnia. The aim of this intervention is to regularize the sleep–wake cycle and strengthen the association between the bed and sleeping by limiting sleep–incompatible behaviors within the bedroom environment (e.g., watching TV, instant messaging), while developing a consistent sleep–wake schedule (Bootzin, 1972). In this intervention the therapist traditionally provides a detailed rationale and assists patients to (1) use the bed only for sleep (i.e., no TV watching or talking on cell phones); (2) go to bed only when sleepy; (3) get out of bed and go to another room when unable to fall asleep or return to sleep within approximately 15–20 minutes, and return to bed only when sleepy again; and (4) arise in the morning at the same time each weekday, and no later than plus 2 hours on weekends (Bootzin & Stevens, 2005). The goal is to gradually move toward a regular schedule 7 days a week. Achieving these steps requires providing a rationale (the therapist), setting goals for bedtime and waketime (the therapist), using a daily sleep diary to monitor progress toward goals, and reviewing the diary at weekly therapy sessions (therapist and patient). The goal is to lower the potential for youth to become engaged in rewarding and arousing activities at bedtime, while at the same time creating an inviting and reinforcing sleep environment.

Sleep Restriction

Sleep restriction aims to reduce the amount of nonsleeping time spent in bed. This approach is particularly effective with persons who spend a lot of time worrying or who are otherwise unable to achieve sleep but remain in bed. Patients are initially asked to keep a sleep diary for 1–2 weeks to determine their minimally necessary sleep duration. Patients are then asked to set a firm wakeup time (e.g., 6:30 A.M.) and to stay awake until a bedtime that will allow only their minimally necessary sleep duration but no more—even if they could sleep more. Youth needing a minimum of 5 hours sleep would therefore initially be asked to stay awake (with no naps) until 1:30 A.M. and awake right at 6:30 A.M. Bright light exposure is often paired with the enforced wakeup to help reset the circadian rhythm. Patients are instructed to gradually increase their allowable sleep period by starting their bedtime 15 minutes earlier each week, and always keeping to the same wake time. Patients are instructed to avoid naps, to keep to this schedule on all nights, and to avoid makeup sleeping on weekends. Sleep restriction is very often integrated with stimulus control in a blended CBT protocol.

Cognitive Therapy

Cognitive therapy, also known as cognitive restructuring, is an established treatment for insomnia as well as for depression (Hollon, Shelton, & Davies, 1993; Weersing & Brent, 2006). Difficulty getting to sleep is highly attributable to excessive worry, rumination, and negative cognitions. Cognitive therapy helps manage bedtime worry, rumination, and anxiety that are counterproductive to sleep onset (Espie, 2002). Cognitive therapy teaches several methods to help patients evaluate worry and rumination:

- Diary writing or scheduling a "worry period" to encourage the processing of worries several hours prior to bedtime
- Creating a "to do" list prior to getting into bed to reduce worry about future plans/events
- Training on how to disengage from presleep worry and redirect attention to pleasant (distracting) imagery
- Demonstrating the adverse consequences of thought suppression while in bed
- Scheduling a presleep "wind down" period prior to bedtime to promote disengagement from daytime concerns.

Dysfunctional beliefs about sleep are important maintainers of insomnia (Edinger. Wohlgemuth, Radtke, Marsh, & Quillian, 2001; Morin et al., 2002). Typical unhelpful beliefs about sleep include "There is no point going to bed earlier because I won't be able to fall asleep," "Sleep is a waste of time," and "Getting more sleep doesn't help me." Cognitive therapy for dysfunctional sleep beliefs involves a four-step process: (1) identification of dysfunctional thoughts; (2) use of guided discovery and Socratic questioning to challenge the beliefs; (3) individualized experiments to test the validity and utility of dysfunctional beliefs and to collect data on new beliefs; and (4) the identification and dropping of safety behaviors that prevent disconfirmation of dysfunctional beliefs. The foundation of this module is manualized (Harvey, 2005; Morin & Espie, 2003; Ree & Harvey, 2004).

Sleep Hygiene Psychoeducation

Sleep hygiene is an inclusive term that refers to a list of sleep-promoting behaviors (e.g., limiting presleep caffeine intake), improvements in the sleep environment (e.g., removal of stimulating activities from the bedroom), education about sleep impacts, and a rationale for therapy changes. Overall, this approach aims to correct unhelpful sleep habits (e.g., surfing the Internet until late), and to develop new healthy sleep habits (e.g., on waking up, be active; if possible, during the day have bright light exposure, such as walking outdoors) (Stepanski & Wyatt, 2003).

Clinical Trials Research

To date there have been no trials attempting to prevent depression in either adolescents or adults by treating or preventing insomnia or sleep disorder. However, there have been two randomized trials with adults that offer some indirect support for this idea, examining the treatment of insomnia simultaneous with treatment of comorbid depression (Fava et al., 2006; Manber et al., 2008). A similar pilot has also been conducted with substance-abusing adolescents (Bootzin & Stevens, 2005). We review each below.

The randomized trial of adult depression (Fava et al., 2006) compared the selective serotonin reuptake inhibitor (SSRI) antidepressant fluoxetine plus placebo versus fluoxetine plus the sleep agent eszopiclone (Lunesta(r)) in adults meeting DSM-IV criteria for both current major depression and insomnia. The joint insomnia–depression treatment condition was associated with significantly more depression response (59 vs. 48%) and remission (42 vs. 32%) relative to the depression-only treatment arm. Similar advantages were observed in clinician-rated depression (Hamilton Depression Rating Scale [HAM-D]), improvement at work, and all major sleep outcomes (sleep latency, wake time after sleep onset [WASO], increased total sleep time [TST], sleep quality, and depth of sleep). Although this study examined *pharmacological* treatments for both depression and insomnia, its general concept and results suggest that other insomnia treatment modalities (e.g., CBT-I) may also achieve similar benefits.

Another recent adult trial (Manber et al., 2008) took a somewhat different approach to treating insomnia in the context of depression. Participants (n = 30) with both major depression and insomnia were all given antidepressant medication (escitalopram). In addition, they were randomized to receive either an attention-control, sham insomnia treatment or CBT-I. Escitalopram + CBT-I resulted in a higher rate of remission of depression and insomnia (62 and 50% remission, respectively) than escitalopram plus the control insomnia treatment (33 and 8%, respectively). Most sleep diary and actigraphy variables showed a similar advantage for the CBT-I plus antidepressant condition. Although the small sample of this pilot study suggests caution (a larger randomized controlled trial [RCT] is underway), the results are very promising and suggest similar approaches may be possible with youth who are actively depressed or are at-risk.

Outcome literature on psychosocial treatment of youth insomnia is nearly nonexistent. Bootzin and Stevens (2005) conducted the first uncontrolled trial of a CBT-I treatment in a sample of sleep-disordered, substance-abusing adolescents, with a focus on improving substance abuse outcomes through improved sleep. This trial enrolled 55 adolescents (ages 13–19) who were just completing substance abuse treatment programs and who had sleep or daytime sleepiness problems. The CBT-I protocol was specifically adapted for adolescents and focused on stimulus control, cognitive therapy, mindfulness-based stress reduction, and sleep hygiene education. Treatment completers showed significant improvements on a wide range of sleep outcomes, including improved sleep efficiency, sleep-onset latency, number of awakenings, total sleep time (by both actigraphy and diary), and sleep quality ratings. Noncompleters generally failed to improve or got worse. Although substance use increased for both completers and noncompleters during the active insomnia treatment, self-reported drug problems at follow-up evaluations declined for the completers but continued to increase for the noncompleters. In a separate report on this same sample, improved sleep was associated with decreased aggression (Haynes et al., 2006). This initial trial was limited by the lack of a randomized control condition, and had a focus on substance abuse and aggression treatment rather than depression. However, the generally positive results are encouraging for this proposed paradigm of preventing depression.

This near dearth of treatment development and evaluation for youth insomnia and related sleep disorder is especially surprising given the consistent recent literature on youth insomnia prevalence and associated morbidity. This is clearly an area of research development needed before depression prevention research can proceed through this mechanism.

OBESITY, DISORDERED EATING PATTERNS, AND PHYSICAL INACTIVITY

Because of its rapidly increasingly prevalence and target as a high-priority public health issue, treating youth obesity and closely associated behaviors (e.g., disordered eating patterns, physical inactivity) may provide an opportunity to prevent consequent conditions such as depression.

Epidemiology

Overweight/obesity among youth has been declared a "public health crisis" in the United States and other Western countries due to its alarming increase in prevalence (Flegal, 1999; Kohn & Booth, 2003; Lobstein, Baur, & Uauy, 2004; Sokol, 2000). In the past two decades, the percentage of overweight adolescents has more than tripled from 5 to 17% (Ogden et al., 2010). Further, in a cross-sectional, nationally representative school-based study, American adolescents had the highest prevalence of overweight of 15 Western countries (Lissau et al., 2004).

Until recently, overweight for children and adolescents was defined by the age- and sex-specific 95th percentile of body mass index (BMI) using the 2000 Centers for Disease Control and Prevention (CDC) BMI-for-age growth charts (Kuczmarski et al., 2000; Berkowitz, & Stunkard, 2002) with those youth between the 85th and 95th percentiles of BMI described as "at risk for overweight." Recently, the American Medical Association, in collaboration with the Department of Health and Human Services Health Resources and Services Administration and the CDC, convened an expert committee that recommended that this classification be modified to better reflect the medical risks associated with excess weight. According to this new classification, those between the 85th and 95th percentile should now be classified as "overweight," and those over the 95th percentile as "obese" (Barlow, 2007), resulting in the classification of 34% of youth as overweight or obese, according to the most recent national statistics (including 38% of those between 6 and 11 years of age and 34% of those from 12 to 19 years of age) (Ogden et al., 2006).

Morbidity

Such trends are particularly troubling given the psychosocial and physical health risks associated with being overweight in childhood and adolescence (Must & Strauss, 1999). Overweight during youth confers longer-term health risks even for those who later achieve normative weight as adults (Must, Jacques, Dallal, Bajema, & Dietz, 1992). Further, both longer-term health risks and the probability of adult obesity is greater for overweight adolescents than for those developing weight problems earlier in childhood (Must et al., 1992; Whitaker, 1992). Although many of the adverse consequences of youth-related obesity do not become manifest until adulthood, obese youth may also suffer more immediate medical sequelae from their condition, including pediatric- or adolescent-onset cardiovascular disease, endocrine and pulmonary problems, orthopedic, gastroenterological, neurological difficulties, and abnormal growth acceleration/early sexual maturation (Slyper, 1998; Strauss, 1999). Further, longitudinal studies have repeatedly shown that obesity in youth is associated with long-term health problems, including a two- to three-fold increase in the rate of adult cardiovascular disease and hypertension (Mossberg, 1989) and early development of type 2 diabetes mellitus (Srinivasan, Bao, Wattigny, & Berenson, 1996). In addition, overweight is associated with a higher prevalence of intermediate metabolic problems such as insulin resistance, elevated blood lipids, increased blood pressure, and impaired glucose tolerance. More than a quarter of overweight adolescents (BMI ≥ 95th percentile) have been found to meet criteria for metabolic syndrome (i.e., at least three of the following: elevated blood pressure, low HDL-cholesterol, high triglyceride level, high fasting glucose, abdominal obesity) (Cook, Weitzman, Auinger, Nguyen, & Dietz, 2003). Further, although obesity is generally not considered the cause of polycystic ovary syndrome (PCOS) in young women per se, it is found at a higher rate among overweight young women. Moreover, excess weight can exacerbate the associated metabolic consequences of PCOS, including infertility, diabetes mellitus, and cardiovascular disease, thus suggesting differential obesity-related morbidity among young women (Orio et al., 2007).

Arguably the most significant immediate and near-term morbidities for overweight adolescents are psychosocial. Severely obese adolescents have been found to have health-related quality of life (QOL) problems that are similar to youth diagnosed with cancer (Schwimmer, Burwinkle, & Varni, 2003). In addition, compared to many other chronic physical conditions, overweight during adolescence has greater social and economic consequences, such as fewer years of education, lower family income, higher poverty rates, and lower marriage rates (Gortmaker et al., 1999; Dietz, 1997). One study estimated that hospital costs alone for obesity-related disorders in youth have more than tripled in the last two decades to more than $127 million in 1997–1999 (Wang & Dietz, 2002), and overall obesity costs have been estimated at $117 billion each year (U.S. Department of Health and Human Services, 2001). The higher level of medical morbidity among overweight adolescents compared to their normal-weight peers (Slyper, 1998; Strauss, 1999; Srinivasan et al., 1996; Cook et al., 2003) increases the likelihood of excess health care service use (Wang & Dietz, 2002). Further, 70–80% of overweight adolescents become obese adults

(Whitaker, Wright, Pepe, Seidel, & Dietz, 1997; Guo, Roche, Chumlea, Gardner, & Siervogel, 1994; Serdula et al., 1993). Obese adults incur more health care costs than either smokers or drinkers—$395 a year per obese individual in excess health care costs (1998 $) (Sturm, 2002). Finally, productivity costs (i.e., cost of lost work days) attributable to obesity have been estimated to be as great or greater than excess health care costs (Wolf & Colditz, 1998; Wang, Yang, Lowry, & Wechsler, 2003; Avenell et al., 2004).

Gender Differences

Substantial increases in youth obesity rates have been seen for both males and females over the past 20 years with slightly higher prevalence rates among boys than girls (34.8 vs. 32.4% for male and female youth, respectively) (Ogden et al., 2006). However, there have been reports that the risk of becoming overweight during adolescence appears to be higher among girls than it is among boys (Daniels et al., 2005), perhaps in part due to the decrease in fat-free mass as a percentage of body weight in adolescent males in comparison to adolescent females, in whom both fat and fat-free masses increase during puberty (Mueller, 1982).

Comorbidity with Depression

A report using the National Health and Nutrition Examination Survey–III (NHANES-III) data suggests that the relationship between body weight and depression levels in adolescents depends on the degree of obesity. This report found depression to be uncommon among those at low or normative weights, whereas among the most obese subjects (in the 95th–100th percentile) the prevalence of major depression was substantial at 20% for boys and 30% for girls (Stunkard, Faith, & Allison, 2003). Youth seeking clinical treatment for obesity have been found to have particularly elevated levels of depressive symptoms (Britz et al., 2000; Epstein, Klein, & Wisniewski, 1994a; Sheslow, Hassink, Wallace, & De Lancey, 1993; Wallace, Sheslow, & Hassink, 1993; Doyle, Le Grange, Goldschmidt, & Wilfley, 2007; Erermis et al., 2004; Zeller, Saelens, Roehrig, Kirk, & Daniels, 2004; Zeller & Modi, 2006).

Importantly, research suggests that female adolescents' psychosocial functioning may be differentially affected by excess weight (Katz et al., 2000; Chu & Powers, 1995; Epstein et al., 1994a; Petersen & Leffert, 1995; Steinberg & Silverberg, 1986; Sheslow et al., 1993; Wallace et al., 1993; Young-Hyman et al., 2006). A recent study by Anderson and colleagues (2007) analyzed a prospective community-based cohort that was assessed multiple times from 9 years of age to early adulthood. They found that adolescent obesity in females (but not males) predicted an increased risk for subsequent MDD (adjusted hazard ratio [HR] = 3.9, 95% confidence interval [CI] = 1.3, 11.8). Similarly, a number of studies with adults have reported relationships between obesity and depression for females but not for males (Carpenter, Hasin, Allison, & Faith, 2000; Faith, Matz, & Jorge, 2002; Istvan, Zavela, & Weidner, 1992). Population-based studies have found high rates of psychological problems, including depression, in obese adolescent girls but not boys (Zametkin, Zoon, Klein, & Munson, 2004; Musante, Costanzo, & Friedman, 1998; Needham & Crosnoe, 2005), although some community-based studies have failed to support this association (Friedman et al., 1995; Mustillo et al., 2003; Stice & Bearman, 2001; Wardle, Williamson, Johnson, & Edwards, 2006).

Females may be at greater risk for weight-related psychosocial problems, including depression, because body image is an important component of their self-esteem (Manus & Killeen, 1995; Pesa, Syre, & Jones, 2000). Indeed, severity of obesity appears to be associated with more impaired self-esteem (Israel & Ivanova, 2002). A number of reports on the association of depression and obesity are cross-sectional, thereby making it difficult to discern the direction of the relationship. Some studies have even explicitly examined whether depression in adolescence appears to be associated with the later development and persistence of obesity (Goodman & Whitaker, 2002; Richardson et al., 2003; Stice, Presnell, Shaw, & Rohde, 2005b). Yet at least some of the research in adolescent and adult populations have investigated this direction of causality and reported findings suggesting that obesity is a risk factor for the subsequent development of depression (Anderson et al., 2007; Roberts, Kaplan, Shema, & Strawbridge, 2000; Roberts, Deleger, Strawbridge, & Kaplan, 2003).

Possible Mechanisms of Risk

What is most consistent among the research conducted to date is that adolescent girls reporting body dissatisfaction, restrictive dieting, and binge–purge behaviors are at higher risk for developing depressive symptoms (Doyle et al., 2007; Erermis et al., 2004; Friedman et al., 1995; Needham & Crosnoe, 2005; Stice, Martinez, Presnell, & Groesz, 2000a; Stice & Bearman, 2001). Although attitudinal factors may be more important than physical factors in the development of body dissatisfaction and disordered eating practices (Stice & Bearman, 2001), weight issues are frequently associated with body dissatisfaction and the adoption of disordered eating practices (Doyle et al., 2007; Erermis et al., 2004; Friedman et al., 1995; Musante et al., 1998; Tanofsky-Kraff et al., 2004). Thus, one possible mechanism for a causal link between youth obesity and subsequent depression may be through the development of body dissatisfaction and disordered eating practices.

Another potentially important mediator of the relationship between childhood obesity and the subsequent development of depressive symptoms is being teased about appearance and body weight. There has been substantial research documenting the increased rate of teasing and peer victimization of overweight youth (Adams & Bukowski, 2008; Hayden-Wade et al., 2005; Neumark-Sztainer, Story, & Faibisch, 1998). In a study of 50 overweight adolescent females, 96% reported stigmatizing experiences because of their weight (Neumark-Sztainer et al., 1998). Further, peer victimization and weight-related teasing from peers or family and resulting experiences of shame among overweight youth have been shown to be associated with low body satisfaction, low self-esteem, high depressive symptoms, and thinking about and attempting suicide (Eisenberg, Neumark-Sztainer, & Story, 2003; Sjoberg, Nilsson, & Leppert, 2005; Thompson, Coovert, Richards, Johnson, & Cattarin, 1995; Thompson, Heinberg, Altabe, & Tantleff-Dunn, 1999).

Prospective studies of adolescents have found that a history of teasing mediates the relationship between obesity status and subsequent levels of depression (Thompson et al., 1995). For example, obese adolescent females in a 4-year prospective study reported higher levels of peer victimization, which in turn led to a worsening in self-concept and further increases in their BMI over time (Adams & Bukowski, 2008). Such relationships were not seen in obese adolescent males or in nonobese adolescents included in the study (Adams & Bukowski, 2008). Research has suggested that obese school-age girls have fewer friends than their nonobese peers (Pierce & Wardle, 1997; Strauss & Pollack, 2003) and studies with clinically overweight children have found that many believe that they had personally caused their obesity, were extremely ashamed of their weight, and attributed their weight to the reason for having few friends and being excluded from social activities (Pierce & Wardle, 1997). Such teasing and social isolation have also been associated with the prospective development of unhealthy dieting practices (Haines, Neumark-Sztainer, Eisenberg, & Hannan, 2006a; Hayden-Wade et al., 2005), which, in turn, may be related to the development of depression, as reviewed above.

Finally, in addition to the possible factors that may mediate the effect of obesity on subsequent depression in youth discussed above, there may be preconditions that increase the risk for both the development of obesity and depression. For example, adverse childhood experiences and child neglect have been found to be associated with both adult obesity (Felitti et al., 1998; Lissau & Sorensen, 1994; Williamson, Thompson, Anda, Dietz, & Felitti, 2002) and the development of depression (Diaz, Simontov, & Rickert, 2002; Harris, 2001), and clinical researchers have suggested that adverse childhood experiences/neglect may play a common moderating role in the development of both conditions (Noll, Zeller, Trickett, & Putnam, 2007; Stunkard et al., 2003).

Period of Greatest Prevention Opportunity

The high rates of childhood obesity (38% in 2003–2004 for school-age girls and 32% among female adolescents, according to NHANES data; Ogden et al., 2006) suggest that prevention efforts aimed at prepubertal young women (i.e., before the onset of increased depression risk) should be feasible. Importantly, a great deal of national attention has been given in the last few years to the need for prevention and early treatment of childhood obesity with resultant efforts underway in schools, community-based agencies, and through health care providers (Eckel, Daniels, Jacobs, & Robertson, 2005; Koplan, Liverman, & Kraak, 2005; Krebs & Jacobson, 2003). These efforts and the concomitant resources marshaled to address the problem may provide previously unrealized opportunities for the prevention of depression that may be secondary to obesity. Research on critical periods for abnormal weight gain suggest that adolescence is among them—a period in which the risks of becoming overweight are higher for females than males (Daniels et al., 2005). Although much of the research on weight control in youth has focused on younger children and their families, adolescents may be an even more important target population for such efforts. Further, healthy eating and exercise patterns established among adolescents may be more likely to be sustained into adulthood than similar efforts aimed at younger children. In contrast to interventions with younger children, in which parents or schools are largely the agent of change, adolescents have established enough independence to maintain such lifestyle changes and thus warrant a focus on the individual factors involved in such an effort.

Evidence-Based Interventions

There has been a great deal of research on both the prevention and treatment of childhood obesity, although somewhat less about addressing these problems during adolescence. Several comprehensive reviews of the interventions involved in this process provide a more complete description of the prevention (Boon & Clydesdale, 2005; Doak, Visscher, Renders, & Seidell, 2006; Flodmark, Marcus, & Btitton, 2006; Sharma, 2006; Stice, Shaw, & Marti, 2006c) and treatment of youth obesity (Whitlock et al., 2010; Wilfley et al., 2007). The largely school-based obesity prevention programs have generally demonstrated modest impact on purported mediators of obesity development, such as improved dietary intake and increased rates of moderately vigorous physical activity and fitness (Caballero et al., 2003; Gortmaker et al., 1999; Luepker et al., 1996), yet they provide only limited evidence that short-term changes in these purported behavioral mediators lead to alterations in body composition/anthropometric measures or sustained changes in the targeted behaviors (Boon & Clydesdale, 2005;

Sharma, 2006; Thomas, 2006). More intensive, clinic-based behavioral programs that target the family for obesity treatment in school-age children have been shown to be efficacious and result in sustained improvements in weight management (Epstein, Valoski, Wing, & McCurley, 1994b; Epstein, Paluch, Roemmich, & Beecher, 2007; Savoye et al., 2007). The prototypical approach of these behaviorally based programs is based on Epstein and colleagues' family-based obesity treatment for school-age children (Wilfley et al., 2007; Goldfield & Epstein, 2002) and has been adapted for use with adolescents (Berkowitz, Wadden, Tershakovec, & Cronquist, 2003; Berkowitz et al., 2006). Treatment generally consists of a minimum of weekly sessions over a 6-month period and combines caloric restriction (1,200–1,500 calories per day) with increased physical activity (120–450 minutes per week) and concomitant reduction in sedentary behaviors/ screen time, use of self-monitoring (food and physical activity logs) to set and evaluate behavior change goals, stimulus control, problem solving, contingency management, cognitive restructuring, and social support. Finally, data supporting the use of pharmacological therapy and bariatric surgery for youth weight problems are limited and inconclusive and, due to concern about side effects, generally limited to extremely overweight youth with substantial comorbidities (Xanthakos, 2008; Velhote & Damiani, 2008; Jones, 2008; Widhalm et al., 2008; Nadler, Youn, Ren, & Fielding, 2008; Daniels et al., 2005; Inge et al., 2004; Yanovski, 2001).

Although obesity treatment strategies for youth, as described above, are important approaches to pursue, such intensive treatment efforts are expensive and time-intensive for those involved. Consequently, it may be equally important to focus on some of the purported mediators of the obesity–depression relationship reviewed in the previous section, because these intermediary factors may require less intensive interventions to address successfully. This "intermediary factors approach" includes interventions aimed at decreasing body dissatisfaction, emerging disordered eating patterns, and peer weight-based teasing.

Eating Disorders Prevention Programs/Reducing Body Dissatisfaction

A recent meta-analysis of eating disorders prevention programs suggests that a number of the empirically tested programs are efficacious and demonstrate the largest effects when targeted to those at risk (i.e., girls with body image concerns) and when interactive rather than psychoeducational in nature (Stice & Shaw, 2003). We describe two programs here that have received strong empirical support for decreasing disordered eating behaviors and cognitions as well as negative affect. The first is a four-session, 3-hour, dissonance-based program for decreasing disordered eating behaviors and cognitions as well as negative affect. Adolescent girls with body image concerns who have internalized the thin ideal (promulgated broadly by the media) engage in verbal, written, and behavioral exercises in which they critique this ideal (Stice, Mazotti, Weibel, & Agras, 2000b; Stice, Chase, Stormer, & Appel, 2001). Engagement in these counterattitudinal activities is theorized to result in psychological discomfort that motivates participants to reduce their thin-ideal internalization, which in turn should decrease eating disorder risk factors as well as disordered eating practices. The results from a number of RCTs have suggested that this low-intensity program consistently results in significantly greater reductions in thin-ideal internalization, body dissatisfaction, dietary restraint scores, bulimic symptoms, obesity onset, as well as negative affect than alternative prevention programs (Stice et al., 2000b; Stice & Bearman, 2001; Stice, Hayward, Cameron, Killen, & Taylor, 2000a). Importantly, these results have been replicated by different investigators, using lay as well as professionally trained facilitators, and with an even more abbreviated intervention (Becker, Smith, & Ciao, 2005; Green, Scott, Diyankova, & Glasser, 2005; Matusek, Wendt, & Wiseman, 2004; Roehrig, Thompson, Brannick, & van den Berg, 2006). These robust findings as well, as the effect of the program in reducing negative affect, suggest its promise for broader dissemination and potentially reducing the risks associated with the development of depression among adolescent girls.

The second promising intervention approach focuses on a healthy weight intervention that has been found to result in modest weight loss as well as significant improvements in dietary restraint scores, bulimic symptoms and negative affect (Stice et al., 2001; Stice, Trost, & Chase, 2003; Stice, Shaw, Burton, & Wade, 2006b). The intervention consists of six sessions focused on teaching healthy, effective weight control behaviors that allow participants to induce a negative energy balance and providing basic nutritional information that may help facilitate these changes. Importantly, although the effect of the dissonance-based program was greater on reducing thin-ideal internalization and body dissatisfaction, there were no differences in the magnitude of the reduction in dietary restraint scores, bulimic symptoms, or negative affect. Given its promise in promoting at least modest weight loss, this intervention is a promising low-intensity approach for addressing obesity and preventing depression. Interestingly, despite the concern among eating disorder prevention advocates that dieting may lead to an increase in disordered eating symptoms, well-designed empirically based weight management interventions appear to be consistent with the focus of eating disorders prevention efforts (Neumark-Sztainer, 2003, 2005), do not appear to contribute to body dissatisfaction in adolescent girls (Huang, Norman, Zabinski, Calfes, & Patrick, 2007), and may actually reduce disordered eating behaviors (Groesz & Stice, 2007; Stice, Presnell, Groesz, & Shaw, 2005a; Stice et al., 2006a).

Reducing Weight-Based Teasing, Creating Positive Peer and Family Environments

Although little research has been done on interventions designed to reduce weight-related teasing, a recent pilot study evaluated a school-based program targeting both peers and families and reported a significant decrease in teasing in the intervention school in comparison to reports of teasing in a school in which only the assessment was conducted (Haines, Neumark-Sztainer, Perry, Hannen, & Levine, 2006b). Further, research has found that familial weight commentary (i.e., weight-based teasing and parental encouragement to diet, particularly paternal encouragement to diet among female adolescents) is associated with depressive symptoms and unhealthy weight control behaviors, and that priority of family meals and positive mealtime environments are inversely related to these negative outcomes (Fulkerson, Strauss, Neumark-Sztainer, Story, & Boutelle, 2007; Mellin, Neumark-Sztainer, Story, Ireland, & Resnick, 2002). Also, there is some suggestion that parental encouragement of very modest changes in diet (e.g., eating breakfast) and physical activity (e.g., increasing steps) may result in substantive improvements in weight and other functional outcomes, which may encourage parents to help their children adopt more healthful lifestyle choices in a more productive and less harmful manner (Rampersaud, Pereira, Girard, Adams, & Metzl, 2005; Rodearmel et al., 2006). Collectively, this research suggests specific targets for possible family-based interventions that may protect against both the development of depressive symptoms and unhealthy weight control behaviors among adolescent girls.

Other Innovative Approaches: Exercise Therapy

Finally, increasing physical activity has long been recognized as an important foundation for effective weight management in both adults and youth, but recently researchers have also reported that such interventions appear to decrease depressive symptomatology as well among youth (Daley, Copeland, Wright, Roalfe, & Wales, 2006; Stella et al., 2005). Studies have shown that regular exercise can have positive effects on psychopathological outcomes (i.e., depression, anxiety, and low self-esteem) in adult and nonobese child populations (Motl, Birnbaum, Kubik, & Dishman, 2004; Steptoe & Butler, 1996). These recent studies suggest that these effects extend to those youth who are already experiencing weight-related difficulties. Thus, increasing opportunities for physical activities for normal and overweight children may help to prevent/improve weight problems as well as decrease the risk for the development of depression. This appears to be a promising approach warranting further investigation.

EFFECTS BEYOND DEPRESSION PREVENTION

Although the primary target reviewed in this chapter is the ultimate prevention of youth depression, successful treatment of youth insomnia and obesity/disordered eating behaviors will likely lead to improved outcomes in other domains as well.

In the case of insomnia successful treatment includes improved educational attainment, given the association of sleep deprivation with reduced school attendance; reduced dropout rates; and improved classroom behavior. Successful sleep disorder treatment for youth might also reduce rates of sleep deprivation-induced motor vehicle accidents (particularly nighttime accidents) and other accidental injuries (Spiegel, Tasali, Penev, & Van Couter, 2004b; Spiegel et al., 2004a; Tasali & Van Cauter, 2002). Finally, insomnia has a possible contributing role in obesity (Scheen & Van Cauter, 1998;, Spiegel, Leproult, & Van Cauter, 1999; Van Cauter, Polonsky, & Scheen, 1997), and metabolic syndrome or diabetes (Spiegel et al., 2002; Taylor et al., 2003). Successful treatment of youth insomnia could ultimately benefit these domains as well.

Preventing excess weight gain or successfully treating youth obesity has been associated with secondary improvements in blood pressure, serum lipids, and insulin resistance (Epstein, Myers, Raynor, & Savoye, 1998; Savoye et al., 2007) as well as improvements in psychosocial outcomes, including increased self-efficacy, and significant reductions in anxiety and depression, withdrawn behavior, attention problems, and somatic complaints (Wilfley et al., 2007; Epstein et al., 1998).

SUMMARY

We believe that adolescent depression, particularly in girls, may be prevented by treating or preventing primary disorders that may play a causal or contributory role in the development of depression. Given the widespread association of depression with so many other psychiatric, behavioral, and medical conditions, the list of candidate primary conditions is extensive. In this chapter we have tried to make the case for two of the less obvious conditions: insomnia and obesity/disordered eating. However, a similar persuasive argument could also be made for a growing list of conditions, such as anxiety, substance abuse, and attention-deficit/hyperactivity disorder (ADHD).

This approach to preventing depression may seem needlessly circuitous when compared to the direct depression-focused approaches studied to date (Clarke et al., 1993, 1995, 2001; Gillham et al., 1995; Horowitz et al., 2007; Possel et al., 2004; Spence et al., 2003; Stice, Burton, Bearman, &

Rohde, 2007; Young et al., 2006). However, we believe that the approach reviewed here has certain advantages. In particular, the societal resources allocated for prevention and health promotion have tended to focus on conditions other than depression and other internalizing disorders. Obesity, in particular, has been a major focus of policy and health promotion efforts in recent years. If we can link successful treatment of obesity/disordered eating (or substance abuse, insomnia, etc.) with the prevention of future depressive episodes, then we have strong reason to make common cause with advocates of these other conditions. Rather than fragmenting our efforts, burdening schools or social service agencies, and targeting youth and families with multiple, narrow-focus interventions for each individual condition, we can increase efficiency by "bundling" our depression prevention efforts with multitarget health promotion and prevention initiatives. This approach increases the chances of garnering funding, makes the approach more adoptable by implementers (thus maximizing dissemination), and may increase youth and parent willingness to participate by focusing broadly on health promotion rather than narrowly on specific (and in some cases, stigmatizing) conditions.

In some circumstances these comorbid disorders may develop after (i.e., be chronologically secondary) or simultaneously with depression, but may still be *clinically* primary with respect to the comorbid depression. In these cases the nonaffective comorbid disorders may be a more appropriate or feasible focus of treatment than depression. There are several situations where another disorder may be clinically primary. First, these other conditions may be more salient or clinically evident than depression, which often goes unrecognized. Youth, parents, and providers may be more likely to recognize and seek treatment for the very evident symptom of insomnia, for instance, than depression. Second, these other conditions or their interventions may be more acceptable and less stigmatizing to patients because of the focus on somatic concerns (as in the case of diet and exercise for obesity) rather the mental–emotional emphasis of depression treatments.

NEXT STEPS

As previously stated, sufficient epidemiological data are essential for identifying candidate primary conditions suitable for this type of approach. Historically, epidemiological studies have been largely cross-sectional. Prospective designs in epidemiological samples, focusing on adolescents with sufficient observation periods extending into adulthood, are needed to gain more information regarding patterns of incidence, relative onset time lines, temporal models, causal mechanisms, distal and proximal factors promoting development of secondary depression, and peak risk phases. There may be other, as yet unidentified underlying mechanisms that are more centrally "causal" for both depression and these other primary conditions. In other words, insomnia and/or obesity/disregulated eating may simply be proxies for the true causal pathway, and treating these primary conditions may yield only modest depression prevention effects because we are not directly addressing the true underlying cause(s).

Additionally, adolescent-specific insomnia and obesity/disordered eating interventions require additional basic efficacy development and testing before launching trials meant to prevent depression. A limited number of intervention trials on these primary conditions in youth has been conducted, as reviewed above. Including secondary measures of depression in these research projects would be an important next step in establishing the viability of the approach described here. Further, the concomitance of these disorders and the similarities in intervention approaches in addressing these conditions suggest that a greater emphasis/recognition by funding sources on the importance of evaluating broader health targets (e.g., mental and physical health simultaneously) is an important prerequisite for fruitful work in this domain.

Ultimately, should controlled trials demonstrate our ability to prevent depression by treating these other conditions, dissemination is a logical next step. It is not too early to consider this future, translational stage. Keeping dissemination in mind now will have implications for how cases are found, designing treatments for the primary conditions with maximum "adoptability," and how these efforts are explained to the hosting community or setting and to participants.

REFERENCES

Adams, R. E., & Bukowski, W. M. (2008). Peer victimization as a predictor of depression and body mass index in obese and non-obese adolescents. *Journal of Child Psychology and Psychiatry, 49*(8), 858–866.

Adrien, J. (2002). Neurobiological bases for the relation between sleep and depression. *Sleep Medicine Reviews, 6*, 341–351.

Agargun, M. Y., Kara, H., & Solmaz, M. (1997). Sleep disturbances and suicidal behavior in patients with major depression. *Journal of Clinical Psychiatry, 58*, 249–251.

Aldrich, M. S. (1989). Automobile accidents in patients with sleep disorders. *Sleep, 12*, 487–494.

Anderson, S. E., Cohen, P., Naumova, E. N., Jacques, P. F., & Must, A. (2007). Adolescent obesity and risk for subsequent major depressive disorder and anxiety disorder: Prospective evidence. *Psychosomatic Medicine, 69*, 740–747.

Avenell, A., Broom, J., Brown, T. J., Poobalan, A., Aucott, L., Stearns, S. C., et al. (2004). Systematic review of the long-term effects and economic consequences of treatments for obesity and implications for health improvement. *Health Technology, 8*(21), iii–182.

Balter, M. B., & Uhlenhuth, E. H. (1992). New epidemiologic findings about insomnia and its treatment. *Journal of Clinical Psychiatry, 53*(Suppl.), 34–39, discussion 40–42.

Barlow, S. E. (2007). Expert committee recommendations regarding the prevention, assessment, and treatment of child and adolescent overweight and obesity: Summary report. *Pediatrics, 120*(Suppl. 4), S164–S192.

Beardslee, W. R., Salt, P., Versage, E. M., Gladstone, T. R., Wright, E. J., & Rothberg, P. C. (1997). Sustained change in parents receiving preventive interventions for families with depression. *American Journal of Psychiatry, 154,* 510–515.

Becker, C. B., Smith, L., & Ciao, A. C. (2005). Reducing eating disorder risk factors in sorority members: A randomized trial. *Behavior Therapy, 36,* 245–254.

Becker, C. B., Smith, L., & Ciao, A. C. (2006). Peer-facilitated eating disorder prevention: A randomized effectiveness trial of cognitive dissonance and media advocacy. *Journal of Counseling Psychology, 53,* 550–555.

Berkowitz, R. I., Fujioka, K., Daniels, S. R., Hoppin, A. G., Owen, S., Perry, A. C., et al. (2006). Effects of sibutramine treatment in obese adolescents: A randomized trial. *Annals of Internal Medicine, 145,* 81–90.

Berkowitz, R. I., & Stunkard, A. J. (2002). Development of childhood obesity. In T.A.Wadden & A. J. Stunkard (Eds.), *Handbook of obesity treatment* New York: Guilford Press.

Berkowitz, R. I., Wadden, T. A., Tershakovec, A. M., & Cronquist, J. L. (2003). Behavior therapy and sibutramine for the treatment of adolescent obesity: A randomized controlled trial. *Journal of the American Medical Association, 289,* 1805–1812.

Bittner, A., Goodwin, R. D., Wittchen, H. U., Beesdo, K., Hofler, M., & Lieb, R. (2004). What characteristics of primary anxiety disorders predict subsequent major depressive disorder? *Journal of Clinical Psychiatry, 65,* 618–626.

Boon, C. S., & Clydesdale, F. M. (2005). A review of childhood and adolescent obesity interventions. *Critical Reviews in Food Science and Nutrition, 45,* 511–525.

Bootzin, R. R. (1972). Stimulus control treatment for insomnia. *Proceedings of the American Psychological Association, 7,* 395–396.

Bootzin, R. R., & Stevens, S. J. (2005). Adolescents, substance abuse, and the treatment of insomnia and daytime sleepiness. *Clinical Psychology Review, 25,* 629–644.

Breslau, N., Roth, T., Rosenthal, L., & Andreski, P. (1996). Sleep disturbance and psychiatric disorders: A longitudinal epidemiological study of young adults. *Biological Psychiatry, 39,* 411–418.

Britz, B., Siegfried, W., Ziegler, A., Lamertz, C., Herpertz-Dahlmann, B. M., Remschmidt, H., et al. (2000). Rates of psychiatric disorders in a clinical study group of adolescents with extreme obesity and in obese adolescents ascertained via a population based study. *International Journal of Obesity and Related Metabolic Disorders, 24,* 1707–1714.

Brunello, N., Armitage, R., Feinberg, I., Holsboer-Trachsler, E., Leger, D.,

Linkowski, P., et al. (2000). Depression and sleep disorders: Clinical relevance, economic burden and pharmacological treatment. *Neuropsychobiology, 42,* 107–119.

Buckley, T. M., & Schatzberg, A. F. (2005). On the interactions of the hypothalamic–pituitary–adrenal (HPA) axis and sleep: Normal HPA axis activity and circadian rhythm, exemplary sleep disorders. *Journal of Clinical Endocrinology and Metabolism, 90,* 3106–3114.

Caballero, B., Clay, T., Davis, S. M., Ethelbah, B., Rock, B. H., Lohman, T., et al. (2003). Pathways: A school-based, randomized controlled trial for the prevention of obesity in American Indian schoolchildren. *American Journal of Clinical Nutrition, 78,* 1030–1038.

Carpenter, K. M., Hasin, D. S., Allison, D. B., & Faith, M. S. (2000). Relationships between obesity and DSM-IV major depressive disorder, suicide ideation, and suicide attempts: Results from a general population study. *American Journal of Public Health, 90,* 251–257.

Carskadon, M. A. (2002). Risks of driving while sleepy in adolescents and young adults. In M.A.Carskadon (Ed.), *Adolescent sleep patterns: Biological, social, and psychological influences* (pp. 148–158). Cambridge, UK: Cambridge University Press.

Carskadon, M. A., Wolfson, A. R., Acebo, C., Tzischinsky, O., & Seifer, R. (1998). Adolescent sleep patterns, circadian timing, and sleepiness at a transition to early school days. *Sleep, 21,* 871–881.

Chang, P. P., Ford, D. E., Mead, L. A., Cooper-Patrick, L., & Klag, M. J. (1997). Insomnia in young men and subsequent depression. The Johns Hopkins Precursors Study. *American Journal of Epidemiology, 146,* 105–114.

Chavira, D. A., Stein, M. B., Bailey, K., & Stein, M. T. (2004). Comorbidity of generalized social anxiety disorder and depression in a pediatric primary care sample. *Journal of Affective Disorders, 80,* 163–171.

Chesson, A. L., Jr., Anderson, W. M., Littner, M., Davila, D., Hartse, K., Johnson, S. et al. (1999). Practice parameters for the nonpharmacologic treatment of chronic insomnia: An American Academy of Sleep Medicine report. *Sleep, 22,* 1128–1133.

Chu, L., & Powers, P. A. (1995). Synchrony in adolescence. *Adolescence, 30,* 453–461.

Clarke, G. N., Hawkins, W., Murphy, M., & Sheeber, L. B. (1993). School-based primary prevention of depressive symptomatology in adolescents: Findings from two studies. *Journal of Adolescent Research, 8,* 183–204.

Clarke, G. N., Hawkins, W., Murphy, M., Sheeber, L. B., Lewinsohn, P. M., & Seeley, J. R. (1995). Targeted prevention of unipolar depressive disorder in an at-risk sample of high school adolescents: A randomized trial of a group cognitive intervention. *Journal of the American Academy of Child and Adolescent Psychiatry, 34,* 312–321.

Clarke, G. N., Hornbrook, M., Lynch, F., Polen, M., Gale, J., Beardslee, W., et al. (2001). A randomized trial of a group cognitive intervention for preventing depression in adolescent offspring of depressed parents. *Archives of General Psychiatry, 58,* 1127–1134.

Cook, S., Weitzman, M., Auinger, P., Nguyen, M., & Dietz, W. H. (2003). Prevalence of a metabolic syndrome phenotype in adolescents: Findings from the third National Health and Nutrition Examination Survey, 1988–1994. *Archives of Pediatrics and Adolescent Medicine, 157,* 821–827.

Coppola, G., Iervolino, G., Mastrosimone, M., La, T. G., Ruiu, F., & Pascotto, A. (2004). Melatonin in wake–sleep disorders in children, adolescents and young adults with mental retardation with or without epilepsy: A double-blind, cross-over, placebo-controlled trial. *Brain and Development, 26,* 373–376.

Costello, E. J., Mustillo, S., Erkanli, A., Keeler, G., & Angold, A. (2003). Prevalence and development of psychiatric disorders in childhood and adolescence. *Archives of General Psychiatry, 60,* 837–844.

Dahl, R. E., & Harvey, A. G. (2007). Sleep disorders. In M. L. Rutter (Ed.), *Oxford textbook of child and adolescent psychiatry.* Oxford, UK: Oford University Press.

Dahl, R. E., & Lewin, D. S. (2002). Pathways to adolescent health sleep regulation and behavior. *Journal of Adolescent Health, 31,* 175–184.

Dahl, R. E., & Ryan, N. D. (1996). The psychobiology of adolescent depression. In D. Cicchetti & S. L. Toth (Eds.), *Adolescence: Opportunities and challenges—Rochester symposium on developmental psychopathology* (pp. 197–232). Rochester, NY: University of Rochester Press.

Daley, A. J., Copeland, R. J., Wright, N. P., Roalfe, A., & Wales, J. K. (2006). Exercise therapy as a treatment for psychopathologic conditions in obese and morbidly obese adolescents: A randomized, controlled trial. *Pediatrics, 118,* 2126–2134.

Daniels, S. R., Arnett, D. K., Eckel, R. H., Gidding, S. S., Hayman, L. L., Kumanyika, S., et al. (2005). Overweight in children and adolescents: Pathophysiology, consequences, prevention, and treatment. *Circulation, 111,* 1999–2012.

De Graaf, R., Bijl, R. V., Ten, H. M., Beekman, A. T., & Vollebergh, W. A. (2004). Pathways to comorbidity: The transition of pure mood, anxiety and substance use disorders into comorbid conditions in a longitudinal population-based study. *Journal of Affective Disorders, 82,* 461–467.

Diaz, A., Simantov, E., & Rickert, V. I. (2002). Effect of abuse on health: Results of a national survey. *Archives of Pediatric and Adolescent Medicine, 156,* 811–817.

Dietz, W. H. (1997). Periods of risk in childhood for the development of adult obesity?: What do we need to learn? *Journal of Nutrition, 127,* 1884S–1886S.

Doak, C. M., Visscher, T. L., Renders, C. M., & Seidell, J. C. (2006). The prevention of overweight and obesity in children and adolescents: A review of interventions and programmes. *Obesity Reviews, 7,* 111–136.

Doyle, A. C., Le Grange, D., Goldschmidt, A., & Wilfley, D. E. (2007). Psychosocial and physical impairment in overweight adolescents at high risk for eating disorders. *Obesity, 15,* 145–154.

Dryman, A., & Eaton, W. W. (1991). Affective symptoms associated with the onset of major depression in the community: Findings from the U.S. National Institute of Mental Health Epidemiologic Catchment Area Program. *Acta Psychiatrica Scandanavica, 84,* 1–5.

Eaton, W. W., Badawi, M., & Melton, B. (1995). Prodromes and precursors: Epidemiologic data for primary prevention of disorders with slow onset. *American Journal of Psychiatry, 152,* 967–972.

Eckel, R. H., Daniels, S. R., Jacobs, A. K., & Robertson, R. M. (2005). America's children: A critical time for prevention. *Circulation, 111,* 1866–1868.

Edinger, J. D., Wohlgemuth, W. K., Radtke, R. A., Marsh, G. R., & Quillian, R. E. (2001). Does cognitive-behavioral insomnia therapy alter dysfunctional beliefs about sleep? *Sleep, 24,* 591–599.

Eisenberg, M. E., Neumark-Sztainer, D., & Story, M. (2003). Associations of weight-based teasing and emotional well-being among adolescents. *Archives of Pediatric and Adolescent Medicine, 157,* 733–738.

Epstein, L. H., Paluch, R. A., Roemmich, J. N., & Beecher, M. D. (2007). Family-based obesity treatment, then and now: Twenty-five years of pediatric obesity treatment. *Health Psychology, 26,* 381–391.

Epstein, L. H., Klein, K. R., & Wisniewski, L. (1994a). Child and parent factors that influence psychological problems in obese children. *International Journal of Eat Disord, 15,* 151–158.

Epstein, L. H., Myers, M. D., Raynor, H. A., & Saelens, B. E. (1998). Treatment of pediatric obesity. *Pediatrics, 101,* 554–570.

Epstein, L. H., Paluch, R. A., Roemmich, J. N., & Beecher, M. D. (2007). Family-based obesity treatment, then and now: Twenty-five years of pediatric obesity treatment. *Health Psychology, 26,* 381–391.

Epstein, L. H., Valoski, A., Wing, R. R., & McCurley, J. (1994b). Ten-year outcomes of behavioral family-based treatment for childhood obesity. *Health Psychology, 13,* 373–383.

Erermis, S., Cetin, N., Tamar, M., Bukusoglu, N., Akdeniz, F., & Goksen, D. (2004). Is obesity a risk factor for psychopathology among adolescents? *Pediatric International, 46,* 296–301.

Espie, C. A. (2002). Insomnia: Conceptual issues in the development, persistence, and treatment of sleep disorder in adults. *Annual Review Psychology, 53,* 215–243.

Faith, M. S., Matz, P. E., & Jorge, M. A. (2002). Obesity–depression associations in the population. *Journal of Psychosomatic Research, 53,* 935–942.

Fallone, G., Acebo, C., Arnedt, J. T., Seifer, R., & Carskadon, M. A. (2001). Effects of acute sleep restriction on behavior, sustained attention, and response inhibition in children. *Perceptual and Motor Skills, 93,* 213–229.

Fava, M., McCall, W. V., Krystal, A., Wessel, T., Rubens, R., Caron, J., et al. (2006). Eszopiclone co-administered with fluoxetine in patients with insomnia coexisting with major depressive disorder. *Biological Psychiatry, 59,* 1052–1060.

Felitti, V. J., Anda, R. F., Nordenberg, D., Williamson, D. F., Spitz, A. M., Edwards, V., et al. (1998). Relationship of childhood abuse and household dysfunction to many of the leading causes of death in adults: The Adverse Childhood Experiences (ACE) Study. *American Journal of Preventive Medicine, 14,* 245–258.

Flegal, K. M. (1999). The obesity epidemic in children and adults: Current evidence and research issues. *Medicine and Science in Sports and Exercise, 31,* S509–S514.

Flodmark, C. E., Marcus, C., & Britton, M. (2006). Interventions to prevent obesity in children and adolescents: A systematic literature review. *International Journal of Obesity (London), 30,* 579–589.

Ford, D. E., & Kamerow, D. B. (1989). Epidemiologic study of sleep disturbances and psychiatric disorders: An opportunity for prevention? *Journal of the American Medical Association, 262,* 1479–1484.

Friedman, M. A., Wilfley, D. E., Pike, K. M., Striegel-Moore, R. H., & Rodin, J. (1995). The relationship between weight and psychological functioning among adolescent girls. *Obesity Research, 3,* 57–62.

Fulkerson, J. A., Strauss, J., Neumark-Sztainer, D., Story, M., & Boutelle, K. (2007). Correlates of psychosocial well-being among overweight adolescents: The role of the family. *Journal of Consulting and Clinical Psychology, 75,* 181–186.

Garcia, J., Rosen, G., & Mahowald, M. (2001). Circadian rhythms and circadian rhythm disorders in children and adolescents. *Seminars in Pediatric Neurology, 8,* 229–240.

Gasquet, I., & Choquet, M. (1994). Hospitalization in a pediatric ward of adolescent suicide attempters admitted to general hospitals. *Journal of Adolescent Health, 15,* 416–422.

Gibson, E. S., Powles, A. C., Thabane, L., O'Brien, S., Molnar, D. S., Trajanovic, N., et al. (2006). "Sleepiness" is serious in adolescence: Two surveys of 3,235 Canadian students. *BMC Public Health, 6,* 116.

Giedke, H., & Schwarzler, F. (2002). Therapeutic use of sleep deprivation in depression. *Sleep Medicine Reviews, 6,* 361–377.

Gillham, J. E., Reivich, K. J., Jaycox, L. H., & Seligman, M. E. P. (1995). Prevention of depressive symptoms in schoolchildren: Two-year follow-up. *Psychological Science, 6,* 343–351.

Glaze, D. G. (2004). Childhood insomnia: Why Chris can't sleep. *Pediatric Clinics of North America, 51,* 33–50.

Goetz, R. R., Puig-Antich, J., Ryan, N., Rabinovich, H., Ambrosini, P. J., Nelson, B., et al. (1987). Electroencephalographic sleep of adolescents with major depression and normal controls. *Archives of General Psychiatry, 44,* 61–68.

Goldfield, G. S., & Epstein, L. H. (2002). Management of obesity in children. In C. G. Fairburn & K. D. Brownell (Eds.), *Eating disorders and obesity: A comprehensive handbook* (2nd ed., pp. 573–577). New York: Guilford Press.

Goodman, E., & Whitaker, R. C. (2002). A prospective study of the role of depression in the development and persistence of adolescent obesity. *Pediatrics, 110,* 497–504.

Gortmaker, S. L., Cheung, L. W., Peterson, K. E., Chomitz, G., Cradle, J. H., Dart, H., et al. (1999). Impact of a school-based interdisciplinary intervention on diet and physical activity among urban primary school children: Eat well and keep moving. *Archives of Pediatric and Adolescent Medicine, 153,* 975–983.

Green, M., Scott, N., Diyankova, I., & Gasser, C. (2005). Eating disorder prevention: An experimental comparison of high level dissonance, low level dissonance, and no-treatment control. *Eating Disorders, 13,* 157–169.

Groesz, L. M., & Stice, E. (2007). An experimental test of the effects of dieting on bulimic symptoms: The impact of eating episode frequency. *Behavior Research Therapy, 45,* 49–62.

Guo, S. S., Roche, A. F., Chumlea, W. C., Gardner, J. D., & Siervogel, R. M. (1994). The predictive value of childhood body mass index values for overweight at age 35 y. *American Journal of Clinical Nutrition, 59,* 810–819.

Haines, J., Neumark-Sztainer, D., Eisenberg, M. E., & Hannan, P. J. (2006a). Weight teasing and disordered eating behaviors in adolescents: Longitudinal findings from Project EAT (Eating Among Teens). *Pediatrics, 117,* e209–e215.

Haines, J., Neumark-Sztainer, D., Perry, C. L., Hannan, P. J., & Levine, M. P. (2006b). V.I.K. (Very Important Kids): A school-based program designed to reduce teasing and unhealthy weight-control behaviors. *Health Education Research, 21,* 884–895.

Hansen, M., Janssen, I., Schiff, A., Zee, P. C., & Dubocovich, M. L. (2005). The impact of school daily schedule on adolescent sleep. *Pediatrics, 115,* 1555–1561.

Harris, T. (2001). Recent developments in understanding the psychosocial aspects of depression. *British Journal of Medical Bulletin, 57,* 17–32.

Harvey, A. G. (2001). Insomnia: Symptom or diagnosis? *Clinical Psychology Review, 21,* 1037–1059.

Harvey, A. G. (2005). A cognitive theory of and therapy for chronic insomnia. *Journal of Cognitive Psychotherapy, 19,* 41–60.

Harvey, A. G. (2006). What about patients who can't sleep?: Case formulation for insomnia. In N. Tarrier (Ed.), *Case formulation in cognitive behaviour therapy: The treatment of challenging and complex clinical cases* (pp. 293–309). New York: Brunner-Routledge.

Hasin, D. S., & Grant, B. F. (2002). Major depression in 6,050 former drinkers: Association with past alcohol dependence. *Archives of General Psychiatry, 59,* 794–800.

Hayden-Wade, H. A., Stein, R. I., Ghaderi, A., Saelens, B. E., Zabinski, M. F., & Wilfley, D. E. (2005). Prevalence, characteristics, and correlates of teasing experiences among overweight children vs. non-overweight peers. *Obesity Research, 13,* 1381–1392.

Haynes, P. L., Bootzin, R. R., Smith, L., Cousins, J., Cameron, M., & Stevens, S. (2006). Sleep and aggression in substance-abusing adolescents: Results from an integrative behavioral sleep-treatment pilot program. *Sleep, 29,* 512–520.

Hollon, S. D., Shelton, R. C., & Davis, D. D. (1993). Cognitive therapy for depression: Conceptual issues and clinical efficacy. *Journal of Consulting and Clinical Psychology, 61,* 270–275.

Horowitz, J. L., & Garber, J. (2006). The prevention of depressive symptoms in children and adolescents: A meta-analytic review. *Journal of Consulting and Clinical Psychology, 74,* 401–415.

Horowitz, J. L., Garber, J., Ciesla, J. A., Young, J. F., & Mufson, L. (2007). Prevention of depressive symptoms in adolescents: A randomized trial of cognitive-behavioral and interpersonal prevention programs. *Journal of Consulting and Clinical Psychology, 75,* 693–706.

Huang, J. S., Norman, G. J., Zabinski, M. F., Calfas, K., & Patrick, K. (2007). Body image and self-esteem among adolescents undergoing an intervention targeting dietary and physical activity behaviors. *Journal of Adolescent Health, 40,* 245–251.

Inge, T. H., Krebs, N. F., Garcia, V. F., Skelton, J. A., Guice, K. S., Strauss, R. S., et al. (2004). Bariatric surgery for severely overweight adolescents: Concerns and recommendations. *Pediatrics, 114,* 217–223.

Israel, A. C., & Ivanova, M. Y. (2002). Global and dimensional self-esteem in pre-adolescent and early adolescent children who are overweight: age and gender differences. *International Journal of Eating Disorders, 31,* 424–429.

Istvan, J., Zavela, K., & Weidner, G. (1992). Body weight and psychological distress in NHANES I. *International Journal of Obesity and Related Metabolic Disorders, 16,* 999–1003.

Jan, J. E., Freeman, R. D., & Fast, D. K. (1999). Melatonin treatment of sleep–wake cycle disorders in children and adolescents. *Developmental Medicine and Child Neurology, 41,* 491–500.

Johnson, E. O., Roth, T., & Breslau, N. (2006a). The association of insomnia with anxiety disorders and depression: Exploration of the direction of risk. *Journal of Psychiatric Research, 40,* 700–708.

Johnson, E. O., Roth, T., Schultz, L., & Breslau, N. (2006b). Epidemiology of DSM-IV insomnia in adolescence: Lifetime prevalence, chronicity, and an emergent gender difference. *Pediatrics, 117,* e247–e256.

Jones, N. (2008). Yes, there is a place for bariatric surgery (and paediatric surgeons) in childhood obesity. *Archives of Disease in Children, 93,* 354.

Judd, L. L., Paulus, M. P., Wells, K. B., & Rapaport, M. H. (1996). Socioeconomic burden of subsyndromal depressive symptoms and major depression in a sample of the general population. *American Journal of Psychiatry, 153*(11), 1411–1417.

Katz, A., Nambi, S. S., Mather, K., Baron, A. D., Follmann, D. A., Sullivan, G., et al. (2000). Quantitative insulin sensitivity check index: A simple, accurate method for assessing insulin sensitivity in humans. *Journal of Clinical Endocrinology and Metabolism, 85,* 2402–2410.

Kendall, P. C., & Kessler, R. C. (2002). The impact of childhood psychopathology interventions on subsequent substance abuse: Policy implications, comments, and recommendations. *Journal of Consulting and Clinical Psychology, 70,* 1303–1306.

Kessler, R. C., & Price, R. H. (1993). Primary prevention of secondary disorders: A proposal and agenda. *American Journal of Community Psychology, 21,* 607–633.

Kessler, R. C., & Walters, E. E. (1998). Epidemiology of DSM-III-R major depression and minor depression among adolescents and young adults in the National Comorbidity Survey. *Depression and Anxiety, 7,* 3–14.

Kimm, S. Y., Barton, B. A., Obarzanek, E., McMahon, R. P., Kronsberg, S. S., Waclawiw, M. A., et al. (2002). Obesity development during adolescence in a biracial cohort: The NHLBI Growth and Health Study. *Pediatrics, 110,* e54.

Kohn, M., & Booth, M. (2003). The worldwide epidemic of obesity in adolescents. *Adolescent Medicine, 14,* 1–19.

Koplan, J. P., Liverman, C. T., & Kraak, V. I. (2005). Preventing childhood obesity: Health in the balance—executive summary. *Journal of the American Dietetic Association, 105,* 131–138.

Krebs, N. F. & Jacobson, M. S. (2003). Prevention of pediatric overweight and obesity. *Pediatrics, 112,* 424–430.

Krishnan, V., & Collop, N. A. (2006). Gender differences in sleep disorders. *Current Opinion in Pulmonary Medicine, 12,* 383–389.

Kuczmarski, R. J., Ogden, C. L., Grummer-Strawn, L. M., Flegal, K. M., Guo, S. S., Wei, R., et al. (2000). CDC growth charts: United States. *Advance Data Report,* No. 314. Vital and Health Statistics of the CDC, 2000.

Leger, D. (1994). The cost of sleep-related accidents: A report for the National Commission on Sleep Disorders Research. *Sleep, 17,* 84–93.

Leger, D. (2000). Public health and insomnia: Economic impact. *Sleep, 23*(Suppl. 3), S69–S76.

Leger, D., Guilleminault, C., Bader, G., Levy, E., & Paillard, M. (2002). Medical and socio-professional impact of insomnia. *Sleep, 25,* 625–629.

Lewinsohn, P. M., Gotlib, I. H., & Seeley, J. R. (1995). Adolescent psychopathology: IV. Specificity of psychosocial risk factors for depression and substance abuse in older adolescents. *Journal of the American Academy of Child and Adolescent Psychiatry, 34,* 1221–1229.

Lissau, I., Overpeck, M. D., Ruan, W. J., Due, P., Holstein, B. E., & Hediger, M. L. (2004). Body mass index and overweight in adolescents in 13 European countries, Israel, and the United States. *Archives of Pediatr Adolesc Med, 158,* 27–33.

Lissau, I., & Sorensen, T. I. (1994). Parental neglect during childhood and increased risk of obesity in young adulthood. *Lancet, 343,* 324–327.

Liu, X., Buysse, D., Gentzler, A. L., Kiss, E., Mayer, L., Kapornai, K., et al. (2007). Insomnia and hypersomnia associated with depressive phenomenology and comorbidity in childhood depression. *Sleep, 30,* 83–90.

Livingston, G., Blizard, B., & Mann, A. (1993). Does sleep disturbance predict depression in elderly people?: A study in inner London. *British Journal of General Practice, 43,* 445–448.

Lobstein, T., Baur, L., & Uauy, R. (2004). Obesity in children and young people: A crisis in public health. *Obesity Review, 5*(Suppl. 1), 4–104.

Luepker, R. V., Perry, C. L., McKinlay, S. M., Nader, P. R., Parcel, G. S., Stone, E. J., et al. (1996). Outcomes of a field trial to improve children's dietary patterns and physical activity: The Child and Adolescent Trial for Cardiovascular Health—CATCH collaborative group. *Journal of the American Medical Association, 275,* 768–776.

Mallon, L., Broman, J. E., & Hetta, J. (2000). Relationship between insomnia, depression, and mortality: A 12-year follow-up of older adults in the community. *International Psychogeriatrics, 12,* 295–306.

Manber, R., Edinger, J. D., Gress, J. L., San Pedro-Salcedo, M. G., Kuo, T. F., & Kalista, T. (2008). Cognitive behavioral therapy for insomnia enhances depression outcome in patients with comorbid major depressive disorder and insomnia. *Sleep, 31,* 489–495.

Manus, H. E., & Killeen, M. R. (1995). Maintenance of self-esteem by obese children. *Journal of Child and Adolescent Psychiatric Nursing, 8,* 17–27.

Matusek, J. A., Wendt, S. J., & Wiseman, C. V. (2004). Dissonance thin-ideal and didactic healthy behavior eating disorder prevention programs: Results from a controlled trial. *International Journal of Eating Disorders, 36,* 376–388.

Mellin, A. E., Neumark-Sztainer, D., Story, M., Ireland, M., & Resnick, M. D. (2002). Unhealthy behaviors and psychosocial difficulties among overweight adolescents: The potential impact of familial factors. *Journal of Adolescent Health, 31,* 145–153.

Merikangas, K. R., Angst, J., Eaton, W., Canino, G., Rubio-Stipec, M., Wacker, H., et al. (1996). Comorbidity and boundaries of affective disorders with anxiety disorders and substance misuse: Results of an international task force. *British Journal of Psychiatry Supplement, 30,* 58–67.

Metlaine, A., Leger, D., & Choudat, D. (2005). Socioeconomic impact of insomnia in working populations. *Industrial Health, 43,* 11–19.

Millman, R. P. (2005). Excessive sleepiness in adolescents and young adults: Causes, consequences, and treatment strategies. *Pediatrics, 115,* 1774–1786.

Mindell, J. A., Owens, J. A., & Carskadon, M. A. (1999). Developmental features of sleep. *Child and Adolescent Psychiatric Clinics of North America, 8,* 695–725.

Morin, C. M., Blais, F., & Savard, J. (2002). Are changes in beliefs and attitudes about sleep related to sleep improvements in the treatment of insomnia? *Behavior Research and Therapy, 40,* 741–752.

Morin, C. M., Bootzin, R. R., Buysse, D. J., Edinger, J. D., Espie, C. A., & Lichstein, K. L. (2006). Psychological and behavioral treatment of insomnia: Update of the recent evidence (1998–2004). *Sleep, 29,* 1398–1414.

Morin, C. M., Colecchi, C., Stone, J., Sood, R., & Brink, D. (1999). Behavioral and pharmacological therapies for late-life insomnia: A randomized controlled trial. *Journal of the American Medical Association, 281,* 991–999.

Morin, C. M., Culbert, J. P., & Schwartz, S. M. (1994). Nonpharmacological interventions for insomnia: A meta-analysis of treatment efficacy. *American Journal of Psychiatry, 151,* 1172–1180.

Morin, C. M., & Espie, C. A. (2003). *Insomnia: A clinical guide to assessment and treatment.* New York: Kluwer Academic/Plenum.

Morin, C. M., Gaulier, B., Barry, T., & Kowatch, R. A. (1992). Patients' acceptance of psychological and pharmacological therapies for insomnia. *Sleep, 15,* 302–305.

Mossberg, H. O. (1989). 40-year follow-up of overweight children. *Lancet, 2,* 491–493.

Motl, R. W., Birnbaum, A. S., Kubik, M. Y., & Dishman, R. K. (2004). Naturally occurring changes in physical activity are inversely related to depressive symptoms during early adolescence. *Psychosomatic Medicine, 66,* 336–342.

Mueller, W. H. (1982). The changes with age of the anatomical distribution of fat. *Social Science and Medicine, 16,* 191–196.

Murtagh, D. R., & Greenwood, K. M. (1995). Identifying effective psychological treatments for insomnia: A meta-analysis. *Journal of Consulting and Clinical Psychology, 63,* 79–89.

Musante, G. J., Costanzo, P. R., & Friedman, K. E. (1998). The comorbidity of depression and eating dysregulation processes in a diet-seeking obese population: A matter of gender specificity. *International Journal of Eating Disorders, 23,* 65–75.

Must, A., Jacques, P. F., Dallal, G. E., Bajema, C. J., & Dietz, W. H. (1992). Long-term morbidity and mortality of overweight adolescents: A follow-up of the Harvard Growth Study of 1922 to 1935. *New England Journal of Medicine, 327,* 1350–1355.

Must, A., & Strauss, R. S. (1999). Risks and consequences of childhood and adolescent obesity. *International Journal of Obesity and Related Metabolic Disorders, 23*(Suppl. 2), S2–S11.

Mustillo, S., Worthman, C., Erkanli, A., Keeler, G., Angold, A., & Costello, E. J. (2003). Obesity and psychiatric disorder: Developmental trajectories. *Pediatrics, 111,* 851–859.

Nadler, E. P., Youn, H. A., Ren, C. J., & Fielding, G. A. (2008). An update on 73 U.S. obese pediatric patients treated with laparoscopic adjustable gastric banding: Comorbidity resolution and compliance data. *Journal of Pediatric Surgery, 43,* 141–146.

National Institutes of Health. (2005). *NIH state-of-the-science conference on manifestations and management of chronic insomnia in adults.* Bethesda, MD: Author.

Needham, B. L., & Crosnoe, R. (2005). Overweight status and depressive symptoms during adolescence. *Journal of Adolescent Health, 36,* 48–55.

Neumark-Sztainer, D. (2003). Obesity and eating disorder prevention: An integrated approach? *Adolescent Medicine: State of the Art Reviews, 14,* 159–173.

Neumark-Sztainer, D. (2005). Can we simultaneously work toward the prevention of obesity and eating disorders in children and adolescents? *International Journal of Eating Disorders, 38,* 220–227.

Neumark-Sztainer, D., Story, M., & Faibisch, L. (1998). Perceived stigmatization among overweight African-American and Caucasian adolescent girls. *Journal of Adolescent Health, 23,* 264–270.

Noll, J. G., Zeller, M. H., Trickett, P. K., & Putnam, F. W. (2007). Obesity risk for female victims of childhood sexual abuse: A prospective study. *Pediatrics, 120,* e61–e67.

Ogden, C. L., Carroll, M. D., Curtin, L. R., Lamb, M. M., & Flegal, K. M. (2010). Prevalence of high body mass index in U.S. children and adolescents. *Journal of the American Medical Association, 303,* 242–249.

Ohayon, M. M., Roberts, R. E., Zulley, J., Smirne, S., & Priest, R. G. (2000). Prevalence and patterns of problematic sleep among older adolescents. *Journal of the American Academy of Child and Adolescent Psychiatry, 39,* 1549–1556.

Ohayon, M. M., & Roth, T. (2003). Place of chronic insomnia in the course of depressive and anxiety disorders. *Journal of Psychiatric Research, 37,* 9–15.

Okawa, M., Uchiyama, M., Ozaki, S., Shibui, K., & Ichikawa, H. (1998). Circadian rhythm sleep disorders in adolescents: Clinical trials of combined treatments based on chronobiology. *Psychiatry and Clinical Neurosciences, 52,* 483–490.

Orio, F. Jr., Palomba, S., Cascella, T., Savastano, S., Lombardi, G., & Colao, A.

(2007). Cardiovascular complications of obesity in adolescents. *Journal of Endocrinological Investigation, 30,* 70–80.

Owens, J. A., Rosen, C. L., & Mindell, J. A. (2003). Medication use in the treatment of pediatric insomnia: Results of a survey of community-based pediatricians. *Pediatrics, 111,* e628–e635.

Paavonen, E. J., Nieminen-von Wendt, T., Vanhala, R., Aronen, E. T., & von Wendt, L. (2003). Effectiveness of melatonin in the treatment of sleep disturbances in children with Asperger disorder. *Journal of Child and Adolescent Psychopharmacology, 13,* 83–95.

Papatheodorou, G., & Kutcher, S. (1995). The effect of adjunctive light therapy on ameliorating breakthrough depressive symptoms in adolescent-onset bipolar disorder. *Journal of Psychiatry and Neuroscience, 20,* 226–232.

Patton, G. C., Coffey, C., & Sawyer, S. M. (2003). The outcome of adolescent eating disorders: Findings from the Victorian Adolescent Health Cohort Study. *European Child and Adolescent Psychiatry, 12*(Suppl. 1), 125–129.

Perlis, M. L., Smith, M., Jungquist, C., & Posner, D. (2005). *The cognitive-behavioral treatment of insomnia: A session by session guide.* New York: Springer Verlag.

Perlis, M. L., Smith, L. J., Lyness, J. M., Matteson, S. R., Pigeon, W. R., Jungquist, C. R., et al. (2006). Insomnia as a risk factor for onset of depression in the elderly. *Behavioral Sleep Medicine, 4,* 104–113.

Pesa, J. A., Syre, T. R., & Jones, E. (2000). Psychosocial differences associated with body weight among female adolescents: The importance of body image. *Journal of Adolescent Health, 26,* 330–337.

Petersen, A. C., & Leffert, N. (1995). Developmental issues influencing guidelines for adolescent health research: A review. *Journal of Adolescent Health, 17,* 298–305.

Pierce, J. W., & Wardle, J. (1997). Cause and effect beliefs and self-esteem of overweight children. *Journal of Child Psychology and Psychiatry, 38,* 645–650.

Pigeon, W. R., & Perlis, M. L. (2007). Insomnia and depression: Birds of a feather? *International Journal of Sleep Disorders, 3,* 82–91.

Pilcher, J. J., & Huffcutt, A. I. (1996). Effects of sleep deprivation on performance: A meta-analysis. *Sleep, 19,* 318–326.

Pine, D. S., Cohen, P., Gurley, D., Brook, J., & Ma, Y. (1998). The risk for early-adulthood anxiety and depressive disorders in adolescents with anxiety and depressive disorders. *Archives of General Psychiatry, 55,* 56–64.

Possel, P., Horn, A. B., Groen, G., & Hautzinger, M. (2004). School-based prevention of depressive symptoms in adolescents: A 6-month follow-up. *Journal of the American Academy of Child and Adolescent Psychiatry, 43,* 1003–1010.

Rampersaud, G. C., Pereira, M. A., Girard, B. L., Adams, J., & Metzl, J. D. (2005). Breakfast habits, nutritional status, body weight, and academic performance in children and adolescents. *Journal of American Dietetic Association, 105,* 743–760.

Ree, M., & Harvey, A. G. (2004). Insomnia. In J. Bennett-Levy, G. Butler, A. Fennell, A. Hackman, & D. Mueller (Eds.), *Oxford guide to behavioural experiments in cognitive therapy* (pp. 287–305). Oxford, UK: Oxford University Press.

Richardson, L. P., Davis, R., Poulton, R., McCauley, E., Moffitt, T. E., Caspi, A., et al. (2003). A longitudinal evaluation of adolescent depression and adult obesity. *Archives of Pediatric and Adolescent Medicine, 157,* 739–745.

Riemann, D., Berger, M., & Voderholzer, U. (2001). Sleep and depression—results from psychobiological studies: An overview. *Biological Psychology, 57,* 67–103.

Riemann, D., & Voderholzer, U. (2003). Primary insomnia: A risk factor to develop depression? *Journal of Affective Disorders, 76,* 255–259.

Roberts, R. E., Deleger, S., Strawbridge, W. J., & Kaplan, G. A. (2003). Prospective association between obesity and depression: Evidence from the Alameda County Study. *International Journal of Obesity and Related Metabolic Disorders, 27,* 514–521.

Roberts, R. E., Kaplan, G. A., Shema, S. J., & Strawbridge, W. J. (2000). Are the obese at greater risk for depression? *American Journal of Epidemiology, 152,* 163–170.

Roberts, R. E., Lee, E. S., Hemandez, M., & Solari, A. C. (2004). Symptoms of insomnia among adolescents in the lower Rio Grande Valley of Texas. *Sleep, 27,* 751–760.

Roberts, R. E., Roberts, C. R., & Chen, I. G. (2002). Impact of insomnia on future functioning of adolescents. *Journal of Psychosomatic Research, 53,* 561–569.

Roberts, R. E., Roberts, C. R., & Xing, Y. (2006). Prevalence of youth-reported DSM-IV psychiatric disorders among African, European, and Mexican American adolescents. *Journal of the American Academy of Child and Adolescent Psychiatry, 45,* 1329–1337.

Rodearmel, S. J., Wyatt, H. R., Barry, M. J., Dong, F., Pan, D., Israel, R. G., et al. (2006). A family-based approach to preventing excessive weight gain. *Obesity, 14,* 1392–1401.

Roehrig, M., Thompson, J. K., Brannick, M., & van den Berg, P. (2006). Dissonance-based eating disorder prevention program: A preliminary dismantling investigation. *International Journal of Eating Disorders, 39,* 1–10.

Rohde, P., Lewinsohn, P. M., Kahler, C. W., Seeley, J. R., & Brown, R. A. (2001). Natural course of alcohol use disorders from adolescence to young adulthood. *Journal of the American Academy of Child and Adolescent Psychiatry, 40,* 83–90.

Rohde, P., Lewinsohn, P. M., & Seeley, J. R. (1991). Comorbidity of unipolar depression: II. Comorbidity with other mental disorders in adolescents and adults. *Journal of Abnormal Psychology, 100,* 214–222.

Sadek, N., & Bona, J. (2000). Subsyndromal symptomatic depression: A new concept. *Depression and Anxiety, 12,* 30–39.

Savoye, M., Shaw, M., Dziura, J., Tamborlane, W. V., Rose, P., Guandalini, C. et al. (2007). Effects of a weight management program on body composition and metabolic parameters in overweight children: A randomized controlled trial. *Journal of the American Medical Association, 297,* 2697–2704.

Scheen, A. J., & Van Cauter, E. (1998). The roles of time of day and sleep quality in modulating glucose regulation: Clinical implications. *Hormone Research, 49,* 191–201.

Schwimmer, J. B., Burwinkle, T. M., & Varni, J. W. (2003). Health-related quality of life of severely obese children and adolescents. *Journal of the American Medical Association, 289,* 1813–1819.

Serdula, M. K., Ivery, D., Coates, R. J., Freedman, D. S., Williamson, D. F., & Byers, T. (1993). Do obese children become obese adults?: A review of the literature. *Preventive Medicine, 22,* 167–177.

Sharma, M. (2006). School-based interventions for childhood and adolescent obesity. *Obesity Review, 7,* 261–269.

Sheslow, D., Hassink, S., Wallace, W., & DeLancey, E. (1993). The relationship between self-esteem and depression in obese children. *Annals of the New York Academy of Science, 699,* 289–291.

Sivertsen, B., Omvik, S., Pallesen, S., Bjorvatn, B., Havik, O. E., Kvale, G., et al. (2006). Cognitive behavioral therapy vs. zopiclone for treatment of chronic primary insomnia in older adults: A randomized controlled trial. *Journal of the American Medical Association, 295,* 2851–2858.

Sjoberg, R. L., Nilsson, K. W., & Leppert, J. (2005). Obesity, shame, and depression in school-aged children: A population-based study. *Pediatrics, 116,* e389–e392.

Slyper, A. H. (1998). Childhood obesity, adipose tissue distribution, and the pediatric practitioner. *Pediatrics, 102,* e4.

Smith, M. T., Perlis, M. L., Park, A., Smith, M. S., Pennington, J., Giles, D. E., et al. (2002). Comparative meta-analysis of pharmacotherapy and behavior therapy for persistent insomnia. *American Journal of Psychiatry, 159,* 5–11.

Smits, M. G., Nagtegaal, E. E., van der Heijden, J., Coenen, A. M., & Kerkhof, G. A. (2001). Melatonin for chronic sleep onset insomnia in children: A randomized placebo-controlled trial. *Journal of Child Neurology, 16,* 86–92.

Sokol, R. J. (2000). The chronic disease of childhood obesity: The sleeping giant has awakened. *Journal of Pediatrics, 136,* 711–713.

Spence, S. H., Sheffield, J. K., & Donovan, C. L. (2003). Preventing adolescent depression: An evaluation of the Problem Solving for Life program. *Journal of Consulting and Clinical Psychology, 71,* 3–13.

Spence, S. H., & Shortt, A. L. (2007). Research review: Can we justify the widespread dissemination of universal, school-based interventions for the prevention of depression among children and adolescents? *Journal of Child Psychology and Psychiatry, 48,* 526–542.

Spiegel, K., Leproult, R., L'hermite-Baleriaux, M., Copinschi, G., Penev, P. D., & Van Cauter, E. (2004a). Leptin levels are dependent on sleep duration: Relationships with sympathovagal balance, carbohydrate regulation, cortisol, and thyrotropin. *Journal of Clinical Endocrinology and Metabolism, 89,* 5762–5771.

Spiegel, K., Leproult, R., & Van Cauter, E. (1999). Impact of sleep debt on metabolic and endocrine function. *Lancet, 354,* 1435–1439.

Spiegel, K., Sheridan, J. F., & Van Cauter, E. (2002). Effect of sleep deprivation on response to immunization. *Journal of the American Medical Association, 288,* 1471–1472.

Spiegel, K., Tasali, E., Penev, P., & Van Cauter, E. (2004b). Brief communication: Sleep curtailment in healthy young men is associated with decreased leptin levels, elevated ghrelin levels, and increased hunger and appetite. *Annals of Internal Medicine, 141,* 846–850.

Srinivasan, S. R., Bao, W., Wattigney, W. A., & Berenson, G. S. (1996). Adolescent overweight is associated with adult overweight and related multiple cardiovascular risk factors: The Bogalusa Heart Study. *Metabolism, 45,* 235–240.

Stein, M. B., Fuetsch, M., Muller, N., Hofler, M., Lieb, R., & Wittchen, H. U. (2001). Social anxiety disorder and the risk of depression: A prospective community study of adolescents and young adults. *Archives of General Psychiatry, 58,* 251–256.

Steinberg, L., & Silverberg, S. B. (1986). The vicissitudes of autonomy in early adolescence. *Child Development, 57,* 841–851.

Stella, S. G., Vilar, A. P., Lacroix, C., Fisberg, M., Santos, R. F., Mello, M. T., et al. (2005). Effects of type of physical exercise and leisure activities on the depression scores of obese Brazilian adolescent girls. *Brazilian Journal of Medical and Biological Research, 38,* 1683–1689.

Stepanski, E. J., & Wyatt, J. K. (2003). Use of sleep hygiene in the treatment of insomnia. *Sleep Medical Reviews, 7,* 215–225.

Steptoe, A., & Butler, N. (1996). Sports participation and emotional wellbeing in adolescents. *Lancet, 347,* 1789–1792.

Stice, E., & Bearman, S. K. (2001). Body-image and eating disturbances prospectively predict increases in depressive symptoms in adolescent girls: A growth curve analysis. *Developmental Psychology, 37,* 597–607.

Stice, E., Burton, E., Bearman, S. K., & Rohde, P. (2007). Randomized trial of a brief depression prevention program: An elusive search for a psychosocial placebo control condition. *Behavior Research Therapy, 45,* 863–876.

Stice, E., Chase, A., Stormer, S., & Appel, A. (2001). A randomized trial of a dissonance-based eating disorder prevention program. *International Journal of Eating Disorders, 29,* 247–262.

Stice, E., Hayward, C., Cameron, R. P., Killen, J. D., & Taylor, C. B. (2000a). Body-image and eating disturbances predict onset of depression among female adolescents: A longitudinal study. *Journal of Abnormal Psychology, 109,* 438–444.

Stice, E., Martinez, E. E., Presnell, K., & Groesz, L. M. (2006a). Relation of successful dietary restriction to change in bulimic symptoms: A prospective study of adolescent girls. *Health Psychology, 25,* 274–281.

Stice, E., Mazotti, L., Weibel, D., & Agras, W. S. (2000b). Dissonance prevention program decreases thin-ideal internalization, body dissatisfaction, dieting, negative affect, and bulimic symptoms: A preliminary experiment. *International Journal of Eating Disorders, 27,* 206–217.

Stice, E., Presnell, K., Groesz, L., & Shaw, H. (2005a). Effects of a weight maintenance diet on bulimic symptoms in adolescent girls: An experimental test of the dietary restraint theory. *Health Psychology, 24,* 402–412.

Stice, E., Presnell, K., Shaw, H., & Rohde, P. (2005b). Psychological and behavioral risk factors for obesity onset in adolescent girls: A prospective study. *Journal of Consulting and Clinical Psychology, 73,* 195–202.

Stice, E., & Shaw, H. (2004). Eating disorder prevention programs: A meta-analytic review. *Psychological Bulletin, 130,* 206–227.

Stice, E., Shaw, H., Burton, E,, & Wade, E. (2006b). Dissonance and healthy weight eating disorder prevention programs: A randomized efficacy trial. *Journal of Consulting and Clinical Psychology, 74*, 263–275.

Stice, E., Shaw, H., & Marti, C. N. (2006c). A meta-analytic review of obesity prevention programs for children and adolescents: The skinny on interventions that work. *Psychological Bulletin, 132*, 667–691.

Stice, E., Trost, A., & Chase, A. (2003). Healthy weight control and dissonance-based eating disorder prevention programs: Results from a controlled trial. *International Journal of Eating Disorders, 33*, 10–21.

Stoller, M. K. (1994). Economic effects of insomnia. *Clinical Therapeutics, 16*, 873–897.

Strauss, R. S. (1999). Childhood obesity. *Currrent Problems in Pediatrics, 29*, 1–29.

Strauss, R. S., & Pollack, H. A. (2003). Social marginalization of overweight children. *Archives of Pediatric and Adolescent Medicine, 157*, 746–752.

Stunkard, A. J., Faith, M. S., & Allison, K. C. (2003). Depression and obesity. *Biological Psychiatry, 54*, 330–337.

Sturm, R. (2002). The effects of obesity, smoking, and drinking on medical problems and costs: Obesity outranks both smoking and drinking in its deleterious effects on health and health costs. *Health Affairs, 21*, 245–253.

Tanofsky-Kraff, M., Yanovski, S. Z., Wilfley, D. E., Marmarosh, C., Morgan, C. M., & Yanovski, J. A. (2004). Eating-disordered behaviors, body fat, and psychopathology in overweight and normal-weight children. *Journal of Consulting and Clinical Psychology, 72*, 53–61.

Tasali, E., & Van Cauter, E. (2002). Sleep-disordered breathing and the current epidemic of obesity: Consequence or contributing factor? *American Journal of Respiratory and Critical Care Medicine, 165*, 562–563.

Taylor, D. J., Lichstein, K. L., & Durrence, H. H. (2003). Insomnia as a health risk factor. *Behavioral Sleep Medicine, 1*, 227–247.

Thomas, H. (2006). Obesity prevention programs for children and youth: Why are their results so modest? *Health Education and Research, 21*, 783–795.

Thompson, J. K., Coovert, M. D., Richards, K. J., Johnson, S., & Cattarin, J. (1995). Development of body image, eating disturbance, and general psychological functioning in female adolescents: Covariance structure modeling and longitudinal investigations. *International Journal of Eating Disorders, 18*, 221–236.

Thompson, J. K., Heinberg, L. J., Altabe, M., & Tantleff-Dunn, S. (1999). *Exacting beauty: Theory, assessment, and treatment of body image disturbance.* Washington, DC: American Psychological Association.

Van Cauter, E., Polonsky, K. S., & Scheen, A. J. (1997). Roles of circadian rhythmicity and sleep in human glucose regulation. *Endocrine Reviews, 18*, 716–738.

Van Dongen, H. P., Maislin, G., Mullington, J. M., & Dinges, D. F. (2003). The cumulative cost of additional wakefulness: Dose–response effects on neurobehavioral functions and sleep physiology from chronic sleep restriction and total sleep deprivation. *Sleep, 26*, 117–126.

Velhote, M. C., & Damiani, D. (2008). Bariatric surgery in adolescents: Preliminary 1-year results with a novel technique (Santoro III). *Obesity Surgery, 6,* 1–6.

Vincent, N., & Lionberg, C. (2001). Treatment preference and patient satisfaction in chronic insomnia. *Sleep, 24,* 411–417.

Voderholzer, U., Al Shajlawi, A., Weske, G., Feige, B., & Riemann, D. (2003). Are there gender differences in objective and subjective sleep measures?: A study of insomniacs and healthy controls. *Depression and Anxiety, 17,* 162–172.

Wallace, W. J., Sheslow, D., & Hassink, S. (1993). Obesity in children: A risk for depression. *Annals of the New York Academy of Sciences, 699,* 301–303.

Wang, G., & Dietz, W. H. (2002). Economic burden of obesity in youths aged 6 to 17 years: 1979–1999. *Pediatrics, 109,* E81.

Wang, L. Y., Yang, Q., Lowry, R., & Wechsler, H. (2003). Economic analysis of a school-based obesity prevention program. *Obesity Research, 11,* 1313–1324.

Wardle, J., Williamson, S., Johnson, F., & Edwards, C. (2006). Depression in adolescent obesity: Cultural moderators of the association between obesity and depressive symptoms. *International Journal of Obesity (London), 30,* 634–643.

Weersing, V. R., & Brent, D. A. (2006). Cognitive behavioral therapy for depression in youth. *Child and Adolescent Psychiatric Clinics of North America, 15,* 939–957, ix.

Weiss, M. D., Wasdell, M. B., Bomben, M. M., Rea, K. J., & Freeman, R. D. (2006). Sleep hygiene and melatonin treatment for children and adolescents with ADHD and initial insomnia. *Journal of the American Academy of Child and Adolescent Psychiatry, 45,* 512–519.

Weissman, M. M., Warner, V., Wickramaratne, P., Moreau, D., & Olfson, M. (1997). Offspring of depressed parents: 10 years later. *Archives of General Psychiatry, 54,* 932–940.

Whitaker, A. H. (1992). An epidemiological study of anorectic and bulimic symptoms in adolescent girls: Implications for pediatricians. *Pediatric Annals, 21,* 752–759.

Whitaker, R. C., Wright, J. A., Pepe, M. S., Seidel, K. D., & Dietz, W. H. (1997). Predicting obesity in young adulthood from childhood and parental obesity. *New England Journal of Medicine, 337,* 869–873.

Whitlock, E. P., O'Connor, E. A., Williams, S. B., Bell, T. L., & Lutz, K. W. (2010). Effectiveness of weight management interventions in children: A targeted systematic review for the USPSTF. *Pediatrics, 125*(2), 396–418.

Widhalm, K., Dietrich, S., Prager, G., Silberhummer, G., Orth, D., & Kispal, Z. F. (2008). Bariatric surgery in morbidly obese adolescents: A 4-year follow-up of ten patients. *International Journal of Pediatric Obesity, 3*(Suppl 1), 78–82.

Wilfley, D. E., Stein, R. I., Saelens, B. E., Mockus, D. S., Matt, G. E., Hayden-Wade, H. A., et al. (2007). Efficacy of maintenance treatment approaches for childhood overweight: A randomized controlled trial. *Journal of the American Medical Association, 298,* 1661–1673.

Wilfley, D. E., Tibbs, T. L., Van Buren, D. J., Reach, K. P., Walker, M. S., & Epstein, L. H. (2007). Lifestyle interventions in the treatment of childhood overweight: A meta-analytic review of randomized controlled trials. *Health Psychology, 26*(5), 521–532.

Williamson, D. F., Thompson, T. J., Anda, R. F., Dietz, W. H., & Felitti, V. (2002). Body weight and obesity in adults and self-reported abuse in childhood. *International Journal of Obesity and Related Metabolic Disorders, 26,* 1075–1082.

Wittchen, H. U., Kessler, R. C., Pfister, H., & Lieb, M. (2000). Why do people with anxiety disorders become depressed?: A prospective-longitudinal community study. *Acta Psychiatrica Scandinavica, 102*(5406), 14–23.

Wolf, A. M., & Colditz, G. A. (1998). Current estimates of the economic cost of obesity in the United States. *Obesity Research, 6,* 97–106.

Wolfson, A. R., & Carskadon, M. A. (1998). Sleep schedules and daytime functioning in adolescents. *Child Development, 69,* 875–887.

Wolfson, A. R., & Carskadon, M. A. (2003). Understanding adolescents' sleep patterns and school performance: A critical appraisal. *Sleep Medicine Reviews, 7,* 491–506.

Xanthakos, S. A. (2008). Bariatric surgery for extreme adolescent obesity: Indications, outcomes, and physiologic effects on the gut–brain axis. *Pathophysiology, 15,* 135–146.

Yamadera, H., Takahashi, K., & Okawa, M. (1996). A multicenter study of sleep–wake rhythm disorders: Therapeutic effects of vitamin B_{12}, bright light therapy, chronotherapy, and hypnotics. *Psychiatry and Clinical Neuroscience, 50,* 203–209.

Yanovski, J. A. (2001). Intensive therapies for pediatric obesity. *Pediatric Clinics of North America, 48,* 1041–1053.

Young, J. F., Mufson, L., & Davies, M. (2006). Efficacy of interpersonal psychotherapy–adolescent skills training: An indicated preventive intervention for depression. *Journal of Child Psychology and Psychiatry, 47,* 1254–1262.

Young-Hyman, D., Tanofsky-Kraff, M., Yanovski, S. Z., Keil, M., Cohen, M. L., Peyrot, M., et al. (2006). Psychological status and weight-related distress in overweight or at-risk-for-overweight children. *Obesity, 14,* 2249–2258.

Younus, M., & Labellarte, M. J. (2002). Insomnia in children: When are hypnotics indicated? *Paediatric Drugs, 4,* 391–403.

Zametkin, A. J., Zoon, C. K., Klein, H. W., & Munson, S. (2004). Psychiatric aspects of child and adolescent obesity: A review of the past 10 years. *Journal of the American Academy of Child and Adolescent Psychiatry, 43,* 134–150.

Zeller, M. H., & Modi, A. C. (2006). Predictors of health-related quality of life in obese youth. *Obesity, 14,* 122–130.

Zeller, M. H., Saelens, B. E., Roehrig, H., Kirk, S., & Daniels, S. R. (2004). Psychological adjustment of obese youth presenting for weight management treatment. *Obesity Research, 12,* 1576–1586.

CHAPTER 11

Preventing Girls' Depression during the Transition to Adolescence

Jane E. Gillham *and* Tara M. Chaplin

The transition to adolescence is a critical period for preventing depression in girls. However, despite the sex difference in depression that emerges during adolescence, little research has focused on developing programs that target gender-related risk factors. Most prevention programs teach cognitive-behavioral skills and use a coeducational group format. Some of these programs, including our research team's program, the Penn Resiliency Program (PRP), appear to reduce and prevent symptoms of depression. However, across the depression prevention literature, average effects are small. Effects of specific programs such as PRP are often inconsistent. In general, girls appear to benefit as much as boys from the existing programs, but programs developed specifically for girls could have more substantial effects. Research on children's social and emotional development identifies a variety of biological, psychological, interpersonal, and contextual risk factors that occur simultaneously during early adolescence, making them ideal targets for interventions aiming to prevent depression in this period. Moreover, many of these factors affect girls more than boys. Yet, many have not yet been targeted by depression prevention efforts. This observation points to a rich and important new area for prevention efforts. We describe our recent work toward developing one such program that targets gender-related risk factors in early adolescent girls.

DEPRESSION IN CHILDREN AND ADOLESCENTS

Rates of depression increase sharply during adolescence. Prior to age 10, depression is relatively rare. By late adolescence it is one of the most common public health problems, affecting 5–10% of youth each year (Office of Applied Studies, 2005; U.S. Department of Health and Human Services, 1999). Even more adolescents suffer from sub-clinical levels of depression that can lead to significant impairment in interpersonal relationships and academic achievement (Gotlib, Lewinsohn, & Seeley, 1995). Rates of depression increase more steeply in girls than in boys, so that by late adolescence a sex difference in depression emerges that will endure through most of adulthood (Hankin & Abramson, 2001; Nolen-Hoeksema & Girgus, 1994). This increase in depression occurs in the context of a developmental period, the transition to adolescence, that is difficult for many children because multiple biological, psychological, and social changes and stressors converge.

There are multiple pathways to depression in children and adolescents. For example, recent research indicates a moderate to strong genetic component to depression (Kendler, Gatz, Gardner, & Pederse, 2006). Depression has also been linked to inhibited temperament, neuroticism, anxiety, pessimistic cognitive styles, and passive and ruminative coping styles (Garber, 2006; Hankin & Abela, 2005; Kendler et al., 2006). Family environments, including parental conflict and parenting characterized by abuse, intrusiveness, and low levels of affection are also linked to depression in children and adolescents (Downey & Coyne, 1990; Garber, 2006) and may interact with biological risk factors for depression (Yap et al., 2008). Parental depression is a particularly strong risk factor for depression in youth (Beardslee, Versage, & Gladstone, 1998; Downey & Coyne, 1990; Weissman et al., 2006b). This finding probably reflects genetic factors, to some degree, but it also appears to be related to the interference of depressive symptoms with parents' interpersonal interactions, including parenting behaviors (Beardslee, 2002; Compas, Langrock, Keller, Merchant, & Copeland, 2002; Garber, 2006; Goodman & Gotlib, 1999). Recent studies indicate that children's psychological adjustment improves when their depressed mothers receive effective treatment (Weissman et al., 2006a). Life stressors such as abuse, loss, and humiliation, as well as stressful contexts such as poverty, increase risk for depression (Bruce, Takeuchi, & Leaf, 1991; Kendler, Gardner, & Prescott, 2002; McLoyd, 1998). Many of these risk factors co-occur (e.g., neuroticism and anxiety, parental depression and parental conflict), and several appear to interact with each other to produce depression (Caspi et al., 2003; Hankin & Abela, 2005; Kendler, Kuhn, & Prescott, 2004). Over the past few years, research has begun to suggest that biological, psychological, and social risk factors do not necessarily lead to depression by themselves (Garber, 2006). Rather, the accumulation of risk factors across multiple domains may be particularly problematic. The variety of risk factors suggests a variety of approaches to treating and preventing depression, including biomedical and psychosocial interventions that target individual, family, and/or community risk factors. Our research group has focused primarily on cognitive-behavioral approaches.

COGNITIVE-BEHAVIORAL APPROACHES

Cognitive-behavioral models of depression are among the most widely researched. These models propose that depression results from, or is exacerbated by, several cognitive factors, including negative self-schema or core beliefs, dysfunctional or perfectionistic standards, biased information processing, and pessimistic or hopeless cognitive styles (Abramson, Metalsky, & Alloy, 1989; Abramson, Seligman, & Teasdale, 1978; Beck, 1967, 1976; Ellis, 1962; Hankin & Abela, 2005). In addition, depression is linked to maladaptive coping and problem-solving strategies, including passive response styles, rumination, and aggression (Abela, Vanderbilt, & Rochon, 2004; Chaplin & Cole, 2005; Keenan & Hipwell, 2005; Nolen-Hoeksema, 1991; Spence, Sheffield, & Donovan, 2002). These cognitive and behavioral risk factors may exacerbate each other and lead to self-fulfilling prophecies or downward spirals. For example, negative core beliefs such as "I'm unlovable" and "Nobody cares about me" make it difficult to start conversations with others or act assertively. These behaviors, in turn, may result in isolation or the continuation of hurtful behavior by others, which may appear to support the original negative beliefs. In theory, these cognitive, coping, and problem-solving difficulties serve as diatheses that may develop earlier in life and set the stage for depression when individuals encounter stressful events or painful emotions. Stressful events include major adversities, such as the breakup of a relationship, as well as day-to-day hassles and challenges that may be particularly common during adolescence (Hankin & Abela, 2005). Recent research supports the diathesis–stress model, indicating that daily hassles increase depressive symptoms in children who have dysfunctional attitudes and low self-esteem (Abela & Skitch, 2007). Individuals who are depressed or who have maladaptive cognitive, coping, or problem-solving styles may also act in ways that precipitate negative events (Hammen, 1991).

In early childhood, depression may be more closely connected to life events such as trauma or separation from caregivers. During late childhood and adolescence, cognitive-behavioral models may become more relevant

(Bemporad, 1994; Garber & Flynn, 1998). For example, in a longitudinal study of children from third to eighth grade, explanatory style began to predict depressive symptoms in sixth grade (Nolen-Hoeksema, Girgus, & Seligman, 1992). In addition, there is some evidence that children's self-concepts and interpretive styles become more negative during adolescence (Gillham, Reivich, & Shatté, 2001; McCauley, Mitchell, Burke, & Moss, 1988; but for exceptions, see Garber, Weiss, & Shanley, 1993; Shapka & Keating, 2005).

Cognitive-behavioral therapy (CBT) targets the negative cognitive, coping, and problem-solving patterns that are associated with depression in adolescents and adults, thereby enabling individuals to manage difficult experiences both during and after therapy. Many studies have demonstrated CBT's effectiveness in treating depression in adults and adolescents (Compton et al., 2004; Hollon & DeRubeis, 2004; Rohde, Lewinsohn, Clarke, Hops, & Seeley, 2005; Stark et al., 2005). Moreover, CBT may prevent depression from recurring. Once therapy has ended, adults who have been treated with CBT are less likely than those treated with medication to experience a recurrence of depression (Hollon et al., 2005).

CBT uses cognitive restructuring techniques (i.e., evaluating the evidence for thoughts and generating alternative interpretations for situations) that rely heavily on metacognitive abilities, which strengthen during adolescence. Thus, although adolescence is a time of increased vulnerability to depression, it is also a period when cognitive abilities and emotional awareness increase and may be channeled toward learning effective coping strategies and skills for challenging maladaptive interpretive styles.

During the past 15 years, several interventions have been developed that use cognitive-behavioral techniques to prevent depression in children and adolescents (Garber, 2006; Horowitz & Garber, 2006; Merry, McDowell, Hetrick, Bir, & Muller, 2004; Spence & Shortt, 2007; Sutton, 2007). Most of these programs are group interventions that can be delivered in schools, clinics, or other community settings. Several have shown positive effects on depressive symptoms. Meta-analytic reviews of depression prevention studies indicate that, on average, programs that target children and adolescents who are at elevated risk for depression have small but significant effects on depressive symptoms (Horowitz & Garber, 2006; Merry et al., 2004; Stice, Shaw, Bohon, Marti, & Rohde, 2009). A few programs have large effects.

In contrast, however, several reviews have found no significant effects for programs that are delivered universally (e.g., to all students within a school) (Horowitz & Garber, 2006; Spence & Shortt, 2007). Stice and colleagues found no significant effects of universal programs at postassessments (conducted soon after the interventions ended). Although universal programs had significant effects at follow-up, effect sizes were considerably smaller than for targeted programs (Stice et al., 2009).

Research on universal interventions is particularly challenging. Participants' average risk for depression is lower than in targeted samples, which means that the average intervention effects will be smaller and more difficult to detect. In addition, universal interventions have often been evaluated under delivery conditions that are far from ideal. They are often delivered to large groups (entire classrooms) of adolescents and by teachers and other community providers who have little background in the intervention model and who receive minimal training (Gillham, 2007; Horowitz & Garber, 2006). Children's attendance is sometimes poor, and programs sometimes need to be shortened because of conflicts with school or after-school activities (e.g., Quayle, Dziurawiec, Roberts, Kane, & Ebsworthy, 2001). If effective universal programs can be developed and disseminated, they could be quite important as part of a comprehensive depression prevention strategy. Schools are particularly promising locations for prevention efforts. Most children in this country attend school, and schools are already major providers of mental health services and programs designed to promote social and emotional well-being.

Research on depression prevention is quite new, and we do not yet know what is possible. Only 12 of the 30 studies included in the Horowitz and Garber (2006) meta-analysis followed participants for more than 6 months postintervention, and most of these suffered from high attrition during follow-up. Thus, it is difficult to determine whether these interventions can prevent depression over time. In addition, in most studies with significant effects, findings resemble treatment more than prevention. That is, depressive symptoms decrease in intervention participants and decrease less steeply or remain constant in controls. Only a few studies report the prevention of increased depressive symptoms over time (Horowitz & Garber, 2006). Most studies have not examined effects on depressive disorders. Of those that have, the Coping with Stress Course (Clarke & Lewinsohn, 1995) has demonstrated the strongest results to date. In three studies it has substantially prevented the onset of depressive disorders in 14- to 19-year-olds with high but subclinical levels of symptoms (Clarke et al., 1995; Clarke et al., 2001; Garber et al., 2009).

THE PENN RESILIENCY PROGRAM

The Penn Resiliency Program (PRP; Gillham, Reivich, & Jaycox, 2008b), developed by our research team, is a group cognitive-behavioral intervention for younger adolescents (ages 10–14). By teaching cognitive and problem-solving skills earlier in life, PRP aims to prevent the increase in depression that occurs in mid- to late adolescence. PRP includes about 18–24 hours of content and is typically delivered in 1- to 2-hour meetings once weekly. PRP was designed for delivery by teachers, counselors, and clinicians who have received training in the cognitive-behavioral model and in PRP, specifically.

PRP consists of two major components. The first component focuses on cognitive skills. Students learn Albert Ellis's adversity–beliefs–consequences (ABC) model: that our beliefs and interpretations of events affect our feelings and behaviors (Ellis, 1962). Students learn to identify maladaptive thinking styles, including styles that fuel pessimistic and catastrophic thinking. Although this program has been found to reduce pessimism in several studies (e.g., Gillham & Reivich, 1999; Gillham, Reivich, Jaycox, & Seligman, 1995; Yu & Seligman, 2002), PRP emphasizes accurate and flexible thinking. Students learn to examine evidence for their beliefs and to consider alternative interpretations. Flexibility and accuracy will lead many students in the direction of optimism, but flexibility and accuracy will also lead some students (especially students who externalize problems) to realize their own contributions to the difficulties they encounter.

The second component of PRP teaches problem-solving and coping skills. Students learn techniques for handling difficult emotions and uncontrollable stressors. These techniques include deep breathing, relaxation, distraction, and seeking social support. Students also learn a variety of skills for handling interpersonal and academic difficulties that are common during adolescence. For example, students learn assertiveness and negotiation techniques, strategies for overcoming procrastination and breaking a large project into manageable chunks, and a multistep approach to interpersonal problem solving that includes perspective taking, creative brainstorming, and decision making. Although the focus of the program becomes more behavioral in later sessions, the link between cognitive and behavioral skills is emphasized throughout. For example, in teaching skills to combat procrastination, group leaders help students identify and evaluate beliefs (e.g., "I'll never be able to do this"; "I do my best work under pressure") that fuel procrastination.

Research on PRP

PRP has been evaluated in at least 19 controlled studies, making it one of the most well-researched cognitive-behavioral prevention programs. Together, these studies have included approximately 2,500 children from a variety of demographic and socioeconomic backgrounds. Although several studies have evaluated PRP with suburban U.S. samples that are predominantly of European American descent (e.g., Jaycox, Reivich, Gillham, & Seligman, 1994; Gillham et al., 2006b), evaluations have also included inner-city African American and Latino samples (Cardemil, Reivich, & Seligman, 2002), as well as children in China (Yu & Seligman, 2002) and

Australia (Pattison & Lynd-Stevenson, 2001; Quayle et al., 2001; Roberts, Kane, Thomson, Bishop, & Hart, 2003).

PRP was originally developed for children at increased risk for depression. Specifically, PRP targeted children who had elevated depressive symptoms or who were experiencing high levels of family conflict. During the past 10 years, however, work on PRP has expanded to include children with few or no symptoms of depression at baseline. In several studies, PRP has been evaluated as a universal intervention, delivered to all children who enroll, regardless of initial symptom level (e.g., Chaplin et al., 2006; Gillham et al., 2007).

A meta-analysis of PRP studies found that the program significantly reduced depressive symptoms relative to control and that these effects endure for at least 12 months following the intervention (Brunwasser, Gillham, & Kim, 2009). In some studies, PRP's effects on depressive symptoms are large and long-lasting. For example, the first evaluation found that PRP participants were half as likely as controls to develop moderate to severe levels of depressive symptoms for 2 years after the program (Gillham et al., 1995). Recent studies suggest that PRP may have positive effects on behavioral problems and anxiety—difficulties that often co-occur with depression in youth. For example, in an evaluation of PRP in Australia, PRP participants reported fewer symptoms of anxiety than controls at postintervention and 6- and 30-month follow-ups, although no effect was found on anxiety at the 18-month follow-up. Parent reports suggested improvements in externalizing behaviors at post-intervention. Interestingly, PRP did not affect depressive symptoms in that study (Roberts et al., 2003; Roberts, Kane, Bishop, Matthews, & Thompson, 2004). In a recent pilot study, the combination of PRP and a cognitive-behavioral parent program prevented the onset of clinically relevant anxiety symptoms in children. Across the 12-month follow-up period, 5% of PRP participants reported clinically relevant levels of anxiety symptoms, as compared to 30% of controls (Gillham et al., 2006b).

An evaluation of PRP in a health maintenance organization (HMO) suggests that PRP may prevent depression- and anxiety-related disorders in children who have high levels of symptoms. Among children with high levels of baseline symptoms, 36% of PRP participants developed depression or anxiety-related disorders during the 2-year follow-up period, as compared with 56% of usual care controls. PRP did not prevent disorders among children with low levels of baseline symptoms (Gillham, Hamilton, Freres, Patton, & Gallop, 2006a).

Several studies have found positive effects on cognitions and cognitive styles related to depression, including explanatory style, hopelessness, and negative automatic thoughts (e.g., Cardemil et al., 2002; Gillham et al., 1995; Yu & Seligman, 2002). Changes in these types of cognitions partially mediate PRP's effects on depressive symptoms in some studies (Gillham et al., 1995; Yu & Seligman, 2002). However, most studies have not evaluated whether PRP works by changing cognitions, problem-solving strategies, or coping behaviors. Important directions for future research are to identify the mechanisms by which PRP works when it is effective.

There is considerable variability in PRP's effects across, and sometimes within, studies. PRP's effects have sometimes varied by school or by participants' gender or ethnicity (e.g., Cardemil et al., 2002; Cardemil, Reivich, Beevers, Seligman, & James, 2007; Gillham et al., 2006a, 2007). However, these moderator effects appear to be inconsistent across studies. A few studies have not found benefits on depressive symptoms (e.g., Pattison & Lynd-Stevenson, 2001; Roberts et al., 2003, 2004). To some degree, differences in PRP's effectiveness across studies appear to reflect differences in group leaders' experience, training, and intervention adherence. For example, a recent evaluation of PRP in a managed care setting found reductions in depressive symptoms relative to control for PRP groups with high intervention fidelity. No benefits were found for groups with lower fidelity (Gillham et al., 2006a).

A recent review of PRP research suggests that effects are strongest when PRP groups are led by members of the PRP research team or by others closely supervised by the team. PRP is often ineffective when group leaders receive minimal training or supervision (Gillham, Brunwasser, & Freres, 2008a). Figure 11.1 summarizes PRP's effect sizes as a function of leader training. The drop-off in effectiveness is disappointing, but common, as psychosocial interventions progress from efficacy trials to community-based implementation. The Resourceful Adolescent Program showed a similar decline in effects when implemented by school staff rather than members of the research team (Harnett & Dadds, 2004; Shochet et al., 2001). Thus, a critical focus of current research is on the development of effective training and dissemination strategies.

Current PRP research aims to make the program's effects stronger and more consistent by including additional intervention components and adapting the program for use with specific populations. For example, current research includes booster sessions that remind students of the PRP skills and help them apply these skills to challenges that emerge later in adolescence. A parent version of PRP can be delivered alongside PRP to teach parents key skills and help them use these skills in their own lives. This training may help parents support their children's use of the PRP skills and model effective coping and problem solving for their children. A pilot study found that the combination of PRP and the parent group prevented symptoms of depression and anxiety through a 12-month follow-up period (Gillham et al., 2006b). A large randomized-controlled study is currently underway that tests these booster and parent intervention components. We

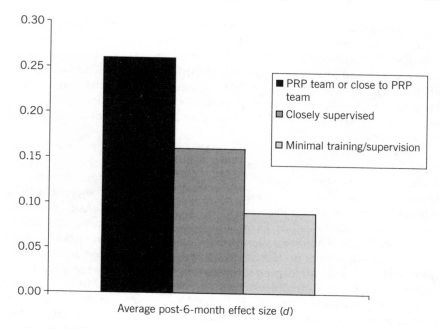

FIGURE 11.1. PRP's effect on depressive symptoms as a function of group leader training.

are also collaborating on a new intervention for depressed mothers and their children that blends family therapy and cognitive-behavioral skills from PRP (Boyd, Diamond, & Bourjolly, 2006).

PRP's Effects for Girls

Given the gender difference in depression, a crucial direction of our current research is the evaluation of PRP's effectiveness in preventing depression in girls. Several researchers and clinicians have suggested that the focus on rationality that underlies cognitive-behavioral interventions, including PRP, may be more appealing to, and more effective with, males. In contrast, interventions that focus on interpersonal relationships, such as interpersonal psychotherapy, may be more appealing to, and effective with, females. In general, however, cognitive-behavioral therapy is an effective treatment for depression in both men and women, and a recent prevention trial found that the effects of cognitive-behavioral and interpersonal prevention programs did not vary by participants' gender (Horowitz, Garber, Ciesla, Young, & Mufson, 2007).

Seven studies have examined gender differences in PRP's effects on depressive symptoms (see Table 11.1). These yield contradictory findings. Three studies found that PRP's effects varied by gender. In two of these, PRP reduced and prevented symptoms in boys but not girls (Reivich, 1996; Shatté, 1997). In the third study, PRP reduced and prevented symptoms in girls but not boys (Gillham et al., 2006a). PRP was also effective in reducing depressive symptoms in an evaluation at an all girls' school (Quayle et al., 2001).

The findings for PRP parallel findings across the literature on cognitive-behavioral depression prevention programs (Garber, 2006). Many studies do not find or report gender differences. Of those that do, a few report stronger effects in boys (e.g., Clarke, Hawkins, Murphy, & Sheeber, 1993), whereas others report stronger effects in girls and women (e.g., Petersen, Leffert, Graham, Alwin, & Ding, 1997; Seligman, Schulman, DeRubeis, & Hollon, 1999). Thus, overall, cognitive-behavioral interventions, including PRP, do not appear to benefit boys more than girls. Nevertheless, given girls' increased risk for depression, it is important to develop prevention programs that are more consistently effective for them. Most cognitive-behavioral prevention programs were developed as coed interventions and do not specifically target gender-related risk factors (Garber, 2006; Le, Muñoz, Ippen, & Stoddard, 2003). Given girls' increased vulnerability to depression, identifying and targeting these risk factors is critical for prevention efforts.

RISK FACTORS FOR DEPRESSION IN GIRLS

Several factors appear to increase risk for depression in girls. There is some evidence that pessimistic cognitive styles and emotion regulation, coping, and problem-solving difficulties that are linked to depression are more common in girls than in boys. Many of these risk factors appear to be more common in girls during childhood, long before the sex difference emerges in adolescence (Nolen-Hoeksema & Girgus, 1994). These risk factors may lead to depression in girls as stressors and contextual challenges increase during adolescence.

Cognitive Styles, Emotion Regulation, and Coping

There is some evidence that girls may have more pessimistic cognitive styles than boys. Most research on explanatory style has not found gender differences (for review, see Gladstone & Kaslow, 1995). However, some studies suggest that girls may explain events more pessimistically than do boys. Some studies have found that girls are more likely than boys to attribute

TABLE 11.1. Penn Resiliency Program Studies That Have Examined Gender Effects

Evaluation	Sample	Conditions and follow-up	Overall effect on depressive symptoms?	Difference in effects for girls versus boys?
Initial evaluation (Gillham et al., 1995; Reivich 1996; Gillham & Reivich, 1999; Jaycox et al., 1994)	143 children (66 girls, 77 boys) in fifth and sixth grades. Ages 10–13 years.	• PRP (3 versions) vs. control • 36-month follow-up	Yes (through 24 months).	Yes; significant effect in boys, not girls.
Effectiveness and specificity study (Reivich, 1996; Shatté, 1997)	152 children (71 girls, 81 boys) in sixth–eighth grades. Mean age 12.7 years.	• PRP vs. alternate intervention vs. control • 12-month follow-up	Yes (through 8 months).	Yes; significant effect in boys, not girls.
First Australian study (Pattison & Lynd-Stevenson, 2001)	66 children (34 girls, 32 boys) in fifth and sixth grades. Ages 9–12 years.	• PRP vs. reverse PRP vs. attention control vs. control • 8-month follow-up	No.	No.
Inner-city study (Cardemil et al., 2002, 2007)	168 children (84 girls, 84 boys) in fifth and sixth grades. Mean age 11.1 years.	• PRP vs. control • 24-month follow-up	Yes (through 24 months) for Latino sample; no for African American sample.	No.
All girls and co-ed PRP study (Chaplin et al., 2006)	208 children (103 girls, 105 boys) in sixth through eighth grades. Ages 11–14 years.	• PRP vs. control (boys randomized to coed PRP vs. control; girls randomized to co-ed PRP vs. all-girls PRP vs. control) • Post	Yes (to post).	No.
HMO study (Gillham, Hamilton, et al., 2006a)	271 children (144 girls, 127 boys). Ages 11–12 years.	• PRP vs. usual care control • 24-month follow-up	No.	Yes; significant effects for girls, not boys.
Effectiveness and specificity study (Gillham et al., 2007)[a]	697 children (321 girls, 376 boys) in grades 6–8. Mean age 12.1 years.	• PRP vs. usual care control • 24-month follow-up	No; moderation by school; yes (through 30 months) in two schools; no for third school.	No.

[a]Analyses of gender differences are not reported in the article. Information in this table is based on recently completed analyses conducted by Jane E. Gillham.

failure on math or spatial relations tests (male sex-typed tasks) to internal/ stable factors (lack of ability), with no gender differences found in explanations for verbal test performance (Gitelson, Petersen, & Tobin-Richards, 1982; Stipek, 1984). Further, a study utilizing a new adolescent-specific measure of explanatory style found that adolescent girls showed a more pessimistic explanatory style overall (for all types of events) than boys (Hankin & Abramson, 2002). Overall, it appears that interventions for girls would benefit from addressing inaccurate explanations for events, with an eye toward events that girls may perceive as being easier for boys, such as math and science.

The ways in which children and adolescents experience, express, and regulate their emotional arousal also have important consequences for the development of depression (for reviews, see Chaplin & Cole, 2005; Cole, Michel, & Teti, 1994; Davidson, Scherer, & Goldsmith, 2003; Garber & Dodge, 1991). Depression may be related to patterns of emotion regulation, including ruminating on sad emotion (Fivush & Buckner, 2000; Nolen-Hoeksema & Girgus, 1994), minimizing anger or lacking assertiveness (Chaplin & Cole, 2005; Izard, 1972; Gross & John, 2003), and experiencing excessive empathy and guilt (Zahn-Waxler, Cole, & Barrett, 1991). Depression may also be related to difficulty in up-regulating positive emotions (Clark & Watson, 1991; Davidson, 2000). Interestingly, girls may be at greater risk for showing all of these patterns of emotion, with the exception of decreased positive emotion.

Rumination is a form of emotion regulation that involves thinking over and over again about one's sadness and problems to the exclusion of making active attempts to remedy the situation. This process of focusing on sadness amplifies it and predicts increases in depressive symptoms in adolescence (Abela, Brozina, & Haigh, 2002; Nolen-Hoeksema, Stice, Wade, & Bohon, 2007; Schwartz & Koenig, 1996). Rumination may also lead youth to neglect more active coping strategies, such as problem solving, that might improve the situation. Thus rumination may lead to more passivity and potentially worse depression (Youngren & Lewinsohn, 1980). Girls tend to ruminate more than do boys, perhaps because sadness tends to be more acceptable for girls than for boys (Brody & Hall, 2000). As young as preschool age, girls are more likely than boys to report feeling sadness and fear (Brody, 1984; Zahn-Waxler, Cole, Welsh, & Fox, 1995) and to express sadness (Chaplin, Cole, & Zahn-Waxler, 2005). In adolescence, girls are more likely than boys to report using rumination as an emotion regulation strategy (Broderick, 1998; Nolen-Hoeksema & Girgus, 1994). In addition, some adolescents co-ruminate—that is, discuss their problems and distressing emotions over and over with a friend. In one study, co-rumination predicted increases in depressive and anxiety symptoms 6 months later for girls, but not for boys. Interestingly, co-rumination also predicted higher perceived quality of friendships, suggesting that it may be important to help girls find alternative ways of responding to stress that can also strengthen their connections to others (Rose, Carlson, & Waller, 2007).

In addition to rumination, girls may be more likely than boys to minimize anger, leading to increased risk for depression. All emotions, even anger, are functional (Barrett & Campos, 1986). In certain contexts, it is appropriate for youth to harness anger in order to push through obstacles, to achieve goals, and perhaps even to resist peer pressure (Izard & Ackerman, 2000). However, some children may develop a tendency to suppress anger displays. Self-reports of "emotional suppression" (including anger suppression) have been associated with depressive symptoms among adults (Cautin, Overholser, & Goetz, 2001; Gross & John, 2003; Riley, Treiber, & Woods, 1989), and observational studies have found that lower anger expression is associated with higher depressive symptoms in adolescents (Chaplin, 2006; Davis, Sheeber, Hops, & Tildesley, 2000). In addition, difficulty expressing anger may inhibit assertive behavior, which may increase depression in children and adolescence (Allen, Hauser, Eickholt, Bell, & O'Connor, 1994). Difficulties with assertiveness and anger expression may be more prevalent for girls than for boys, perhaps because anger is more acceptable for males than females in mainstream U.S. culture (Brody & Hall, 2000). An over-controlled, unassertive presentation at age 7 has been found to predict adolescent depression in girls, whereas an aggressive, undercontrolled presentation predicted depressive symptoms for boys (Block, Gjerde, & Block, 1991).

Excessive empathy or concern for others is another emotional pattern that has been linked to depression and may be more common for girls. Concern for others' distress is part of prosocial development and can be a protective factor for youth (Hoffman, 1982; Kochanska, DeVet, Goldman, Murray, & Putnam, 1994). However, feeling excessive empathy for others, to the exclusion of caring for one's own needs, can create risk for depression and other internalizing disorders (Keenan & Hipwell, 2005; Zahn-Waxler, 2001; Zahn-Waxler, Cole, & Barrett, 1991). An exaggerated sense of responsibility for others can lead to inappropriate feelings of guilt (tied to others' transgressions) and may interfere with the development of a strong sense of self and self-esteem, which may, in turn, contribute to depression.

Girls may be more likely than boys to show excessive empathy and concern for others (Keenan & Hipwell, 2005), perhaps due to girls' theorized orientation toward interpersonal relationships (Cyranowski, Frank, Young, & Shear, 2000; Gilligan, 1982; Jordan, Kaplan, Miller, Stiver, & Surrey, 1991). Starting in early childhood, girls are more likely than boys to show empathic responding to those who are hurt, such as in paradigms in which their mothers feign an injury (Hastings, Zahn-Waxler, Robinson, Usher, &

Bridges, 2000). On teacher and parent reports, girls are rated as being more concerned for others than are boys (e.g., Denham, McKinley, Couchoud, & Holt, 1990; for review, see Zahn-Waxler, 2001). We recently found that higher feelings of worry and oversensitivity (including worry about others) predicted increases in depressive symptoms 1 year later for early adolescent girls, but not for boys (Chaplin, Gillham, & Seligman, 2009). Thus, over-concern for others may be more common for, and possibly more detrimental for, girls than for boys in terms of risk for depression.

Depression prevention programs for early adolescent girls would benefit from addressing potential patterns of emotion regulation related to depression, including ruminating on sad feelings, minimizing angry feelings to the exclusion of appropriate (assertive) expressions of anger, and experiencing excessive concern for others that may lead to a high level of worry or guilt. Intervention leaders will need to take care to understand the complex cultural systems and gender roles that reinforce these patterns in girls.

Social and Contextual Changes

As they enter adolescence, youth, and particularly girls, face several new stressors and challenges. Changes occur in the structure of school class-rooms and in peer interactions. As compared to elementary school, middle school classrooms are less positive and more competitive (Eccles et al., 1993). This change is disruptive for both boys and girls, but may be particularly difficult for girls for several reasons. First, the competitive atmo-sphere is at odds with socialized gender roles for females to emphasize cooperation over competition (Gilligan, 1982; Jordan et al., 1991). Second, girls are more likely than boys to transition to middle school at the same time as the onset of puberty, creating an accumulation of risk (Simmons & Blythe, 1987).

The middle school transition also brings an increase in the adolescents' social sphere, with youth beginning to spend more time with peers and less with parents (Csikszentmihalyi & Larson, 1984). Friendships become more intimate and salient (Berndt, 1987). Yet, at the same time that adolescents begin to value their friends more, the change to middle school disrupts peer networks. This disruption may be especially challenging for girls, who tend to have more intimate friendships than boys (Rose & Rudolph, 2006). In addition, middle school and junior high school peer culture often emphasizes popularity rather than close friendships (LeCroy & Daley, 2001). This emphasis may contribute to relational aggression—a type of aggression that is more common in girls than in boys and that increases in adolescence (Rose, Swenson, & Waller, 2004). Several studies suggest that children who perceive or experience rejection and victimization by others

are at increased risk for depression (La Greca & Harrison, 2005; Nolan, Flynn, & Garber, 2003).

As they enter adolescence, youth also become increasingly aware of the larger society, and girls may begin to attend to cultural messages about their possible roles in society (Hill & Lynch, 1983). Although opportunities for girls and women have increased dramatically in this country in the past 50 years, even today, girls are bombarded with images that convey limited career options for women or show women in stereotypical roles. Limitations to their future aspirations may lead to feelings of depression (Nolen-Hoeksema, 2001).

At the same time that these contextual stressors occur during early adolescence, girls experience the onset of puberty. With pubertal development, early adolescent girls may begin to wrestle with emerging sexuality. Interest in romantic relationships increases, and many girls begin dating. Although there are many positive aspects to romantic interests and relationships, they are a new area of anxiety and stress for many adolescents. For example, breakups of romantic relationships are predictive of first onset of depressive disorders during adolescence (Monroe, Rohde, Seeley, & Lewinsohn, 1999). Moreover, recent research suggests that dating itself may increase risk for depression in adolescents, particularly for girls (Joyner & Udry, 2000; La Greca & Harrison, 2005). Girls who have difficulties with emotion regulation or assertiveness, or who are overly concerned about the feelings of others, may be particularly vulnerable to the ups and downs of romantic relationships in adolescence (Davila, Steinberg, Kachadourian, Cobb, & Fincham, 2004; Rizzo, Daley, & Gunderson, 2006). In addition, girls are at least two to three times more likely as boys to be the victims of sexual abuse, and sexual abuse rates increase for girls in adolescence, making the development of sexuality and romantic relationships a highly complex and emotional process for some girls (Nolen-Hoeksema & Girgus, 1994).

The physiological aspects of puberty may also contribute to depression. Some research suggests that increases in estrogen (and testosterone) levels in girls that occur during puberty may be related to depression (Angold, Costello, Erklani, & Worthman, 1999), although other work suggests that this relationship may be accounted for, at least in part, by the associated morphological changes of puberty (e.g., increase in body fat) and associated increases in stress for girls (Angold, Costello, & Worthman, 1998; Brooks-Gunn & Warren, 1989).

Interventions for early adolescent girls must address the complex simultaneous contextual and biological stressors, providing a safe environment in which girls may open up about these many life changes and find coping skills. Interpersonal relationships, especially romantic relationships, appear to be a crucial focus for prevention efforts.

Body Image

Physical changes associated with puberty may also lead to disruptions in adolescents' body image, particularly for girls, as the changes to girls' bodies (increases in body fat, larger hips) bring them further from the thin body shape that is the ideal in American culture (at least for European Americans), whereas the changes to boys' bodies (increases in muscle, deeper voice, growing taller) bring them closer to the cultural ideal for a man. Indeed, adolescent girls view their changing bodies more negatively than do boys (Petersen, Sarigiani, & Kennedy, 1991). These changes in body image, combined with increasing self-consciousness during adolescence, can lead to low self-image and potentially to feelings of depression (Stice & Bearman, 2001). Body image concerns, then, may be another reason the transition to puberty is more closely linked to depression in girls than boys (Ge, Conger, & Elder, 2001; Petersen et al., 1991).

Exposure to messages and images that emphasize physical attractiveness also increases in early adolescence. Girls' reading of teen magazines increases. Many of these magazines (and some television shows and advertisements) emphasize physical appearance and unrealistic standards of attractiveness, as well as traditional roles for women (LeCroy & Daley, 2001; Fredrickson & Roberts, 1997; Malkin, Wornian, & Chrisler, 1999; Smith, 1994). This emphasis may contribute to body dissatisfaction and hopelessness about future goals (Stice, Hayward, Cameron, Killen, & Taylor, 2000; Stice, Spangler, & Agras, 2001). Media images also may lead to "objectification," wherein girls view themselves increasingly from the observer's perspective and become overly concerned with their appearance (Fredrickson & Roberts, 1997). Perhaps because the thin ideal is more often presented as an ideal for European Americans, body image concerns do not appear to be as severe for African American girls as for European American girls, and this may help to buffer them from depressive symptoms (Parker, Nichter, Nichter, & Vuckovic, 1995). However, even among African American girls, body image concerns are on the rise, with one study finding half of African American girls reporting a desire to lose weight (Grant et al., 1999). In this study, low body image was associated with greater depression, suggesting that body image is an important target for depression prevention programs for African American girls, as it likely is for girls of other ethnic groups.

Family Factors

Within the family system are several factors that may contribute to the development of depression in youth, including parental depression and parental conflict (Downey & Coyne, 1990). Some of these factors may affect girls more than boys.

The transition to adolescence can be a difficult time for families. Conflict between adolescents and their parents increases (Saab, 2004), and many parents feel challenged as they struggle to balance their adolescents' increasing need for autonomy with their own concerns about safety or the need for appropriate rules and limits. Despite the increased conflict between parents and adolescents, most adolescents also report valuing what their parents think of them (Saab, 2004).

The Health Behaviour of School-Aged Children (HBSC) study of 6th-through 10th-grade students in Canada documents several changes in parent–child relationships that occur during adolescence (Boyce, 2004). For example, younger children were more likely than older children to report that their parents are easy to talk to. Similarly, younger children were more likely to report feeling understood by their parents. Interestingly, findings on several indices suggest that girls are more likely than boys to report strained relationships with their parents during this developmental phase. For example, across all grades, girls were less likely than boys to report that their fathers were easy to talk to, and girls were less likely to report feeling understood by their parents. In grades 8–10, girls tended to report having more arguments than boys with their parents, and they were more likely to report that they considered leaving home at times (Saab, 2004).

Girls also may be more affected by parental depression than boys. Mothers are more likely than fathers to be depressed, as a function of the gender difference in depression, and mothers may be more likely to pass on depression to their adolescent daughters (Sheeber, Davis, & Hops, 2002). Several studies find that maternal depression is more strongly linked to depressive symptoms in adolescent daughters than in sons (Fergusson, Horwood, & Lynskey, 1995; Hops, 1996; but for an exception, see Ge, Conger, Lorenz, Shanahan, & Elder, 1995). Daughters are more likely than sons to imitate their mothers' depressive behaviors. Research has found greater synchrony of negative emotional displays (e.g., crying) between mother–daughter pairs than mother–son pairs starting in early childhood (Radke-Yarrow, Nottelmann, Belmont, & Welsh, 1993). In addition, mothers may have the role of socializing girls to adopt female gender roles (Sheeber et al., 2002), some of which promote a passive style that may increase girls' vulnerability to depression (Gilligan, 1982). Research suggests that parental depression is a particularly challenging stressor for children who have limited coping skills and ruminative response styles (Compas et al., 2002).

Interventions that treat parental depression, help parents and children cope more effectively, and strengthen attachments within the family may be especially helpful for preventing depression in girls. At a minimum, educating parents about the content of programs in which their children participate may help them to support the positive changes their children are making.

GIRLS' PRP AND THE GIRLS IN TRANSITION PROGRAM

After we found greater benefits for boys than for girls in the initial PRP study, our research team began to explore possible explanations and methods for improving PRP's effects with girls. We became concerned about possible limits to the coed format that is typically used for the intervention. In the period of early adolescence, girls experience different challenges than boys. As a result, girls may have different topics to discuss in PRP groups. At the same time, they may feel particularly hesitant to discuss these concerns in a coed environment. Although body image concerns are common in early adolescence, in the coed groups these concerns were mentioned rarely, if at all.

Another reason that girls may benefit from an all-girls format is that boys often receive more attention than girls in coed group settings, including classrooms (Bailey, 1993; Jones, 1989; Krupnick, 1985). There are likely several reasons for this imbalance. Boys may be more comfortable expressing their opinions in groups, and they are more likely than girls to call out in class (Altermatt, Jovanovic, & Perry, 1998). Further, boys are more likely than girls to have aggressive and disruptive behavior problems (Achenbach, 1991), which may lead them to act out in group situations. Over the years, many of our PRP group leaders have noted this difference in attentional and behavioral difficulties in boys. These leaders often report that they work harder to engage the boys in their groups and direct more attention to boys so that their groups can stay on task and cover the intervention content. Some leaders worry that girls, who are generally more cooperative and compliant, receive less attention as a result.

Girls' PRP

There is some empirical evidence that girls may benefit more from delivery in an all-girls format. An evaluation of PRP in a girls' school in Australia found significant and substantial reductions in depressive symptoms 6 months after the intervention ended (Quayle et al., 2001). The effect size at the 6-month follow-up ($d = 0.60$) is among the largest in the literature on PRP, especially when samples have not been selected on the basis of elevated symptoms. PRP also tended to prevent mild to moderate symptoms. At the 6-month follow-up, 5% of PRP participants and 31% of controls reported symptoms that were at least mild to moderate in intensity. These findings should be interpreted cautiously, however, given the small sample size ($N = 47$).

A recent study compared PRP's effectiveness for girls when delivered in an all-girls versus coed format (Chaplin et al., 2006). Girls were randomly assigned to coed PRP groups, all-girls PRP groups, or a usual care control. The content of the intervention was the same in the girls and coed groups; both groups participated in PRP. The only difference was whether the setting was single sex or coed. Findings showed that both all-girls and coed PRP prevented depressive symptoms from pre- to postintervention. However, girls in the all-girls groups had better attendance and showed greater improvements in hopelessness than those in the coed groups. The transition to an all-girls format was a relatively small change. A further step would be to design an intervention that not only is in an all-girls setting but that also contains *content* that explicitly addresses gender-specific concerns.

Targeting Gender-Related Risk Factors: The Girls in Transition Program

Educators, clinicians, and researchers have expressed the need for school curricula and interventions that help girls address the social–contextual risk factors that may undermine their self-esteem, achievement, and emotional well-being (e.g., Denmark, 1999; Garber, 2006; Hawkins, Catalano, Kosterman, Abbott, & Hill, 1999; Le et al., 2003; LeCroy & Daley, 2001; Machoian, 2005). Although several community-based interventions (e.g., Girls Incorporated, Girls on the Run International) are designed to promote girls' development, the effect of these interventions on psychological well-being has rarely been evaluated empirically. In contrast, most of the existing depression prevention programs are coed group interventions that are not specifically designed for girls and do not target gender-related risk factors. One exception is a cognitive-behavioral intervention targeting body dissatisfaction in undergraduate women that was evaluated by Bearman and colleagues. This intervention reduced body dissatisfaction and symptoms of depression and bulimia through a 3-month follow-up period (Bearman, Stice, & Chase, 2003). Another promising intervention is the Go Grrrls program (LeCroy & Daley, 2001). Although not specifically designed to prevent depression, this program strives to enhance well-being in early adolescent girls by helping them reflect on societal messages, develop positive self-images, set goals, and establish and maintain friendships. An evaluation found that, relative to control, the Go Grrrls curriculum improved girls' scores on measures of body image satisfaction, assertiveness, self-efficacy, self-liking, and competence. The program also tended ($p < .10$) to improve hopelessness, which is closely linked to depression (LeCroy, 2004).

The Girls in Transition (GT) program is a new intervention for early adolescent girls. GT includes key cognitive-behavioral concepts and skills from PRP, but focuses more on emotion regulation, interpersonal relationships and conflicts, and contextual risk factors. New activities target rumination, body image concerns, media messages, and relational aggression, as well as other risk factors that may be particularly relevant to depression in girls. Like PRP, GT is designed to be delivered in twelve, 90- to 120-minute lessons, but can easily be divided into shorter sessions to fit with school schedules. A GT leader's manual contains lesson plans and in-class activities. The student workbook contains summaries of the main points as well as activities designed to help students apply the concepts and skills to their day-to-day lives. In addition to the girls' program, the GT program offers two 90-minute parent sessions, which share information on girls' development in early adolescence and on skills taught in the program so that they can be reinforced at home. The GT program is designed to be delivered by teachers or school counselors.

GT is divided into four units (summaries of individual lessons are included in Appendix 11.1). The first unit, "Thinking Skills," is based on CBT for depression (Beck, 1967; Beck, Rush, Shaw, & Emery, 1979; Ellis, 1962) and adapted, in part, from the PRP (Gillham, Reivich, & Jaycox, 1998). It teaches many of the cognitive and problem-solving skills in PRP described above, but applies these skills to problems that are common for early adolescent girls, such as unrealistic negative thoughts about one's appearance (negative body image) and changing relationships/conflicts with peers. The second component, "Problem Solving and Coping," includes several problem-solving and assertiveness skills that can be particularly beneficial in day-to-day interactions with peers and friends and for dealing with relational aggression problems (Crick & Grotpeter, 1995). In this unit, we include a discussion of difficulties that some girls may experience with acting assertively as well as gender roles around assertiveness. The unit also includes several strategies for managing sadness, anxiety, and anger, and for breaking the cycle of rumination. Girls are taught, for example, to identify situations in which they ruminate and to brainstorm short-term strategies for distraction (e.g., "I can play with my dog") so that they can calm down and later regroup to solve the problem. They list the distraction strategies on a worksheet labeled "Changing the Channel," to which they can refer when they experience strong negative emotions or uncontrollable stressors in the future. The third unit, "Challenging Media Messages; Identifying Strengths and Goals," encourages girls to think critically about societal and media messages that place limits on women's abilities or place great importance on popularity or unrealistic ideals for physical appearance. Girls are encouraged to put these messages in perspective by thinking about the qualities that are important in their lives, particularly in their close relationships (e.g., Wilgosh, 2002). GT helps girls identify their strengths, work toward their aspirations, and identify positive role models (e.g., Wilgosh, 2002). The fourth unit reviews the major concepts and skills and helps girls anticipate situations in which the skills may be helpful.

There is considerable overlap between units because the cognitive, problem-solving, coping, and social factors are conceptualized as interacting with, and influencing, each other. For example, social factors can influence the development of negative cognitive styles and beliefs about assertiveness. Conversely, cognitive restructuring skills can be used to critique media messages about physical attractiveness in girls and women. As in PRP, skits and hypothetical examples are included to illustrate a wide variety of problems and concerns that are typical in this age group. The GT girls' group also includes examples related to concerns about body image, popularity and cliques, relational aggression, and other issues that may be particularly relevant to girls during the middle and early high school years. The cognitive, problem-solving, coping, and goal-setting skills are applied to these experiences.

We are piloting a slightly condensed (10-session) version of the GT intervention as an optional after-school program with groups of sixth-, seventh-, and eighth-grade girls. The project is open to all girls who enroll (participants are not screened into the groups based on elevated depressive symptoms or other risk factors). The project is using a wait-list controlled design. About half of the girls participate in GT groups during their first year in the project, and the remainder will participate in the groups at the end of the study. This study is ongoing and will include several cohorts of participants. We recently completed the intervention groups with first cohort of participants.

Our impressions as group leaders are that the all-girls format influenced the topics that group members discussed and enabled girls to focus on gender-related challenges that occur during early adolescence. This was apparent from the first session. When asked about problems that are common during the middle school years, many girls brought up concerns about physical attractiveness, including concerns about aspects of their appearance or clothing. Several sixth-grade girls discussed feeling pressure to wear clothing that was more revealing or "more sexy."

A study examining transcripts from the initial sessions supports these impressions (Adams-Deutsch, 2006). Most girls seemed to feel that they experience different stressors than boys during middle school. A quote from one of the sixth-grade girls illustrates this nicely.

"Like guys, they just put on whatever's on top in their drawers and make sure it's not like orange and red pants. And we spend hours trying to figure out what to wear. . . . So we always have to kind of deal with that and how our hair looks, and my hair's a mess right now because I just came back from gym." (inAdams-Deutsch, 2006, p. 4)

Whether or not the girls' impressions about this gender difference is correct, it was clear that many of them worried about their appearance, and some felt that others judged their appearance negatively. Even girls who were aware that their physical development was within normal ranges reported these kinds of concerns. One sixth-grade girl reported being teased because her breasts hadn't developed yet. Other girls worked hard to control their weight or limited their interactions and achievements.

"People last year, they would always say, 'Put some cream on those mosquito bites,' because I'm pretty much flat. Another girl said, 'Is your head on backwards?' and another person called me 'the walking board.'" (in Adams-Deutsch, 2006, p. 5)

"I've been called fat a lot . . . I mean, I know I'm not skinny, and I've worked on that really hard, and I've never thought about being anorexic or bulimic, or whatever. But it really is hard because you think to yourself, 'Oh I wish I could be skinny, maybe I could feel more confident about myself!'" (in Adams-Deutsch, 2006, pp. 6–7)

"I'm not a confident person. I won't go in front of the class because kids will laugh at me. I'm not skinny, but I'm not obese, you know, in the middle, *normal*. It's really hard. People are always like, 'You're fat,' and I can't tolerate it." (in Adams-Deutsch, 2006, p. 9)

Given the close connection between body dissatisfaction, eating disorders, and depression, programs that target body image concerns could be particularly important for preventing depression in girls. Conversations with the girls in our groups indicated that concerns about physical appearance are already quite common by sixth grade. Although we did not formally examine other types of concerns, our impressions are that interpersonal conflicts, particularly handling transgressions and rejection by friends, were also common themes across the sessions. Interventions such as GT can provide a safe place for these kinds of discussions and teach skills for dealing with the challenges that are particularly relevant to girls during the transition to adolescence.

Girls' and mothers' attendance and feedback support the feasibility of the program. Due to conflicts that emerged with other after-school activities, 3 of the 17 girls assigned to the program did not attend any sessions. The 14 other girls attended 8 of the 10 sessions, on average. Twelve of their mothers attended at least one of the two parent meetings. Feedback at the end of the program indicated that girls enjoyed the program and believed it was helpful. Girls' average likert scale ratings fell between "very true" and "mostly true" for items assessing their general impressions ("I liked the program a lot"; "I learned a lot from GT that will help me solve problems"; "I learned a lot from GT that will help me feel happier in my life"; "I would recommend the program to other girls"). Girls also reported that they were using many of the GT skills, particularly attending to self-talk, analyzing problems to figure out why they are upset, and using relaxation techniques when upset. An important next step for future research is to evaluate whether GT improves coping, reduces body image concerns, and prevents symptoms of depression.

OTHER ROUTES TO PREVENTION FOR GIRLS

Research on girls' development suggests many routes to depression prevention. GT focuses on only a few of these and only one age group. There are many exciting directions for future work in this area. For example, interventions with a stronger interpersonal focus (Young, Mufson, & Davies, 2006) or that blend cognitive-behavioral and interpersonal approaches may be particularly helpful for girls as they navigate interactions with peers, close friends, romantic partners, and family members that may become increasingly complex and stressful.

The variety of risk factors and high prevalence of depression in girls suggest a multileveled approach to intervention that includes both targeted and universal interventions (Garber, 2006). Psychosocial interventions that teach cognitive, coping, and problem-solving skills may be helpful for most children and could begin long before adolescence. Interventions that normalize body image concerns or help girls become more comfortable expressing themselves in interpersonal relationships might be beneficial to most girls during adolescence. Such programs could also encourage girls to reflect on the costs and benefits of gender-related responses to stress in interpersonal relationships, especially at their extremes. Interventions could help girls identify unhelpful emotional and behavioral patterns, such as extreme empathy, overconcern for others, and co-rumination, and help girls interact in ways that preserve the best aspects of their capacity for connections without harming themselves in the process.

Currently, some of the most promising interventions target youth who have high levels of symptoms or who are affected by parental depression, parental divorce, or bereavement (e.g., Beardslee, 2002; Clarke et al., 2001; Sandler et al., 2003; Wolchik et al., 2000). Targeted programs could be helpful for adolescents who are experiencing other kinds of stressful interpersonal experiences. For example, programs might be helpful for girls who are dating or who have experienced the breakup of a relationship recently. Programs that help peers or friends support each other through such stressors could be particularly helpful. Given the close relationship between depression in mothers and daughters, interventions that target this dyad could be especially important for interrupting the intergenerational transmission of depression. Although harder to evaluate, community- or societal-level interventions that counteract negative media messages, prevent discrimination or abuse, promote positive images, and increase opportunities for girls and women could have a large impact on girls' vulnerability to depression.

CONCLUSION

In conclusion, there appear to be several promising routes to preventing the increase in depression that occurs among early adolescent girls. We have incorporated the cognitive, emotional, interpersonal, and contextual risk factors that are common among girls in early adolescence into our existing cognitive-behavioral prevention program in order to tailor it for girls at this age. By doing this, we use knowledge gathered through basic developmental science on girls' cognitive, emotional and social development to inform the development of our prevention program. We hope that through developmentally informed intervention delivered within a caring environment, we will be able to attenuate the trajectory toward depression and other internalizing disorders among adolescent girls.

APPENDIX 11.1. SUMMARY OF GIRLS GROUP LESSONS

Unit 1. Thinking Skills

The thinking skills component teaches girls to identify negative interpretations and negative or pessimistic thinking styles and to challenge these beliefs by examining evidence and considering more realistic alternatives. These complex skills are simplified to be appropriate to the developmental level of early adolescence. The program uses cartoons, skits, videos, and stories to make concepts such as pessimistic thinking more concrete and understandable. The program encourages girls to think flexibly about day-to-day problems that are common in the middle school years. The thinking skills are introduced in Lessons 1 through 4 and are reviewed and practiced throughout the remainder of the program.

Lesson 1. Introduction

Major goals are to:

- Introduce group members to the GT program.
- Build group rapport and create an environment that encourages girls to discuss their thoughts, feelings, goals, and day-to-day problems they may be experiencing.
- Introduce the elements of the cognitive model (events, interpretations, and emotions).

Overview: The group leaders discuss the goals of the GT program and engage the group members in activities designed to introduce them to each other and increase their comfort in talking about day-to-day experiences in the group setting. Logistical issues such as the group schedule, group rules, and confidentiality are discussed. In addition, leaders engage the group in discussions and activities that cover the elements of the cognitive model. For example, one discussion focuses on problems and challenges that are common during middle school, including challenges that may be particularly relevant to girls. Typically, this focus leads to discussions about peer acceptance, popularity, and experiences of rejection. In addition, girls often discuss the pressures they feel to achieve, be popular, and conform to certain standards of attractiveness (e.g., wear certain types of clothes). Group members also discuss emotional experiences, including the quality and intensity of different emotions. Finally, the notion of self-talk (or automatic thoughts) is introduced. For homework, girls pay attention to their emotions and self-talk during the following week.

Lesson 2. Cognitive Model

Major goals are to:

- Introduce the cognitive model.
- Practice identifying beliefs and interpretations.

Overview: Leaders introduce the cognitive model—the theory that when events occur, our emotional and behavioral reactions are determined, to a large extent, by our beliefs and interpretations. Girls practice identifying interpretations using both hypothetical and real-life examples, and they also practice generating alternative beliefs and interpretations. Leaders facilitate a discussion about how alternative interpretations can dramatically change our emotional and behavioral responses following an event. For homework, girls apply the cognitive model to events in their own lives and try to note any times in which they feel sad, worried, or angry and the kinds of beliefs that seem to be involved.

Lesson 3. Thinking Styles

Major goals are to:

- Teach girls about thinking styles, particularly pessimistic thinking styles that are linked to depression, anxiety, and behavioral problems.
- Help girls recognize the effects of thinking styles.
- Help girls identify their own thinking styles, especially pessimistic thinking styles that may lead to distress and make it difficult to achieve their goals.

Overview: Leaders use skits, role plays, and videos to illustrate different thinking styles and to launch a discussion of the consequences of these styles. For example, some of the characters in skits display pessimistic styles that lead to hopelessness or hostile styles that lead them to unrealistically blame others for the setbacks they encounter. Leaders discusses Aaron Beck's concept of self-fulfilling prophecy—the idea that negative beliefs (e.g., "No one likes me") can lead to behaviors (e.g., withdrawing from friends) that create events (e.g., no one calls) that seem to confirm the initial negative beliefs. These self-fulfilling prophecies operate in achievement contexts as well. Negative beliefs (e.g., "I can't do math") lead to behaviors (e.g., stop studying) that create events (e.g., do poorly on exam) that seem to confirm the initial negative beliefs. The group discusses the ways in which self-fulfilling prophecies can affect a variety of life domains. Girls consider experiences in their own lives, identify situations in which they may be vulnerable to these kinds of negative thoughts, and generate alternative interpretations that are more realistic. For homework, girls attend to the interpretations they make and practice generating more realistic alternatives to any unrealistic negative interpretations they identify.

Lesson 4. Identifying and Challenging Negative Assumptions

Major goals are to:

- Teach girls about unrealistic assumptions and standards (e.g., perfectionism) and help them recognize how these standards may be operating in their own lives.
- Continue to encourage girls to challenge negative beliefs by examining evidence and considering alternatives.

Overview: Leaders facilitate a discussion about unrealistic standards and assumptions and their consequences. Examples of these standards/assumptions include: "If I'm not good at everything, I'm a failure"; "I have to be liked by everyone"; "In order to be happy, I need to be very popular." Leaders facilitate a discussion about these beliefs, especially beliefs about physical attractiveness or self-expression that may be more common in girls than boys. Leaders point out that some of these beliefs are tied to important values but create problems because they are too rigid or conflict with other important goals and values. The group discusses the consequences of these beliefs. Leaders help students identify any of these beliefs that may be operating in their lives. The group engages in several activities designed to help students dispute unrealistic beliefs by examining evidence and by generating more realistic alternatives. Group members coach each other on the use of these disputation techniques. For homework, girls try to identify unrealistic standards and assumptions that may be operating in their own lives and practice applying disputation skills.

Unit 2. Problem Solving and Coping

This section of the curriculum teaches girls several strategies for solving day-to-day problems in their lives. Group members share the strategies they use for solving problems and coping with stress. The group leaders teach assertiveness, problem-solving, and decision-making strategies. The group also discusses strategies for coping with uncontrollable stressors and strong negative emotions. Group leaders teach several strategies that may help students feel better when they have little control over the events in their lives. These skills are presented in Lessons 5, 6, and 7, and are reviewed and practiced throughout the remainder of the program.

Lesson 5. Assertiveness

Major goals are to:

- Discuss a variety of effective techniques the group members are already using for solving interpersonal problems in their lives.
- Teach girls a strategy for assertiveness.

Overview: The lesson begins with videotaped scenarios and role plays in which one eighth-grade girl does something that upsets a second girl. Leaders encourage group members to discuss the scenarios and how they might respond if these situations happened to them. Through this discussion, the group considers the pros and cons of a variety of interpersonal responses, including those that are aggressive, passive, and assertive. Leaders encourage girls to reflect on their own beliefs about these different styles of responding, especially beliefs that may make it hard to respond assertively. The group examines and critiques negative beliefs about what it means for girls to be assertive ("Girls who are assertive are bossy"; "It's not nice to be assertive"). Leaders encourage girls to apply the disputation skills to these beliefs (to think of alternatives and evidence) and to consider positive examples of assertiveness that they have observed in others. Following this discussion, leaders present a structured technique for assertiveness that includes (1) describing the problem objectively, (2) expressing how one feels, and (3) asking for a change. Using role plays, group members practice applying this technique to hypothetical situations and then to situations in their own lives. For homework, girls try out the assertiveness technique if an appropriate situation emerges during the week.

Lesson 6. Interpersonal Problem-Solving

Major goals are to:

- Provide girls with more practice and coaching in the assertiveness technique.
- Introduce a four-step approach to problem solving.

Overview: In the first part of the lesson, girls discuss their experiences using the assertiveness technique. Leaders encourage girls to describe what they did as well as what happened and any obstacles they faced. Leaders provide coaching and help students refine their use of the assertiveness skill. The remainder of the lesson presents a four-step approach to interpersonal problem solving that includes goal setting, creative brainstorming, decision making, and enacting and evaluating the solution. The group applies this approach to a few hypothetical and real-life examples and generates a list of solutions (e.g., assertiveness, seeking support or advice) that may be helpful to consider across a variety of situations. For homework, girls apply problem-solving steps to challenges in their own lives. Girls also keep a journal about their responses to negative emotions in preparation for the next session.

Lesson 7. Coping with Strong Emotions

Major goals are to:

- Help girls identify the strategies they use to help themselves feel better.
- Teach girls specific strategies for relaxation, distraction, and engaging in pleasant events.

Overview: Leaders facilitate a discussion about the ways in which group members cope when they are feeling very sad, worried, or angry, or when something upsetting happens that they can't control. Leaders encourage girls to talk about responses that help them feel better as well as responses that don't seem to help. Group members work together to make a list of things that they can do to feel better. During this discussion, leaders introduce the concept of rumination (i.e., repeatedly dwelling on negative emotional experiences in a way that prolongs and amplifies the negative emotion). Leaders encourage girls to reflect on times when they may have ruminated (either alone or with a friend) and to describe what happened. The group discusses some of the beliefs that may fuel rumination ("There's nothing I can do to feel better"; "This helps me get in touch with my emotions"). The group discusses the negative consequences of rumination, including the amplification of negative emotion. Leaders help group members generate a variety of strategies for coping with negative emotion. Leaders also walk members through two relaxation procedures (progressive muscle relaxation and relaxation using imagery). These relaxation exercises are practiced again in later lessons. For homework, girls develop an individualized list of strategies that they can use to cope with difficult emotions or experiences. Leaders encourage girls to practice these strategies during the week.

Unit 3. Challenging Media Messages; Identifying Strengths, and Goals

Leaders introduce a conceptual framework to help girls apply the skills they have learned. Throughout the remainder of the program, girls engage in several activities and discussions designed to consolidate these skills. Group members also consider media and other cultural messages to which they are increasingly exposed as they enter adolescence, particularly messages about the characteristics and roles of girls and women and the importance of popularity as opposed to close friendships. Leaders encourage group members to think critically about negative messages and to reflect on their goals and the personal qualities that are most important in their lives.

Lesson 8. Skills Consolidation and Social Context

Major goals are to:

- Help girls consolidate the skills they have learned.
- Begin a discussion of cultural images and messages, particularly messages related to gender, that students may have internalized.

Overview: The first half of the lesson is devoted to practicing the skills that have been covered so far in the program. Leaders present a conceptual framework that emphasizes the "thinking," "doing," and "feeling" skills and help girls determine when each type of skill may be most useful. Leaders encourage girls to discuss difficult situations they are facing, or situations they anticipate facing in the near future. The group members practice applying the different skills to these situations. In the second half of the lesson, leaders introduce the idea that our negative beliefs and interpretations are sometimes internalized from the messages we receive from others around us and from cultural products such as books, television shows, websites, advertisements, etc. Although we often don't question these messages, they can convey harmful beliefs and unrealistic standards. Group members reflect on messages and unrealistic standards they have noticed, particularly standards for girls and women. For homework, girls record positive and negative images of women they observe in the media over the week.

Lesson 9. Critiquing Media Messages, Identifying Strengths and Goals

Major goals are to:

- Help girls become aware of media images and messages that may be harmful to their self-image.
- Help girls counter concerns about body image.
- Help girls identify the personal qualities that are related to their most important relationships and goals.

Overview: Leaders facilitate a discussion about the images group members observed during the past week. Leaders ask group members for their observations about positive and negative images of girls and women, and about the standards or expectations these messages convey. Leaders discuss the emphasis in the media on physical attractiveness and the unrealistic models of attractiveness. Through discussion and activities, leaders encourage girls to reflect on the personal qualities that are more important in friendships and other significant relationships, and for achieving their goals. Leaders discuss the concept of personality strengths, emphasizing that we each have a unique pattern of strengths. For homework, group members engage in activities designed to help them identify their own personal strengths. Girls also reflect on positive role models, including women they admire in their family or community. Girls interview their mothers or other women in their families about their role models and goals.

Lesson 10. Positive Role Models and Goals

Major goals are to:

- Help girls identify positive female role models.
- Help girls reflect on their goals and develop strategies for achieving these goals.

Overview: Group members talk about their personal strengths and develop plans for using their strengths on a daily basis. Group members also talk about the positive female role models they have identified, and the qualities that they most admire in these women. If possible, the group leaders arrange for two or three women in the community to come to this lesson and talk about their work, their goals, and their thoughts about the qualities that are most important in life, including their work and relationships. A particular effort is made to include at least one woman whose profession is in the sciences. If it is not possible for community members to attend, the leaders present videos and written excerpts from interviews, articles, and biographies about women who are prominent in their fields or whose work is having a beneficial impact in the community. Girls then participate in an activity that encourages them to identify short- and long-term goals and to apply the problem-solving skills (particularly creative brainstorming and enacting solutions) to these goals. For homework, girls take a step (or steps) toward one of their goals. They also try to identify and address any roadblocks, including negative beliefs that may make it difficult to reach their goals at times.

Unit 4. Planning Ahead and Review

During the final unit of the program, group members review the concepts and skills from the program and anticipate situations in the future when these skills may be particularly useful.

Lessons 11. Goals, Review, and Future Use of Skills

Major goals are to:

- Help girls develop strategies for achieving goals.
- Encourage girls to consider how the skills they have learned in the program will help them achieve their goals.

Overview: Girls discuss the goals on which they worked for homework, including the steps they took and any obstacles they encountered. Leaders encourage the girls to consider all of the skills they have learned in the program that can help them achieve goals and deal with any obstacles that they may encounter along the way. Following this discussion, leaders encourage girls to think about their future aspirations and longer-term goals. Girls discuss the skills that may be helpful in achieving these goals. The one-step-at-a-time technique is reviewed as a strategy for breaking large projects and/or long-term goals into smaller, manageable steps. In the last part of the session, leaders begin a review of the GT program. For homework, girls make a list of the skills and activities that they found most helpful in the program, in preparation for a more detailed program review in lesson 12. If they choose, girls can develop activities (e.g., skits) that will help them to review concepts and skills in the final lesson.

Lesson 12. Review, Future Use of Skills, and Celebration

Major goals are to:

- Review the skills from the program.
- Help girls anticipate future situations in which the use of skills may be helpful.
- Acknowledge and celebrate the accomplishments of the group and say goodbye.

Overview: In this lesson, leaders encourage girls to think about their aspirations and some of the difficult situations they may encounter in the future, particularly during the next few months. Girls share the lists of skills they generated for homework. They then work together to create a list of take-home messages and reminders—what they found most helpful about the program and what might be most helpful to take with them for the future. Girls complete a brief (anonymous) feedback survey about their experiences in the program. The last part of the lesson is devoted to celebrating the completion of the group and to saying goodbye.

REFERENCES

Abela, J. R. Z., Brozina, K., & Haigh, E. (2002). An examination of the response styles theory of depression in third- and seventh-grade children: A short-term longitudinal study. *Journal of Abnormal Child Psychology, 30,* 515–527.

Abela, J. R. Z., & Skitch, S. A. (2007). Dysfunctional attitudes, self-esteem, and hassles: Cognitive vulnerability to depression in children of affectively ill parents. *Behaviour Research and Therapy, 45,* 1127–1140.

Abela, J. R. Z., Vanderbilt, E., & Rochon, A. (2004). A test of the integration of response styles and social support theories of depression in third- and seventh-grade children. *Journal of Social and Clinical Psychology, 23,* 653–674.

Abramson, L. Y., Metalsky, G. I., & Alloy, L. B. (1989). Hopelessness depression: A theory based subtype of depression. *Psychological Review, 96,* 358–372.

Abramson, L. Y., Seligman, M. E. P., & Teasdale, J. E. (1978). Learned helplessness in humans: Critique and reformulation. *Journal of Abnormal Psychology, 87,* 49–74.

Achenbach, T. M. (1991). *Manual for the Child Behavior Checklist.* Burlington: University of Vermont.

Adams-Deutsch, Z. (2006). *Girls in Transition: Preventing distorted body images and depression.* Unpublished manuscript, Swarthmore College, Swarthmore, PA.

Allen, J. P., Hauser, S. T., Eickholt, C., Bell, K. L., & O'Connor, T. G. (1994). Autonomy and relatedness in family interactions as predictors of expressions of negative adolescent affect. *Journal of Research on Adolescence, 4,* 535–552.

Altermatt, E. R., Jovanovic, J., & Perry, M. (1998). Bias or responsivity? Sex and achievement level effects on teachers' classroom questioning practices. *Journal of Educational Psychology, 90,* 516–527.

Angold, A., Costello, E. J., Erklani, A., & Worthman, C. M. (1999). Pubertal changes in hormone levels and depression in girls. *Psychological Medicine, 29,* 1043–1053.

Angold, A., Costello, E. J., & Worthman, C. M. (1998). Puberty and depression: The roles of age, pubertal status, and pubertal timing. *Psychological Medicine 28,* 51–61.

Bailey, S. M. (1993). The current status of gender equity research in American schools. *Educational Psychologist, 28,* 321–339.

Barrett, K. C., & Campos, J. J. (1987). Perspectives on emotional development: II. A functionalist approach to emotions. In J. Osofsky (Ed.), *Handbook of infant development* (pp. 555–578). New York: Wiley.

Beardslee, W. R. (2002). *Out of the darkened room: When a parent is depressed— protecting the children and strengthening the family.* Boston: Little, Brown.

Beardslee, W. R., Versage, E. M., & Gladstone, T. R. G. (1998). Children of affectively ill parents: A review of the past 10 years. *Journal of the American Academy of Child and Adolescent Psychiatry, 31,* 1134–1141.

Bearman, S. K., Stice, E., & Chase, A. (2003). Evaluation of an intervention targeting both depressive and bulimic pathology: A randomized prevention trial. *Behavior Therapy, 34,* 277–293.

Beck, A. T. (1967). *Depression: Clinical, experimental, and theoretical aspects.* New York: Harper & Row.

Beck, A. T. (1976). *Cognitive therapy and the emotional disorders.* New York: New American Library.

Beck, A. T., Rush, A. J., Shaw, B. F., & Emery, G. (1979). *Cognitive therapy of depression: A treatment manual*. New York: Guilford Press.

Bemporad, J. (1994). Dynamic and interpersonal theories of depression. In W. M. Reynolds & H. F. Johnston (Eds.), *Handbook of depression in children and adolescents* (pp. 81–95). New York: Plenum Press.

Berndt, T. J. (1987). The distinctive features of conversations between friends: Theories, research, and implications for sociomoral development. In W. M. Kurtines & J. L. Gewirtz (Eds.), *Moral development through social interaction* (pp. 281–300). Oxford, UK: Wiley.

Block, J., Gjerde, P. F., & Block, J. H. (1991). Personality antecedents of depressive tendencies in 18-year-olds: A prospective study. *Journal of Personality and Social Psychology, 60*, 726–738.

Boyce, W. (2004). *Young people in Canada: Their health and well being*. Report of the HBSC study. Available at *www.phac-aspc.gc.ca/dca-dea/publications/hbsc-2004/index_e.html*.

Boyd, R. C., Diamond, G. S., & Bourjolly, J. (2006). Developing a family-based depression prevention program in urban community mental health clinics: A qualitative investigation. *Family Process, 45*(2), 187–203.

Broderick, P. C. (1998). Early adolescent gender differences in the use of ruminative and distracting coping strategies. *Journal of Early Adolescence, 18*, 173–191.

Brody, L. R. (1984). Sex and age variations in the quality and intensity of children's emotional attributions to hypothetical situations. *Sex Roles, 11*, 51–59.

Brody, L. R., & Hall, J. (2000). Gender, emotion, and expression. In M. Lewis & J. Haviland-Jones (Eds.), *Handbook of emotions* (2nd ed., pp. 325–414). New York: Guilford Press.

Brooks-Gunn, J., & Warren, M. P. (1989). Biological and social contributions to negative affect in young adolescent girls. *Child Development 60*, 40–55.

Bruce, M. L., Takeuchi, D. T., & Leaf, P. J. (1991). Poverty and psychiatric status: Longitudinal evidence from the New Haven Epidemiologic Catchment Area Study. *Archives of General Psychiatry, 48*, 470–474.

Brunwasser, S. M., Gillham, J. E., & Kim, E. (2009). A meta-analytic review of the Penn Resiliency Program's effects on depressive symptoms. *Journal of Consulting and Clinical Psychology, 77*, 1042–1054.

Cardemil, E. V., Reivich, K. J., Beevers, C. J., Seligman, M. E. P., & James, J. (2007). The prevention of depressive symptoms in low-income, minority children: Two-year follow-up. *Behaviour Research and Therapy, 45*, 313–327.

Cardemil, E. V., Reivich, K. J., & Seligman, M. E. P. (2002). The prevention of depressive symptoms in low-income minority middle school students. *Prevention and Treatment, 5*,.

Caspi, A., Sugden, K., Moffit, T. E., Taylor, A., Craig, I. W., & Harrington, H. (2003). Influence of life stress on depression: Moderation by a polymorphism in the 5-HTT gene. *Science, 301*, 386–389.

Cautin, R. L., Overholser, J. C., & Goetz, P. (2001). Assessment of mode of anger expression in adolescent psychiatric inpatients. *Adolescence, 36*, 163–170.

Chaplin, T. M. (2006). Anger, happiness, and sadness: Associations with depressive symptoms in late adolescence. *Journal of Youth and Adolescence, 35,* 977–986.

Chaplin, T. M., & Cole, P. M. (2005). The role of emotion regulation in the development of psychopathology. In B. L. Hankin & J. R. Z. Abela (Eds.), *Development of psychopathology: A vulnerability-stress perspective* (pp. 49–74). Thousand Oaks, CA: Sage.

Chaplin, T. M., Cole, P. M., & Zahn-Waxler, C. (2005). Parental socialization of emotion expression: Gender differences and relations to child adjustment. *Emotion, 5,* 80–88.

Chaplin, T. M., Gillham, J. E., Reivich, K., Elkon, A. G. L., Samuels, B., Freres, D. R., Winder, B., & Seligman, M. E. P. (2006). Depression prevention for early adolescent girls: A pilot study of all-girls versus co-ed groups. *Journal of Early Adolescence, 26,* 110–126.

Chaplin, T. M., Gillham, J. E., & Seligman, M. E. P. (2009). Gender, anxiety, and depressive symptoms: A longitudinal study of early adolescents. *Journal of Early Adolescence, 29,* 307–327.

Clark, L. A., & Watson, D. (1991). Tripartite model of anxiety and depression: Psychometric evidence and taxonomic implications. *Journal of Abnormal Psychology, 100,* 316–336.

Clarke, G. N., Hawkins, W., Murphy, M., & Sheeber, L. (1993). School-based primary prevention of depressive symptomatology in adolescents: Findings from two studies. *Journal of Adolescent Research, 8,* 183–204.

Clarke, G. N., Hawkins, W., Murphy, M., Sheeber, L. B., Lewinsohn, P. M., & Seeley, J. R. (1995). Targeted prevention of unipolar depressive disorder in an at-risk sample of high school adolescents: A randomized trial of a group cognitive intervention. *Journal of the American Academy of Child and Adolescent Psychiatry, 34,* 312–321.

Clarke, G. N., Hornbrook, M., Lynch, F., Polen, M., Gale, J., Beardslee, W., et al. (2001). A randomized trial of a group cognitive intervention for preventing depression in adolescent offspring of depressed parents. *Archives of General Psychiatry, 58,* 1127–1134.

Clarke, G. N., & Lewinsohn, P. M. (1995). *Instructor's manual for the Adolescent Coping with Stress Course.* Portland, OR: Kaiser Permanente Center for Health Research. Available at *www.kpchr.org/acwd/acwd.html.*

Cole, P. M., Michel, M. K., & Teti, L. O. (1994). The development of emotion regulation and dysregulation: A clinical perspective. In N. A. Fox (Ed.), *The development of emotion regulation: Biological and behavioral considerations. Monographs of the Society for Research in Child Development, 59*(2–3, Serial No. 240), 73–100.

Compas, B. E., Langrock, A. M., Keller, G., Merchant, M. J., & Copeland, M. E. (2002). Children coping with parental depression: Processes of adaptation to family stress. In S. H. Goodman & I. H. Gotlib (Eds.), *Children of depressed parents: Mechanisms of risk and implications for treatment* (pp. 227–252). Washington, DC: American Psychological Association.

Compton, S. N., March, J. S., Brent, D., Albano, A. M., Weersing, V. R., & Curry, J. (2004). Cognitive-behavioral psychotherapy for anxiety and depressive disorders in children and adolescents: An evidence-based medicine review. *Journal of the American Academy of Child and Adolescent Psychiatry, 43,* 930–959.

Csikszentmihalyi, M., & Larson, R. (1984). *Being adolescent.* New York: Basic Books.

Crick, N. R., & Grotpeter, J. K. (1995). Relational aggression, gender and social-psychological adjustment. *Child Development, 66,* 710–722.

Cyranowski, J. M., Frank, E., Young, E., & Shear, K. (2000). Adolescent onset of the gender difference in lifetime rates of major depression. *Archives of General Psychiatry, 57,* 21–27.

Davidson, R. J. (2000). Affective style, psychopathology, and resilience: Brain mechanisms and plasticity. *American Psychologist, 55,* 1196–1214.

Davidson, R. J., Scherer, K. R., & Goldsmith, H. H. (Eds.). (2003). *Handbook of affective sciences.* Oxford, UK: Oxford University Press.

Davila, J., Steinberg, S. J., Kachadourian, L., Cobb, R., & Fincham, F. (2004). Romantic involvement and depressive symptoms in early and late adolescence: The role of a preoccupied relational style. *Personal Relationships, 11,* 161–178.

Davis, B., Sheeber, L., Hops, H., & Tildesley, E. (2000). Adolescent responses to depressive parental behaviors in problem-solving interactions: Implications for depressive symptoms. *Journal of Abnormal Child Psychology, 28,* 451–65.

Denham, S. A., McKinley, M., Couchoud, E. A., & Holt, R. (1990). Emotional and behavioral predictors of preschool peer ratings. *Child Development, 61,* 1145–1152.

Denmark, F. L. (1999). Enhancing the development of adolescent girls. In N. G. Johnson, M. C. Roberts, & J. Worell (Eds.), *Beyond Appearance: A new look at adolescent girls* (pp. 377–404). Washington, DC: American Psychological Association.

Downey, G., & Coyne, J. C. (1990). Children of depressed parents: An integrative review. *Psychological Bulletin, 108,* 50–76.

Eccles, J. S., Midgley, C., Wigfield, A., Buchanan, C. M., Reuman, D., Flanagan, C., et al. (1993). Development during adolescence: The impact of stage-environment fit on young adolescents' experiences in schools and in families. *American Psychologist, 48,* 90–101.

Ellis, A. (1962). *Reason and emotion in psychotherapy.* New York: Lyle Stuart.

Fergusson, D. M., Horwood, L. J., & Lynskey, M. T. (1995). Maternal depressive symptoms and depressive symptoms in adolescents. *Journal of Child Psychology and Psychiatry, 36,* 1161–1198.

Fergusson, D. M., Horwood, J., Ridder, E. M., & Beautrais, A. L. (2005). Subthreshold depression in adolescence and mental health outcomes in adulthood. *Archives of General Psychiatry, 62,* 66–72.

Fivush, R., & Buckner, J. P. (2000). Gender, sadness, and depression: The development of emotional focus through gendered discourse. In A. H. Fischer (Ed.), *Gender and emotion: Social psychological perspectives* (pp. 232–253). Paris: Cambridge University Press & Editions de la Maison des Sciences de l'Homme.

Fredrickson, B. L., & Roberts, T. (1997). Objectification theory: Toward understanding women's lived experiences and mental health risks. *Psychology of Women Quarterly, 21,* 173–206.

Garber, J. (2006). Depression in children and adolescents: Linking risk research and prevention. *American Journal of Preventive Medicine, 31*(6SI), S104–S125.

Garber, J., Clarke, G. N., Weersing, V. R., Beardslee, W. R., Brent, D. A., Gladstone, T. R. G., et al. (2009). Prevention of depression in at-risk adolescents: A randomized controlled trial. *Journal of the American Medical Association, 301,* 2215–2224.

Garber, J., & Dodge, K. A. (1991). *The development of emotion regulation and dysregulation.* New York: Cambridge University Press.

Garber, J., & Flynn, C. (1998). Origins of depressive cognitive style. In D. K. Routh & R. J. DeRubeis (Eds.), *The science of clinical psychology: Accomplishments and future directions* (pp. 53–93). Washington, DC: American Psychological Association.

Garber, J., Weiss, B., & Shanley, N. (1993). Cognitions, depressive symptoms, and development in adolescents. *Journal of Abnormal Psychology, 102,* 47–57.

Ge, X., Conger, R. D., & Elder, G. H. (2001). Pubertal transition, stressful life events, and the emergence of gender differences in adolescent depressive symptoms. *Developmental Psychology, 37,* 404–417.

Ge, X., Conger, R. D., Lorenz, F. O., Shanahan, M., & Elder, H. (1995). Mutual influences in parent and adolescent psychological distress. *Developmental Psychology, 31,* 406–419.

Gillham, J. E. (2007). Commentary on the prevention of depressive symptoms in children and adolescents: A meta-analytic review. *Evidence-Based Mental Health, 10,* 52.

Gillham, J. E., Brunwasser, S. M., & Freres, D. R. (2008a). Preventing depression early in adolescence: The Penn Resiliency Program. In J. R. Z. Abela & B. L. Hankin (Eds.), *Depression in children and adolescents: Causes, treatment, and prevention* (pp. 309–332). New York: Guilford Press.

Gillham, J. E., Hamilton, J., Freres, D. R., Patton, K., & Gallop, R. (2006a). Preventing depression among early adolescents in the primary care setting: A randomized controlled study of the Penn Resiliency Program. *Journal of Abnormal Child Psychology, 34,* 203–219.

Gillham, J. E., & Reivich, K. J. (1999). Prevention of depressive symptoms in school children: A research update. *Psychological Science, 10,* 461–462.

Gillham, J. E., Reivich, K. J., Freres, D. R., Chaplin, T. M., Shatté, A. J., Samuels, B., et al. (2007). School-based prevention of depressive symptoms: A randomized controlled study of the effectiveness and specificity of the Penn Resiliency Program. *Journal of Consulting and Clinical Psychology, 75,* 9–19.

Gillham, J. E., Reivich, K. J., Freres, D. R., Lascher, M., Litzinger, S., Shatté, A., et al. (2006b). School-based prevention of depression and anxiety symptoms in early adolescence: A pilot of a parent intervention component. *School Psychology Quarterly, 21,* 323–348.

Gillham, J. E., Reivich, K. J., & Jaycox, L. H. (2008a). *The Penn Resiliency Program.* Unpublished manual, University of Pennsylvania, Philadelphia, PA.

Gillham, J. E., Reivich, K. J., Jaycox, L. H., & Seligman, M. E. P. (1995). Preventing depressive symptoms in schoolchildren: Two-year follow-up. *Psychological Science, 6*, 343–351.

Gillham, J. E., Reivich, K. J., & Shatté, A. J. (2001). Building optimism and preventing depressive symptoms in children. In E. C. Chang (Ed.), *Optimism and pessimism* (pp. 301–320). Washington, DC: American Psychological Association.

Gilligan, C. (1982). *In a different voice: Psychological theory and women's development.* Cambridge, MA: Harvard University Press.

Gitelson, I. B., Petersen, A. C., & Tobin-Richards, M. H. (1982). Adolescents' expectancies of success, self-evaluations, and attributions about performance on spatial and verbal tasks. *Sex Roles, 8*, 411–419.

Gladstone, T. R. G., & Kaslow, N. J. (1995). Depression and attributions in children and adolescents: A meta-analytic review. *Journal of Abnormal Child Psychology, 23*, 597–606.

Goodman, S. H., & Gotlib, I. H. (1999). Risk for psychopathology in the children of depressed mothers: A developmental model for understanding mechanisms of transmission. *Psychological Review, 106*, 458–490.

Gotlib, I. H., Lewinsohn, P. M., & Seeley, J. R. (1995). Symptoms versus a diagnosis of depression: Differences in psychosocial functioning. *Journal of Consulting and Clinical Psychology, 63*, 90–100.

Grant, K., Lyons, A., Landis, D., Cho, M., Scudiero, M., Reynolds, L., et al. (1999). Gender, body image, and depressive symptoms among low-income African American adolescents. *Journal of Social Issues, 55*, 299–315.

Gross, J. J., & John, O. P. (2003). Individual differences in two emotion regulation processes: Implications for affect, relationships, and well-being. *Journal of Personality and Social Psychology, 85*, 348–362.

Hammen, C. L. (1991). The generation of stress in the course of unipolar depression. *Journal of Abnormal Psychology, 100*, 555–561.

Hankin, B. L., & Abela, J. R. Z. (2005). Depression from childhood through adolescence and adulthood: A developmental vulnerability and stress perspective. In B. L. Hankin & J. R. Z. Abela (Eds.), *Development of psychopathology: A vulnerability–stress perspective* (pp. 245–288). Thousand Oaks, CA: Sage.

Hankin, B. L., & Abramson, L. Y. (2001). Development of gender differences in depression: An elaborated cognitive vulnerability–transactional stress theory. *Psychological Bulletin, 127*, 773–796.

Hankin, B. L., & Abramson, L. Y. (2002). Measuring cognitive vulnerability to depression in adolescence: Reliability, validity and gender differences. *Journal of Clinical Child and Adolescent Psychology, 31*, 491–504.

Harnett, P. H., & Dadds, M. R. (2004). Training school personnel to implement a universal school-based prevention of depression program under real-world conditions. *Journal of School Psychology, 42*, 343–357.

Hastings, P. D., Zahn-Waxler, C., Robinson, J., Usher, B., & Bridges, D. (2000). The development of concern for others in children with behavior problems. *Developmental Psychology, 36*, 531–546.

Hawkins, J. D., Catalano, R. F., Kosterman, R., Abbott, R., & Hill, K. G. (1999). Preventing adolescent health-risk behavior by strengthening protection during childhood. *Archives of Pediatrics and Adolescent Medicine, 153*, 226–334.

Hill, J. P., & Lynch, M. E. (1983). The intensification of gender-related role expectations during early adolescence. In J. Brooks-Gunn & A. C. Petersen (Eds.), *Girls at puberty: Biological and psychosocial perspectives* (pp. 201–288). New York: Plenum Press.

Hoffman, M. L. (1982). Development of prosocial motivation: Empathy and guilt. In N. Eisenberg (Ed.), *The development of prosocial behavior* (pp. 281–313). New York: Academic Press.

Hollon, S. D., & DeRubeis, R. J. (2004). Effectiveness of treatment for depression. In R. L. Leahy (Ed.), *Contemporary cognitive therapy: Theory, research and practice* (pp. 45–61). New York: Guilford Press.

Hollon, S. D., DeRubeis, R. J., Shelton, R. C., Amsterdam, J. D., Salomon, R. M., O'Reardon, J. P., et al. (2005). Prevention of relapse following cognitive therapy vs. medications in moderate to severe depression. *Archives of General Psychiatry, 62*, 417–422.

Hops, H. (1996). Intergenerational transmission of depressive symptoms: Gender and developmental considerations. In C. Mundt, M. J. Goldstein, K. Hahlweg, & P. Fiedler (Eds.) *Interpersonal factors in the origin and course of affective disorders* (pp. 113–129). London: Gaskell/Royal College of Psychiatrists.

Horowitz, J. L., & Garber, J. (2006). The prevention of depressive symptoms in children and adolescents: A meta-analytic review. *Journal of Consulting and Clinical Psychology, 74*, 401–415.

Horowitz, J. L., Garber, J., Ciesla, J. A., Young, J. F., & Mufson, L. (2007). Prevention of depressive symptoms in adolescents: A randomized trial of cognitive-behavioral and interpersonal prevention programs. *Journal of Consulting and Clinical Psychology, 75*, 693–706.

Izard, C. E. (1972). *Patterns of emotions: A new analysis of anxiety and depression.* New York: Academic Press.

Izard, C. E., & Ackerman, B. P. (2000). Motivational, organizational, and regulatory functions of discrete emotions. In M. Lewis & J. Haviland-Jones (Eds.). *Handbook of emotions* (2nd ed., pp. 253–322). New York: Guilford Press.

Jaycox, L. H., Reivich, K. J., Gillham, J., & Seligman, M. E. P. (1994). Prevention of depressive symptoms in school children. *Behaviour Research and Therapy, 32*(8), 801–816.

Jones, G. (1989). Gender bias in classroom interactions. *Contemporary Education, 60*, 216–222.

Jordan, J. V., Kaplan, A. G., Miller, J. B., Stiver, I. P., & Surrey, J. L. (1991). *Women's growth in connection: Writings from the Stone Center.* New York: Guilford Press.

Joyner, K., & Udry, J. R. (2000). You don't bring me anything but down: Adolescent romance and depression. *Journal of Health and Social Behavior, 41*, 369–391.

Keenan, K., & Hipwell, A. E. (2005). Preadolescent clues to understanding depression in girls. *Clinical Child and Family Psychology Review, 8*, 89–105.

Kendler, K. S., Gardner, C. O., & Prescott, C. A. (2002). Toward a comprehensive developmental model for major depression in women. *American Journal of Psychiatry, 159*, 133–1145.

Kendler, K. S., Gatz, M., Gardner, C. O., & Pederse, N. L. (2006). Personality and major depression. *Archives of General Psychiatry, 63*, 1113–1120.

Kendler, K. S., Kuhn, J. P., & Prescott, C. A. (2004). The interrelationship of neuroticism, sex, and stressful life events in the prediction of episodes of major depression. *American Journal of Psychiatry, 161*, 631–636.

Kochanska, G., DeVet, K., Goldman, M., Murray, K., Putnam, S. P. (1994). Maternal reports of conscience development and temperament in young children. *Child Development, 65*, 852–868.

Krupnick, C. (1985). Women and men in the classroom. *On Teaching and Learning, 12*, 18–25.

La Greca, A. M., & Harrison, H. M. (2005). Adolescent peer relations, friendships, and romantic relationships: Do they predict social anxiety and depression? *Journal of Clinical Child and Adolescent Psychology, 34*, 49–61.

Le, H., Muñoz, R. F., Ippen, C. G., & Stoddard, J. L. (2003). Treatment is not enough: We must prevent major depression in women. *Prevention and Treatment, 6*,.

LeCroy, C. W. (2004). Experimental evaluation of "Go Grrrls" preventive intervention for early adolescent girls. *Journal of Primary Prevention, 25*, 457–473.

LeCroy, C. W., & Daley, J. (2001). *Empowering adolescent girls: Examining the present and building skills for the future with the Go Grrrls Program.* New York: Norton.

Machoian, L. (2005). *The disappearing girl.* New York: Dutton.

Malkin, A. R., Wornian, K., & Chrisler, J. C. (1999). Women and weight: Gendered messages on magazine covers. *Sex Roles, 40*, 647–656.

McCauley, E., Mitchell, J. R., Burke, P., & Moss, S. (1988). Cognitive attributes of depression in children and adolescents. *Journal of Consulting and Clinical Psychology, 56*, 903–908.

McLoyd, V. C. (1998). Socioeconomic disadvantage and child development. *American Psychologist, 53*, 185–204.

Merry, S. N., McDowell, H. H., Hetrick, S. E., Bir, J. J., & Muller, N. (2004). Psychological and/or educational interventions for the prevention of depression in children and adolescents. *The Cochrane Library, 2*.

Monroe, S. M., Rohde, P., Seeley, J. R., & Lewinsohn, P. M. (1999). Life events and depression in adolescence: Relationship loss as a prospective risk factor for first onset of major depressive disorder. *Journal of Abnormal Psychology, 108*, 606–614.

Nolan, S., Flynn, C., & Garber, J. (2003). Prospective relations between rejection and depression in young adolescents. *Journal of Personality and Social Psychology, 85*, 745–755.

Nolen-Hoeksema, S. (1991). Responses to depression and their effects on the duration of depressive episodes. *Journal of Abnormal Psychology, 100*, 569–582.

Nolen-Hoeksema, S. (2001). Gender differences in depression. *Current Directions in Psychological Science, 10*, 173–176.

Nolen-Hoeksema, S., & Girgus, J. S. (1994). The emergence of gender differences in depression during adolescence. *Psychological Bulletin, 115*, 424–443.

Nolen-Hoeksema, S., Girgus, J. S., & Seligman, M. E. P. (1992). Predictors and consequences of childhood depressive symptoms: A five-year longitudinal study. *Journal of Abnormal Psychology, 101,* 405–422.

Nolen-Hoeksema, S., Stice, E., Wade, E., & Bohon, C. (2007). Reciprocal relations between rumination and bulimic, substance abuse, and depressive symptoms in female adolescents. *Journal of Abnormal Psychology, 116,* 198–207.

Office of Applied Studies. (2005). *Results from the 2004 National Survey on Drug Use and Health: National findings* (DHHS Publication No. SMA 05-4062, NSDUH Series H-28). Rockville, MD: Substance Abuse and Mental Health Services Administration.

Parker, S., Nichter, M., Nichter, M., & Vuckovic, N. (1995). Body image and weight concerns among African American and white adolescent females: Differences that make a difference. *Human Organization, 54,* 103–114.

Pattison, C., & Lynd-Stevenson, R. M. (2001). The prevention of depressive symptoms in children: The immediate and long-term outcomes of a school based program. *Behaviour Change, 18,* 92–102.

Petersen, A. C., Leffert, N., Graham, B., Alwin, J., & Ding, S. (1997). Promoting mental health during the transition into adolescence. In J. Schulenberg, J. L. Maggs, & A. K. Hierrelmann (Eds.), *Health risks and developmental transitions during adolescence* (pp. 471–497). New York: Cambridge University Press.

Petersen, A. C., Sarigiani, P. A., & Kennedy, R. E. (1991). Adolescent depression: Why more girls? *Journal of Youth and Adolescence, 20,* 247–271.

Quayle, D., Dziurawiec, S., Roberts, C., Kane, R., & Ebsworthy, G. (2001). The effect of an optimism and lifeskills program on depressive symptoms in preadolescence. *Behaviour Change, 18,* 194–203.

Radke-Yarrow, M., & Klimes-Dougan, B. (2002). Parental depression and offspring disorders: A developmental perspective. In S. H. Goodman & I. H. Gotlib (Eds.), *Children of depressed parents: Mechanisms of risk and implications for treatment* (pp. 155–173). Washington, DC: American Psychological Association.

Radke-Yarrow, M., Nottelmann, E., Belmont, B., & Welsh, J. D. (2003). Affective interactions of depressed and nondepressed mothers with their children. *Journal of Abnormal Child Psychology, 21,* 683–695.

Reivich, K. J. (1996). *The prevention of depressive symptoms in adolescents.* Unpublished doctoral dissertation, University of Pennsylvania, Philadelphia.

Riley, W. T., Treiber, F. A., & Woods, M. G. (1989). Anger and hostility in depression. *Journal of Nervous and Mental Disease, 177,* 668–674.

Rizzo, C. J., Daley, S. E., & Gunderson, B. H. (2006). Interpersonal sensitivity, romantic stress, and the prediction of depression: A study of inner-city minority adolescent girls. *Journal of Youth and Adolescence, 35,* 469–478.

Roberts, C., Kane, R., Bishop, B., Matthews, H., & Thompson, H. (2004). The prevention of depressive symptoms in rural children: A follow-up study. *International Journal of Mental Health Promotion, 6,* 4–16.

Roberts, C., Kane, R., Thomson, H., Bishop, B., & Hart, B. (2003). The prevention of depressive symptoms in rural school children: A randomized controlled trial. *Journal of Consulting and Clinical Psychology, 71,* 622–628.

Rohde, P., Lewinsohn, P. M., Clarke, G. N., Hops, H., & Seeley, J. R. (2005). The Adolescent Coping with Depression Course: A cognitive-behavioral approach to the treatment of adolescent depression. In E. D. Hibbs & P. S. Jensen (Eds.), *Psychosocial treatments for child and adolescent disorders: Empirically based strategies for clinical practice* (2nd ed., pp. 218–237). Washington, DC: American Psychological Association.

Rose, A. J., Carlson, W., & Waller, E. M. (2007). Prospective associations of co-rumination with friendship and emotional adjustment: Considering the socioemotional trade-offs of co-rumination. *Developmental Psychology, 43,* 1019–1031.

Rose, A. J., & Rudolph, K. D. (2006). A review of sex differences in peer relationship processes: Potential trade-offs for the emotional and behavioral development of girls and boys. *Psychological Bulletin, 132,* 98–131.

Rose, A. J., Swenson, L. P, & Waller, E. M. (2004). Overt and relational aggression and perceived popularity: Developmental differences in concurrent and prospective relations. *Developmental Psychology, 40,* 378–387.

Saab, H. (2004). The home. In W. Boyce (Ed.), *Young people in Canada: Their health and well being.* Report of the HBSC study (pp. 17–24). Available at *www.phac-aspc.gc.ca/dca-dea/publications/hbsc-2004/index_e.html.*

Sandler, I. N., Ayers, T. S., Wolchik, S. A., Tein, J., Kwok, O., Haine, R. A., et al. (2003). The family bereavement program: Efficacy evaluation of a theory-based prevention program for parentally bereaved children and adolescents. *Journal of Consulting and Clinical Psychology, 71,* 587–600.

Schwartz, J. A., & Koenig, L. J. (1996). Response styles and negative affect among adolescents. *Cognitive Therapy and Research, 20,* 13–36.

Seligman, M. E. P., Schulman, P., DeRubeis, R. J., & Hollon, S. D. (1999). The prevention of depression and anxiety. *Prevention and Treatment, 2.*

Shapka, J. D., & Keating, D. P. (2005). Structure and change in self-concept during adolescence. *Canadian Journal of Behavioural Science, 37,* 83–96.

Shatté, A. J. (1997). *Prevention of depressive symptoms in adolescents: Issues of dissemination and mechanisms of change.* Unpublished doctoral dissertation, University of Pennsylvania, Philadelphia.

Sheeber, L., Davis, B., & Hops, H. (2002). Gender-specific vulnerability to depression in children of depressed mothers. In S. H. Goodman & I. H. Gotlib (Eds.), *Children of depressed parents: Mechanisms of risk and implications for treatment* (pp. 253–274). Washington, DC: American Psychological Association.

Shochet, I. M., Dadds, M. R., Holland, D., Whitefield, K., Harnett, P. H., & Osgarby, S. M. (2001). The efficacy of a universal school-based program to prevent adolescent depression. *Journal of Clinical Child Psychology, 30,* 303–315.

Simmons, R. G., & Blythe, D. A. (1987*). Moving into adolescence: The impact of pubertal change and school context.* Hawthorne, NY: Aldine de Gruyter.

Smith, L. J. (1994, Spring). A content analysis of gender differences in children's advertising. *Journal of Broadcasting and Electronic Media,* 323–337.

Spence, S. H., Sheffield, J., & Donovan, C. (2002). Problem-solving orientation and attributional style: Moderators of the impact of negative life events on the development of depressive symptoms in adolescence? *Journal of Clinical Child and Adolescent Psychology, 31,* 219–222.

Spence, S. H., & Shortt, A. L. (2007). Research review: Can we justify the widespread dissemination of universal, school-based interventions for the prevention of depression among children and adolescents? *Journal of Child Psychology and Psychiatry, 48,* 526–542.

Stark, K. D., Hoke, J., Ballatore, M., Valdez, C., Scammaca, N., & Griffin, J. (2005). Treatment of child and adolescent depressive disorders. In E. D. Hibbs & P. S. Jensen (Eds.), *Psychosocial treatments for child and adolescent disorders: Empirically based strategies for clinical practice* (2nd ed., pp. 239–265). Washington, DC: American Psychological Association.

Stice, E., & Bearman, S. K. (2001). Body-image and eating disturbances prospectively predict increases in depressive symptoms in adolescent girls: A growth-curve analysis. *Developmental Psychology, 37,* 597–607.

Stice, E., Hayward, C., Cameron, R. P., Killen, J. D., & Taylor, C. B. (2000). Body-image and eating disturbances predict onset of depression among female adolescents: A longitudinal study. *Journal of Abnormal Psychology, 109,* 438–444.

Stice, E., Shaw, H., Bohon, C., Marti, C. N., & Rohde, P. (2009). A meta-analytic review of depression programs for children and adolescents: Factors that predict magnitude of intervention effects. *Journal of Consulting and Clinical Psychology, 77,* 486–503.

Stice, E., Spangler, D., & Agras, W. S. (2001). Exposure to media-portrayed thin-ideal messages adversely affects vulnerable girls: A longitudinal experiment. *Journal of Social & Clinical Psychology, 20,* 270–288.

Stipek, D. J. (1984). Sex differences in children's attributions for success and failure on math and spelling tests. *Sex Roles, 11,* 969–981.

Sutton, J. (2007). Prevention of depression in youth: A qualitative review and future suggestions. *Clinical Psychology Review, 27,* 252–271.

U. S. Department of Health and Human Services. (1999). *Mental health: A report of the Surgeon General.* Rockville, MD: U.S. Department of Health and Human Services, Substance Abuse and Mental Health Services Administration, Center for Mental Health Services, National Institutes of Health, National Institute of Mental Health.

Weissman, M. M., Pilowsky, D. J., Wickramaratne, P. J., Talati, A., Wisniewski, S. R., Fava, M., et al. (2006a). Remissions in maternal depression and child psychopathology: A STAR*D—child report. *Journal of the American Medical Association, 295,* 1389–1398.

Weissman, M. M., Wickramaratne, P. J., Nomura, Y., Warner, V., Pilowsky, D., & Verdeli, H. (2006b). Offspring of depressed parents: 20 years later. *American Journal of Psychiatry, 163,* 1001–1008.

Wilgosh, L. (2002). Examining gender images, expectations, and competence as perceived impediments to personal, academic and career development. *International Journal for the Advancement of Counselling, 24,* 239–260.

Wolchik, S. A., West, S. G., Sandler, I. N., Tein, J., Coatsworth, D., Lengua, L., et al. (2000). An experimental evaluation of theory-based mother and mother–child programs for children of divorce. *Journal of Consulting and Clinical Psychology, 68,* 843–856.

Yap, M. B., Whittle, S., Yucel, M., Sheeber, L., Pantelis, C., Simmons, J. G., et al. (2008). Interaction of parenting experiences and brain structure in the prediction of depressive symptoms in adolescents. *Archives of General Psychiatry, 65,* 1377–1385.

Young, J. F., Mufson, L., & Davies, M. (2006). *Journal of Child Psychology and Psychiatry, 47,* 1254–1262.

Youngren, M. A., & Lewinsohn, P. M. (1980). The functional relation between depression and problematic interpersonal behavior. *Journal of Abnormal Psychology, 89,* 333–341.

Yu, D. L., & Seligman, M. E. P. (2002). Preventing depressive symptoms in Chinese Children. *Prevention and Treatment, 5.*

Zahn-Waxler, C. (2001). The development of empathy, guilt, and internalization of distress: Implications for gender differences in internalizing and externalizing problems. In R. Davidson (Ed.), *Anxiety, depression, and emotion: Wisconsin Symposium on Emotion* (Vol. I). New York: Oxford University Press.

Zahn-Waxler, C., Cole, P. M., & Barrett, K. C. (1991). Guilt and empathy: Sex differences and implications for the development of depression. In J. Garber & K. A. Dodge (Eds.), *The development of emotion regulation and dysregulation* (pp. 243–272). Cambridge, UK: Cambridge University Press.

Zahn-Waxler, C., Cole, P. M., Welsh, J. D., & Fox, N. A. (1995). Psychophysiological correlates of empathy and prosocial behaviors in preschool children with behavior problems. *Development and Psychopathology, 7,* 27–48.

CHAPTER 12

Preventive Intervention in Families of Depressed Parents

A Family Cognitive-Behavioral Intervention

Bruce E. Compas
Gary Keller
Rex Forehand

Parental depression is one of the strongest risk factors for depression and other forms of psychopathology in children (e.g., Goodman, 2007; Goodman & Gotlib, 1999). Compared with children of nondepressed parents, children and adolescents of parents with current or past major depression have problems in multiple areas of functioning, including higher levels of internalizing and externalizing problems, impaired school performance, lower social competence, lower levels of self-esteem, and higher rates of affective and nonaffective psychiatric diagnoses (Goodman & Tully, 2006). Children of depressed parents are also at increased risk for higher levels of medical utilization, suicide attempts, and substance abuse disorders (e.g., Hammen, Burge, Burney, & Adrian, 1990; Kramer et al., 1998; Weissman, Warner, Wickramaratner, Moreau, & Olfson, 1997). Research has focused primarily on depression in mothers, but some effects also have been found for paternal depression (Connell & Goodman, 2002), suggesting that the effects of depression of both mothers and fathers on children's mental health are important to consider. Previous research has been mixed with regard to rates of emotional and behavioral problems in daughters and sons of parents with depression. Some studies suggest that girls are more adversely affected (e.g., Hopps, 1995), others have found evidence of more

problems in boys (e.g., Rhode et al., 2005), and still others have reported
no gender differences (e.g., Ohannessian et al., 2005).

Given the high risk for negative developmental outcomes among offspring of depressed parents, the development and evaluation of preventive
interventions for this population is a high priority (Beardslee & Gladstone,
2001). In this chapter we describe the rationale and evidence for a family-
based cognitive-behavioral preventive intervention for families faced with
the stress of a parent suffering from depression. Following the guidelines
in the report of the Institute of Medicine (Mrazek & Haggerty, 1994) on
the prevention of mental disorders, we first outline some of the risk and
protective factors in children of depressed parents. We then describe the
development of a preventive intervention designed to address these processes in families of parents with a history of, or current, major depressive
disorder (MDD). Next we report on preliminary findings from an open
trial examining the feasibility, acceptability, and initial effects of this intervention. Finally, we describe the results of a randomized clinical trial to test
the efficacy of this intervention compared with a self-study, written information intervention condition and highlight directions for future research.
Throughout this chapter and consistent with the theme of this volume, we
note the role of gender in offspring of depressed parents.

MECHANISMS OF RISK IN OFFSPRING
OF DEPRESSED PARENTS

Although the effects of parental depression on child and adolescent development are well documented, the mechanisms that account for these effects
are less clear. This is due in part to the complex set of biological, psychological, and interpersonal processes involved in conferring risk from depression in a parent to children in these families. Goodman and Gotlib (1999)
have provided a framework to guide research in this area, highlighting four
mechanisms through which risk may be transmitted from depressed parents to their children: (1) heritability of depression; (2) innate dysfunctional
neuroregulatory mechanisms; (3) exposure to negative maternal cognitions,
behaviors, and affect; and (4) the stressful context of the children's lives.
Furthermore, they identify three factors that might moderate this risk,
including a spouse's health and involvement with the child, the course and
timing of a parent's depression, and characteristics of the child.

Our research has been guided by a model that is focused on three
processes: exposure to stressful parent–child interactions that are the result
of the symptoms of parental depression, the ways that children react to
these stressors, and the ways that children cope with these stressful interactions. We have selected these mechanisms because research has shown that

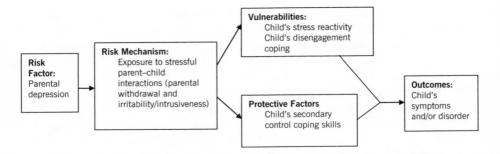

FIGURE 12.1. Heuristic model of effects of parental depression on children.

(1) they are important influences on the emotional and behavioral health of children of depressed parents, (2) they are closely linked to one another, and, most importantly, (3) they are potentially changeable through psychological intervention. Based on these findings and drawing on the framework of Goodman and Gotlib (1999), we have developed a heuristic model focused on these specific risk and protective mechanisms for children of depressed parents (see Figure 12.1).

The occurrence of episodes of MDD in a parent during the life of a child constitutes the primary risk factor, and exposure to stressful parent–child interactions (in the form of parental withdrawal and irritability/intrusiveness) is the primary psychosocial mechanism through which parental depression exerts its effects on children. Parental depression and parent–child stress are further mediated by vulnerabilities (children's stress reactivity and use of disengagement coping) and by protective factors (children's use of secondary control coping skills). We propose that preventive interventions can reduce risk by enhancing the parenting skills of depressed parents, reduce vulnerabilities by teaching children skills to modulate their reactivity to stress, and enhance protective factors by teaching children adaptive coping skills.

Stressful Parent–Child Interactions

A central aspect of the stress of living with a depressed parent is characterized by increased negative and unpredictable parental behaviors (e.g., irritability, inconsistent discipline), decreased supportive parental behaviors (e.g., less warmth, praise, nurturance), and heightened marital conflict (e.g., Cummings, DeArth-Pendley, DuRocher-Schudlich, & Smith, 2001; McKee et al., 2008). The core symptoms of MDD can lead to disruptions in parenting as a result of parental sadness and withdrawal (e.g., social withdrawal, avoidance, unresponsiveness to their children's needs) and parental

intrusiveness and irritability (e.g., irritability toward their children, over-involvement in their children's lives; e.g., Forehand, McCombs, & Brody, 1987; Gelfand & Teti, 1990; Malphurs et al., 1996), and parents' use of guilt induction with these children (Rakow, Forehand, Champion, Fear, & Compas 2009; Rakow et al., in press). Exposure to these types of parental behaviors contributes to a chronically stressful environment for children. For example, Adrian and Hammen (1993) found that children of depressed mothers were exposed to stressful events within their families because of increased interpersonal conflict, and that family stress was an important predictor of both internalizing and externalizing problems in children. Goodman and Brumley (1990), in a home observation study, found that depressed mothers were emotionally unavailable and withdrawn and were less sensitive to child behavior.

It is noteworthy that disrupted parenting has also been documented in parents of children and adolescents who are depressed. For example, research by Cole and colleagues suggests that parents who reward their children at very low rates and who withhold positive reinforcement until very high levels of performance are reached have children who evince a variety of depressive cognitions (Cole & Rehm, 1986). High levels of parent–child conflict, rejection, parental control, and noncontingent responding, coupled with low levels of parent–child cohesion, may contribute to depressive thinking and self-criticism in children (Cole & McPherson, 1993). Pineda, Cole, and Bruce (2007) found that mothers of adolescents with higher levels of depressive symptoms provided less positive reinforcement than mothers of adolescents with low levels of depressive symptoms, and they were less likely to respond to adolescents' displays of sadness with supportive parenting behavior.

Further evidence of the role of stressful parent–child interactions comes from studies using direct observations of parents and children in families of depressed parents. In a meta-analysis of this research, Lovejoy, Graczyk, O'Hare, and Neuman (2000) found significant and moderate effect sizes for the effects of maternal depressive symptoms and disorder on hostile negative parenting (e.g., negative affect, coercive, hostile behavior; mean $d = 0.40$), disengaged (withdrawn) parenting (e.g., neutral affect, ignoring; mean $d = 0.29$), and a small but significant adverse effect on positive parenting behaviors (engaging child in a pleasant or affectionate way; mean $d = 0.16$). These studies reflect the significance of disrupted parenting in families of depressed parents and underscore the usefulness of direct observations of parent–child interactions in these families. The authors conclude that depressed mothers are more likely to become angry when children misbehave or make normal demands on them. Lovejoy et al. argue that the "findings support the need for intervention with depressed mothers, as their parenting behaviors are a component of the risk associated with living with a depressed mother" (p. 588). Negative parenting persists even after controlling for presence of current MDD, suggesting that depressed parents continue to parent poorly after an episode has ended (Seifer, Dickstein, Sameroff, Magee, & Hayden, 2001).

In a series of studies we have examined children's exposure to stressful parent–child interactions in the form of disrupted parenting behaviors in families of depressed parents. First, Jones, Beach, and Forehand (2001) studied the role of maternal depressive symptoms and family relationship stress in a community sample. Mother's initial depressive symptoms generated perceived stress in both marital and mother–adolescent relationships a year later. In turn, mother-reported family relationship stress exacerbated her depressive symptoms. Mother-reported stressful family interactions also contributed to higher levels of depressive symptoms in both adolescent girls and boys. Although no evidence of a stress generation process for fathers was found, father-reported family relationship stress was associated with greater adolescent depressive symptoms.

We have further examined parents' and adolescents' reports of stressful parent–child interactions in a sample of parents with a history of MDD (Jaser et al., 2005, 2007; Langrock, Compas, Keller, Merchant, & Copeland, 2002). Parents with a history of major depression reported on their children's coping and reactivity to parental stressors and anxiety/depression and on their aggressive behavior symptoms; self-reports were obtained from children in these families who were old enough (age 10 years or older) to complete standardized questionnaires. Based on parent reports, Langrock et al. found that children were exposed to moderate levels of stress related to parental withdrawal, intrusiveness, and marital conflict in the previous 6 months. All children were faced with parental withdrawal, and almost all children were exposed to parental intrusiveness in the past 6 months. Comparison exposure to stressors related to withdrawn and intrusive parenting styles revealed that children were equally exposed to both types. The two types of stress also were positively correlated with parents' current depressive symptoms.

Based on parents' and adolescents' reports, Jaser et al. (2005) found that stressors related to parental withdrawal and parental intrusiveness were significantly correlated with adolescents' symptoms of anxiety/depression and aggression. Specifically, parent reports of adolescents' anxiety/depression and aggressive symptoms on the Child Behavior Checklist (CBCL; Achenbach & Rescorla, 2001) were significantly positively correlated with parent reports of their own withdrawn and intrusive parenting behaviors and with adolescents' reports of their parents' intrusiveness. Adolescents' reports of their own anxiety/depression and aggressive symptoms on the Youth Self-Report (YSR; Achenbach & Recorla, 2001) were significantly positively correlated with their reports of their parents' intrusive (but not withdrawn) behaviors. Thus, Jaser et al. (2005) provide support for the association between stressful parent–child interactions and children's internalizing and externalizing symptoms, above and beyond the effects of shared method variance that result in the reliance on single sources of information for both of these constructs.

More recently we have used direct observations in the laboratory of parent–child interactions in families of mothers with and without a history of MDD to further assess the characteristics of stress related to parental depression (Jaser, Reeslund, Champion, Reising, & Compas, 2008). Mothers with a history of depression were significantly more likely to exhibit sad affect and disengaged and antisocial parenting behaviors than mothers with no history of depression across the two interactions, but these differences were largely accounted for by mothers' current depressive symptoms. Mothers' self-reports of their current depressive symptoms were also related to higher levels of observed sadness and antisocial behaviors, and to child and mother reports of maternal intrusive and withdrawn parent behaviors. Mothers' prior histories of depression and their current depressive symptoms were associated with higher levels of parent and self-reported internalizing problems in adolescents. Regression analyses indicated that the relationship between current maternal depressive symptoms and adolescents' internalizing and externalizing problems was mediated by the presence of sadness in mothers' interactions with their children (Jaser er al., 2008).

To summarize, children of depressed parents are faced with the demands of stress related to both parental withdrawal and parental intrusiveness. These two factors of parental withdrawal and intrusiveness are moderately positively correlated, suggesting that children are faced with stress related to *both* types of parental behaviors, rather than either a withdrawn or intrusive parent. Consistent with a model in which stressful parent–child interactions mediate the effects of parental depression, parents' self-reports of depressive symptoms were positively associated with parental withdrawal and intrusiveness. Most importantly, stressful parent–child interactions characterized by parental withdrawal and parental intrusiveness were significantly correlated with higher levels of children's symptoms of anxiety/depression and aggression. It is noteworthy that we have not found evidence in any of these studies for gender differences among children of depressed parents in their exposure to stressful parent–child interactions or in their rates of internalizing or externalizing problems.

Children's Coping and Stress Reactivity

In spite of the evidence implicating stress processes as a risk factor for children in families of depressed parents, relatively little research has examined the ways that children react to and cope with family stress. In the first research on this issue, Radke-Yarrow and colleagues (Radke-Yarrow, 1998; Radke-Yarrow & Brown, 1993) examined the general coping styles of children of depressed parents, and Klimes-Dougan and Bolger (1998) compared the coping styles of children of depressed and well mothers, including social support and distancing coping. These studies are limited, however, in that they did not examine the ways that children cope specifically with stressors associated with parental depression or the relationship of coping with children's internalizing and externalizing problems.

To address this issue, we have examined children's coping and stress responses as possible mediators of the relation between parental withdrawal and intrusiveness and children's symptoms of anxiety/depression and aggressive behavior (Champion et al., 2009; Fear et al., 2009; Jaser et al., 2005, 2007, 2008; Langrock et al., 2002). Across these studies our findings suggest that children's use of secondary control engagement coping (positive thinking, cognitive restructuring, acceptance, distraction; see Compas et al., 2001) is correlated with lower symptoms of anxiety/depression and aggressive behavior problems. Conversely, higher levels of stress reactivity (e.g., emotional arousal, physiological arousal, intrusive thoughts, rumination) are correlated with higher symptoms of anxiety/depression and more aggression. Secondary control coping and involuntary engagement stress responses partially mediate the relation between parent–child interaction stress (parental withdrawal and intrusiveness) and children's anxiety/depression. Furthermore, Jaser et al. (2007) found that adolescents' self-reports of coping with stressful parent–child interactions were significantly correlated with their reports of coping with peer-related stressors, suggesting that adolescents' coping generalizes across contexts. Although this study was cross-sectional, these are the first data that we are aware of that show the potentially important role of children's coping and stress responses in adaptation to family stress related to parental depression.

We examined parents' reports of stressful parent–child interactions, children's coping and stress responses, and children's internalizing and externalizing symptoms in a series of nested path models to test for mediation (Langrock et al., 2002). The full model achieved an excellent fit, and a mediated model (without direct paths from parental withdrawal and intrusiveness to child symptoms) also attained an excellent fit. The model explained 25% of the variance in symptoms of anxiety/depression symptoms and 17% of the variance in aggressive behavior problems. Parental withdrawal predicted less secondary control engagement coping and higher stress reactivity. In turn, stress reactivity predicted more anxiety/depression symptoms and aggressive behavior problems, whereas secondary control engagement coping predicted fewer anxiety/depression symptoms, but did not significantly account for aggressive behavior problems.

As a more stringent test of the associations among stress, coping, and symptoms, we examined cross-informant correlations between parent reports and children's self-reports (Jaser et al., 2005). Cross-informant convergent validity correlations for parents' and children's reports of children's coping and stress responses were all positive and significant (r's ranged from .34 to .52, mean $r = .45$), indicating that parents and children were moderately consistent in their reports of the ways in which children responded to stressful parent–child interactions. Parents' reports of children's secondary control coping and involuntary engagement stress responses were significantly correlated with children's self-reports of anxiety/depression on the YSR ($r = -.26$ and .25, respectively). Similarly, children's self-reports of secondary control coping and involuntary engagement stress responses were significantly correlated with parents' reports of anxiety/depression and aggression on the CBCL ($r = -.36$ and $r = .29$, respectively). These correlations establish important associations between the ways in which children cope with and respond to stressful parent–child interactions and children's symptoms, and these associations are independent of method (informant) effects.

We have also examined children's and adolescents' responses to their mothers' depression, which take the form of caretaking for their mothers (Champion et al., 2009). Specifically, two types of caretaking behaviors were examined: emotional caretaking (e.g., caring for a mother's emotional distress) and instrumental caretaking (e.g., looking after younger siblings). We found support for an independent effects model in which maternal depression history, intrusive parenting, and both instrumental and emotional caretaking were found to function as separate risk factors for symptoms of anxiety/depression in adolescents of parents with a history of depression. The two types of caretaking behavior were significantly correlated and, when entered in a regression model together, instrumental and emotional caretaking accounted for shared variance in adolescents' symptoms of anxiety/depression.

Finally, we have examined adolescents' coping with an additional source of stress that is associated with parental depression, interparental conflict, in families containing a parent with current or past MDD (Fear et al., 2009). Higher levels of interparental conflict were associated with more anxiety/depression and aggressive symptoms, greater perceived coping inefficacy, and greater use of primary control coping and disengagement coping by children (as reported by the parent). Furthermore, higher levels of interparental conflict, more perceived self-blame, and greater use of disengagement coping were all associated with more symptoms of both anxiety/depression and aggression. In contrast, greater use of primary control and secondary control coping were associated with fewer anxious/depressed and aggressive symptoms, suggesting that these forms of coping may be protective factors for children in this sample who were coping with interparental conflict. Children's attributions of self-blame were also significantly negatively correlated with their use of secondary control coping responses. Consistent across all regression models tested and regardless of informant of coping (parent vs. child), children's perceptions of self-blame and use of secondary control coping were significant, independent predictors of both anxious/depressed and aggressive symptoms in children.

Taken together, these findings indicate that coping is a mediator of the relation between stressful parent–child interactions and child symptoms. That is, increased levels of stress are related to decreased use of adaptive coping, in this case, secondary control coping. This pattern is consistent with previous research showing that as stressor load increases, complex cognitive functions, including those that comprise secondary control coping, are impaired (e.g., Matthews & Wells, 1996). Those children who most need to mobilize secondary control coping (i.e., those under the highest level of stress) are least able to generate these responses. Similar to our studies of stressful parent–child interactions, we did not find gender differences in coping or stress reactivity in any of these studies.

DEVELOPMENT OF A FAMILY COGNITIVE-BEHAVIORAL INTERVENTION FOR CHILDREN OF DEPRESSED PARENTS

Guided by these findings of risk and protective processes in children of depressed parents, we have developed a preventive intervention designed to (1) reduce stressful parent–child interactions that are associated with parental withdrawal and irritability/intrusiveness, (2) reduce children's reactivity to these stressors, and (3) enhance children's and parents' use of secondary control engagement coping strategies to reduce the risk for symptoms and disorder in these children (Compas, Langrock, Keller, Merchant, & Copeland, 2002). The intervention includes several basic skills, including secondary control engagement coping (acceptance, cognitive restructuring, distraction through pleasant activities) and parenting skills (parental involvement, warmth, and family structure). Pilot research has been conducted to establish the feasibility of recruitment of families and delivery of the intervention, acceptability of the intervention to participants, and initial effects on child and parent functioning.

The family cognitive-behavioral intervention is a manualized 12-session program (eight weekly and four monthly follow-up sessions) that is designed to teach coping skills to families with a parent who has a history of a mood disorder (MDD, dysthymia, or depression NOS) in a small family group format. Each family group includes four families and is co-led by a mental health professional with a master's degree or extensive training in group facilitation and a doctoral student in clinical psychology. All group leaders receive intensive training in the implementation of the intervention protocol.

The program is designed for participation by both parents and children. Goals are to educate families about depressive disorders, increase family awareness of the impact of stress and depression on functioning, help families recognize and monitor stress, facilitate the development of adaptive coping responses to stress, and improve parenting skills. Information is presented to group members during sessions, practice and discussion of skills are facilitated during the sessions, and all members are given weekly home practice exercises. Four monthly follow-up booster sessions are included to provide additional practice and support in continued development and refinement of the skills learned in the initial eight sessions.

The intervention is designed to address the hypothesized mediators of the effects of parental depression on children: parental depressive symptoms and negative affect, stressful parent–child interactions, and children's coping with and reactivity to these stressors. The intervention sessions include separate modules targeting parenting skills and children's coping skills. Specifically, the parenting component of the intervention includes building skills to increase parental warmth and involvement with their children, as well as increasing structure and consequences for positive and problem behavior. Children are taught skills to cope with their parents' depression, including the use of acceptance, distraction, and cognitive reappraisal. The core coping skills are summarized for families with the acronym ADAPT: Acceptance, Distraction, Activities, and Positive Thinking.

During the first three sessions parents and children participate in the same in-session activities; during sessions 4 through 7 children and adolescents meet in separate groups for the majority of the session to practice the skills that have been introduced as adaptive for coping with their parents' depression. Parents also meet as a group during these sessions to learn parenting skills. During session 8, parents and children meet together for a review of materials covered in prior sessions and a discussion of challenges they are likely to face in the future. Follow-up sessions (9–12) include components for the families to work together and breakout sessions for the children and the parents separately.

The design of this intervention is based on research of empirically supported cognitive-behavioral interventions for depression designed for children, adolescents, and adults (e.g., Clarke et al., 1995, 2001; Garber, Clarke, Weersing, Beardslee, Brent, Gladstone, et al., 2009; Lewinsohn, Clarke, Hops, & Andrews, 1990). Many of these interventions are "full package" approaches that include elements of behavioral activation, self-monitoring, and cognitive restructuring approaches. In our focus on working with the whole family and providing education about depression and its effects on families, we draw on the pioneering work of Beardslee and colleagues (Beardslee et al., 1992, 1997). Beardslee's work has highlighted the importance of destigmatizing depression and facilitating open communication within families about the disorder.

The coping skills that are taught and practiced as part of the program are designed to enhance the development of secondary control coping strategies (cognitive restructuring, acceptance, distraction) in participants. Our research, summarized above, has shown that these strategies are effective in coping with stressful parent–child interactions associated with parental depression (e.g., Jaser et al., 2005; Langrock et al., 2002). One goal of the intervention is to increase these skills in the children and adolescents coping with depression in their family. Parents are taught to support their children's use of these skills, and they also are encouraged to practice these skills themselves.

The parenting modules of this intervention are drawn from well-established, empirically supported programs for parenting training designed to address issues of oppositional behavior in children and adolescents (e.g., Forehand & McMahon, 1981; McMahon & Forehand, 2003), and are similar to modules used in parenting interventions for the treatment of childhood anxiety (e.g., Barrett, Dadds, & Rapee, 1996; Dadds, Spencer, Holland, Barrett, & Laurens, 1997: Dadds et al., 1999). The parenting sessions focus on the teaching of basic parenting skills, with an emphasis on areas that are likely to be impacted by depression such as consistency, structure, parental responsiveness, parent–child communication, and involvement in family activities.

Throughout the intervention, in addition to teaching separate skills to the parents and children, there is a focus on the family as a whole. This approach is intended to reduce guilt and to help family members begin to problem solve together, including breaking the "stigma of silence" (Focht & Beardslee, 1996) of discussing a parent's depression within the family. Individual, family, and group exercises and discussions are included to facilitate individual skill acquisition. Socratic questioning and role-playing during the sessions and homework assignments are employed to build skills and to help family members address the specific stresses they experience. The multifamily group format with families that share a common experience with depression is intended to reduce isolation, provide alternatives to one's own family interactions, and provide group support and encouragement. We now describe the content and format of the sessions in more detail.

Sessions 1–3

The initial session is designed to provide participants with an opportunity to become acquainted, provide an overview of the intervention program, and to educate participants about the nature of depression and the effects of parental depression on children. The concept of parent–child stress is introduced, and family members begin the process of identifying sources and effects of stress in their family. These goals are achieved both through the presentation of didactic information and in-session exercises.

The second and third sessions provide an introduction to the concepts of stress and coping. Parents and children identify ongoing sources of stress in their families and the ways that they typically try to cope with these stressors. These sessions also draw on extensive research on the effective treatment of depression and are focused on increasing children's involvement in pleasant activities, both as a method of increasing positive mood and as a means of achieving relief and distraction from stress within the family. Parents and children read through a list of pleasant activities and discuss the kinds they have done together in the past and which ones they would like to increase in the near future. Children also generate pleasant activities in which they can be involved outside the family (e.g., school, sports, clubs, peers).

Sessions 4–7

As noted, the fourth through the seventh sessions are characterized by separate breakout meetings for parents and for children. The goal of this portion of the intervention is to teach, and provide the opportunity for practicing, the skills that children need to cope with their parents' depression and the skills that parents need to learn to be more effective despite their depression.

Children's Coping Skills

Session 4 begins a series of sessions focused on teaching secondary control coping skills to children and adolescents. First, the skill of acceptance is taught. The discussion centers on the issue of control, and the idea of accepting the things we cannot control. A major goal of this session is to help children understand that their parents' depression is not something they can control and that they are not responsible for making their parents better. Next, the importance of practices and participating in fun activities is presented (session 5). Subsequently, skills in positive (but realistic) thinking and cognitive restructuring (session 6) are taught. This session begins to challenge and change negative ways of thinking by allowing parents and children to discuss the pros and cons of negative thinking versus more opti-mistic thinking. Participants discuss stressful scenarios and begin to find alternative, positive ways to think about such events. Finally, in session 7 children are taught to use distraction as a coping skill.

Parenting Skills

Parents focus on engaging in positive time with their children, praising appropriate behavior, and ignoring minor inappropriate behavior in ses-sions 4 and 5. Skills are presented, role playing occurs, homework assigned, and, at the end of the sessions, parents practice the skills with their chil-dren. In session 6, parents learn to set up rules and behavior charts, as well as use positive consequences for following rules and accomplishing behaviors which are being charted. Session 7 involves parents learning to monitor their children (i.e., knowing where they are, who they are with, when they will be home, and what they are doing) and utilizing conse-quences for inappropriate behaviors. As in sessions 4 and 5, sessions 6 and 7 involve presentation of skills, role playing, homework, and practice the new parenting skills.

Session 8

The final session includes a review of the material covered in the previous session, discussion of the importance of providing and receiving social sup-port from within and outside the family, and a discussion of challenges and stresses that families are likely to face the in the future. This gives families the opportunity to mentally prepare for future stressors by generating ideas for how to cope with them.

Booster Sessions (9–12)

Four monthly booster sessions are included to enhance the learning of cop-ing and parenting skills that are taught in the initial eight sessions. Booster sessions include reviews of children's coping skills and parenting skills that were introduced in sessions 1 through 8, and problem-solving regarding any difficulties that families have had in implementing the skills. A major focus is on the continued development of positive parenting skills, as these skills require repeated practice.

Homework

Sessions 1–7 include substantial homework assignments for both parents and children/adolescents. Because prior research has established that the amount and quality of homework completed are associated with better outcomes in cognitive-behavioral interventions (e.g., Weisz, Jensen-Doss, & Jawley, 2006), all homework assignments are turned into the group leaders after each session, copied, and returned to the families the following session. Trained raters evaluate the quantity and quality of homework for each participant per session. Homework assignments increase self-observation of each subject area to be covered in the next class, thereby encouraging participants to relate their own experience to the material to be taught. The assignments also reinforce practicing new skills.

INITIAL EVALUATION OF INTERVENTION

As a first step in examining this program, we conducted an open-trial pilot study to establish the feasibility, acceptability, and initial effects of an earlier version of this family intervention.

Feasibility

We recruited and enrolled 34 families to participate in 10 small-group interventions (a mean of 3.4 families per group intervention). All 34 depressed parents from these families participated in the intervention, along with 18 spouses, and 42 children (23 girls and 19 boys; 28 preadolescent and 14 adolescent children). Diagnostic interviews were conducted with the depressed parent to establish a diagnosis of MDD or dysthymia, according to DSM-IV criteria. All parents had at least one episode of depression during the lifetime of their child, and half the sample met criteria for a current depressive episode at the time of assessment. Families were recruited from several sources, including newspaper advertisements, posters and brochures placed in medical offices, referrals from mental health professionals providing treatment for adult depression, and managed care agency enrollment mailings.

Acceptability

We examined the acceptability of the intervention program to the participants in two ways. First, we monitored the attendance of parents and children at the sessions as a rough index of their commitment to the program. Out of the eight sessions in each intervention, the depressed parents attended a mean of 5.1 sessions, and children attended a mean of 5.6 sessions. Second, parents' and children/adolescents' level of satisfaction with the program was assessed at the end of each intervention session. Participants rated their overall satisfaction with the sessions and their level of comfort participating in the program, as well as rating their satisfaction with specific components of the program. In general, the ratings indicate that the participants were moderately to highly satisfied with the quality of the program and felt comfortable participating in the sessions. One exception was participants' relatively lower rating of satisfaction with learning relaxation skills, a component that was subsequently dropped from the 12-session intervention program we previously described.

Initial Effects

Pre- and postintervention data were collected on a number of relevant variables for families who participated in the intervention, including children's internalizing and externalizing problems, parents' depressive symptoms, parenting skills, and children's coping responses. The initial findings were encouraging as significant decreases occurred from pre- to postintervention for measures in all three of the following areas: child outcome; the hypothesized mediators of change (child coping and parenting); and parent depressive symptoms. The findings suggested the intervention is capable of producing the intended effects.

RANDOMIZED CONTROLLED TRIAL

The initial evaluation laid the foundation for a randomized clinical trial to examine the efficacy of the intervention as compared with a control condition and to examine mechanisms that account for changes in rates of symptoms and disorder in children of depressed parents. We conducted a two-site evaluation in which we randomly assigned 111 families with 155 9–15-year-old children (70 girls and 85 boys) to the intervention or a comparison condition. All parents had current and/or past MDD during the lifetime of their child(ren) as determined by a structured clinical interview. Among the constructs assessed were children's rates of MDD, depressive symptoms, anxiety/depression, internalizing problems, and externalizing problems; children's secondary control coping skills (acceptance, positive thinking, cognitive restructuring, distraction); positive and negative parenting; and parental depressive symptoms. Most constructs were assessed from the perspective of both the parent and child, with parenting being a noteworthy exception as it was assessed by behavioral observations of parent–child interactions. Assessments were conducted at baseline, postintervention and 6-, 12-, 18-, and 24-month follow-ups.

The 12 session intervention (eight weekly sessions and four monthly sessions) was described earlier. The comparison group was a self-study written information condition modeled after Wolchik et al.'s (2000) preventive intervention trial for families coping with parental divorce. Families were mailed written materials to provide education about the nature of depression, the effects of parental depression on families, and the signs of depression in children. Separate materials were developed for parents and children. Materials for children were based on age, with children 9–11 years of age receiving materials written at a lower reading level than for adolescents 12–15 years of age. Following the method used by Wolchik and colleagues, materials were sent in three sets over an 8-week interval to correspond with the first eight sessions in the group intervention. Families were provided with a schedule for reading these materials.

Our findings provide support for the effectiveness of the intervention. In an initial study examining data to the 12-month follow-up, Compas, Forehand, Keller, Champion, Rakow, Reeslund, et al. (2009) found that, relative to the comparison condition, the family cognitive-behavioral preventive intervention was associated with lower levels of child and parent report of child internalizing and, to a lesser extent, externalizing problem measures after intervention. The strongest support emerged at the 12-month follow-up. Although not directly addressed in the intervention program, parent depressive symptoms also decreased following intervention.

In a subsequent study, Compas, Forehand, Champion, Keller, Hardcastle, Cole, et al. (2011) examined follow-up data from 18 and 24 months. Relative to children in the comparison condition, those in the family cognitive-behavioral preventive intervention condition were significantly lower in self-reports of anxiety/depression symptoms and internalizing symptoms at 18 months and significantly lower in externalizing symptoms at 18 and 24 months. Relative to the comparison condition, rates of MDD were significantly lower in children in the intervention over the 24-month follow-up and the effect for any nonaffective diagnosis approached significance. No significant effects were found for parents' symptoms of depression or episodes of MDD. The findings provide some evidence for the long-term effectiveness of the intervention program for children living in families with a parent with a history of depression.

Compas, Champion, Forehand, Cole, Reeslund, Fear, et al. (2010) examined the roles of child coping and parenting skills as mediators of children's outcomes at the 12-month follow-up. Significant differences favoring the family intervention compared with the written information comparison condition were found for changes in composite measures of parent–adolescent reports of adolescents' use of secondary control coping skills and direct observations of parents' positive parenting skills. Changes in adolescents' secondary control coping and positive parenting mediated the effects of the intervention on depressive, internalizing, and externalizing symptoms, accounting for approximately half of the effect of the intervention on the outcome. These findings indicate that both child coping and parenting skills are important components of the intervention.

Finally, we have begun preliminary analyses examining moderators of the outcome of the intervention program. Of particular relevance to this volume, these analyses have not revealed that gender of child moderates treatment outcome for three outcome measures (child depressive symptoms, anxiety/depression, internalizing problems) we have examined thus far in moderational analyses. Although preliminary, these findings suggest our family cognitive-behavioral preventive intervention is effective with both boys and girls.

SUMMARY

Parental depression represents a significant source of risk for child mental health problems, and this risk is conveyed through multiple pathways. We have emphasized two important risk processes: stressful parent–child interactions triggered by parental withdrawal and irritability/intrusiveness and children's stress reactivity. Further, we have demonstrated that children's use of secondary control coping and parents' parenting skills can be protective mechanisms to reduce the risk associated with parental depression. The absence of gender differences in our analyses of stressful parent–child interactions, children's coping, and the effects of our intervention are noteworthy. Although statistical power may have been somewhat limited, our failure to identify gender differences is consistent with some previous studies (e.g., Ohannessian et al., 2005). It is possible that depression in parents contributes to a sufficiently stressful and problematic family environment to exert an equally adverse effect on girls and boys in these families. Further, the development of coping skills of girls and boys may be similarly compromised by parents who model poor emotion regulation and coping skills. Therefore, we would tentatively conclude that preventive interventions for children of parents with depression should include both daughters and sons in these families.

ACKNOWLEDGMENTS

Preparation of this chapter was supported by Grant Nos. R01MH069940 and R01MH69928 from the National Institute of Mental Health.

REFERENCES

Achenbach, T. M., & Rescorla, L. A. (2001). *Manual for ASEBA school-age forms and profiles*. Burlington, VT: University of Vermont, Research Center for Children, Youth, and Families.

Adrian, C., & Hammen, C. (1993). Stress exposure and stress generation in children of depressed mothers. *Journal of Consulting and Clinical Psychology*, *61*, 354–359.

Barrett, P. M., Dadds, M. R., & Rapee, R. M. (1996). Family treatment of childhood anxiety: A controlled trial. *Journal of Consulting and Clinical Psychology*, *64*, 333–342.

Beardslee, W. R., & Gladstone, T. T. G. (2001). Prevention of childhood depression: Recent findings and future prospects. *Biological Psychiatry*, *49*, 1101–1110.

Beardslee, W. R., Hoke, L., Wheelock, I., Rothberg, P. C. et al. (1992). Initial findings on preventive intervention for families with parental affective disorders. *American Journal of Psychiatry*, *149*, 1335–1340.

Beardslee, W. R., Salt, P., Versage, E. M., Gladstone, T. R. G. et al. (1997). Sustained change in parents receiving preventive interventions for families with depression. *American Journal of Psychiatry*, *154*, 510–515.

Beardslee, W. R., Wright, E., Rothberg, P. C., Salt, P. et al. (1996). Response of families to two preventive intervention strategies: Long-term differences in behavior and attitude change. *Journal of the American Academy of Child and Adolescent Psychiatry*, *35*, 774–782.

Beck, A. T., Steer, R. A., Ball, R., & Ranieri, W. F. (1996). Comparison of Beck Depression Inventories IA and –II in psychiatric outpatients. *Journal of Personality Assessment*, *67*, 588–597.

Champion, J. E., Jaser, S. S., Reeslund, K. L., Simmons, L., Potts, J. E., Shears, A. R., et al. (2009). Caretaking behaviors by adolescent children of mothers with and without a history of depression. *Journal of Family Psychology*, *23*, 156–166.

Clarke, G. N., Hawkins, W., Murphy, M., & Sheeber, L. (1993). School-based primary prevention of depressive symptomatology in adolescents: Findings from two studies. *Journal of Adolescent Research*, *8*, 183–204.

Clarke, G. N., Hawkins, W., Lewinsohm, P. M., Murphy, M., & Sheeber, L. et al. (1995). Targeted prevention of unipolar depressive disorder in an at-risk sample of high school adolescents: A randomized trial of group cognitive intervention. *Journal of the American Academy of Child and Adolescent Psychiatry*, *34*, 312–321.

Clarke, G. N., Hornbrook, M., Lynch, F., Polen, M., Gale, J., Beardslee, W., et al. (2001). A randomized trial of a group cognitive intervention for preventing depression in adolescent offspring of depressed parents. *Archives of General Psychiatry*, *58*, 1127–1134.

Cole, D. A., & McPherson, A. (1993). Relation of family subsystems to adolescent depression: Implementing a new family assessment strategy. *Journal of Family Psychology*, *7*, 119–133.

Cole, D. A., & Rehm, L. P. (1986). Family interaction patterns and childhood depression. *Journal of Abnormal Child Psychology*, *14*, 297–314.

Compas, B. E., Champion, J. E., Forehand, R., Cole, D. A., Reeslund, K. L., Fear, J., et al. (2010). Mediators of 12-month outcomes of a family group cognitive-behavioral preventive intervention with families of depressed parents. *Journal of Consulting and Clinical Psychology*, *78*, 623–634.

Compas, B. E., Connor-Smith, J. K., Saltzman, H., Thomsen, A. H., & Wadsworth, M. (2001). Coping with stress during childhood and adolescence: Progress, problems, and potential. *Psychological Bulletin, 127,* 87–127.

Compas, B. E., Forehand, R., Keller, G., Champion, J. E., Rakow, A., Reeslund, K. L., et al. (2009). Randomized controlled trial of a family cognitive-behavioral preventive intervention for children of depressed parents. *Journal of Consulting and Clinical Psychology, 77,* 1007–1020.

Compas, B. E., Forehand, R., Champion, J. E., Keller, G., Hardcastle, E. J., Cole, D. A., et al. (2011). *Family group cognitive-behavioral preventive intervention for families of depressed parents: 18– and 24–month outcomes.* Manuscript submitted for publication.

Compas, B. E., Langrock, A. M., Keller, G., Merchant, M-J., & Copeland, M-E. (2002). Children coping with parental depression: Processes of adaptation to family stress. In S. H. Goodman & I. H. Gotlib (Eds.), *Children of depressed parents: Mechanisms of risk and implications for treatment.* Pp. Washington, DC: American Psychological Association.

Connell, A. M., & Goodman, S. H. (2002). The association between psychopathology in fathers versus mothers and children's internalizing and externalizing behavior problems: a meta-analysis. *Psychological Bulletin, 128,* 746–773.

Connor-Smith, J. K., Compas, B. E., Wadsworth, M. E., Thomsen, A. H., & Saltzman, H. (2000). Responses to stress in adolescence: Measurement of coping and involuntary responses to stress. *Journal of Consulting and Clinical Psychology, 68,* 976–992.

Cummings, M. E., & Davies, P. T. (1994). Maternal depression and child development. *Journal of Child Psychology and Psychiatry and Allied Disciplines, 35,* 73–112.

Cummings, M. E., DeArth-Pendley, G., Du-Rocher-Schudlich, T., & Smith, D. A. (2001). Parental depression and family functioning: Toward a process-oriented model of children's adjustment. In S. R. H. Beach (Ed.), *Marital and family processes in depression: A scientific foundation for clinical practice.* Washington, DC: American Psychological Association.

Dadds, M. R., Holland, D. E., Laurens, K. R., Mullins, M., Barrett, P. M., & Spence, S. (1999). Early intervention and prevention of anxiety disorders in children: Results at 2–year follow-up. *Journal of Consulting and Clinical Psychology, 67,* 145–150.

Dadds, M. R., Spence, S. H., Holland, D., Barrett, P. H., & Laurens, K. (1997). Early intervention and prevention of anxiety disorders: A controlled trial. *Journal of Consulting and Clinical Psychology, 65,* 627–635.

Fear, J., Forehand, R., Colletti, C., Roberts, L., Champion, J., Reeslund, K., & Compas, B. E. (2009). Parental depression and interparental conflict: Adolescents' self-blame and coping responses. *Journal of Family Psychology, 23,* 762–766.

Forehand, R., & McMahon, R. J. (1981). *Helping the noncompliant child.* New York: Guilford Press.

Forehand, R., McCombs, A., & Brody, G. (1987). The relationship of parental depressive mood states to child functioning: An analysis by type of sample and area of child functioning. *Advances in Behaviour Research and Therapy, 9,* 1–20.

Garber, J., Clarke, G. N, Weersing, V. R., Beardslee, W. R., Brent, D. A., Gladstone, T., et al. (2009). Prevention of depression in at-risk adolescents: A randomized controlled trial. *Journal of the American Medical Association, 301*, 2215–2224.

Gelfand, D. M., & Teti, D. M. (1990). The effects of maternal depression on children. *Clinical Psychology Review, 10*, 329–353.

Gladstone, T. R. G., & Beardslee, W. R. (2002). Treatment, intervention, and prevention with children of depressed parents: A developmental perspective. In S. H. Goodman & I. H. Gotlib (Eds.), *Children of depressed parents: Mechanisms of risk and implications for treatment*. Washington, DC: American Psychological Association.

Goodman, S. H. (2007). Depression in mothers. *Annual Review of Clinical Psychology, 3*, 107–135.

Goodman, S. H., & Brumley, H. E. (1990). Schizophrenic and depressed mothers: Relational deficits in parenting. *Developmental Psychology, 26*, 31–39.

Goodman, S. H., & Gotlib, I. H. (1999). Risk for psychopathology in the children of depressed mothers: A developmental model for understanding mechanisms of transmission. *Psychological Review, 106*, 458–490.

Goodman, S. H., & Gotlib, I. H. (2002). *Children of depressed parents: Mechanisms of risk and implications for treatment*. Washington, DC: American Psychological Association.

Goodman S. H., & Tully E. C. (2006). Depression in women who are mothers: an integrative model of risk for the development of psychopathology in their sons and daughters. In *Women and depression: A handbook for the social, behavioral, and biomedical sciences* (pp. 241–282). New York: Cambridge University Press.

Hammen, C., Burge, D., Burney, E., & Adrian, C. (1990). Longitudinal study of diagnoses in children of women with unipolar and bipolar affective disorder. *Archives of General Psychiatry, 47*, 1112–1117.

Jaser, S. S., Champion, J. E., Reeslund, K. L., Keller, G., Merchant, M. J., Benson, M., et al. (2007). Cross-situational coping with peer and family stressors in adolescent offspring of depressed parents. *Journal of Adolescence, 30*, 917–932.

Jaser, S. S., Fear, J. M., Reeslund, K. L., Champion, J. E. Reising, M. M., & Compas, B. E. (2008). Maternal sadness and adolescents' responses to stress in offspring of mothers with and without a history of depression. *Journal of Clinical Child and Adolescent Psychology, 37*, 736–746.

Jaser, S. S., Langrock, A. M., Keller, G., Merchant, M. J., Benson, M. A., Reeslund, K. L., et al. (2005). Coping with the stress of parental depression II: Adolescent and parent reports of coping and adjustment. *Journal of Clinical Child and Adolescent Psychology, 34*, 193–205.

Jaser, S. S., Reeslund, K. L., Champion, J. E., Reising, M. M., & Compas, B. E. (2008). *Parent behavior in mothers with and without a history of depression: Association with adolescent internalizing and externalizing symptoms*. Manuscript submitted for publication.

Jones, D. J., Beach, S. R. H., & Forehand, R. (2001). Stress generation in intact community families: Depressive symptoms, perceived family relationship stress, and implications for adolescent adjustment. *Journal of Social and Personal Relationships, 18*, 443–462.

Klimes-Dougan, B., & Bolger, A. K. (1998). Coping with maternal depressed affect and depression: Adolescent children of depressed and well mothers. *Journal of Youth and Adolescence, 27*, 1–15.

Kramer, R. A., Warner, V., Olfson, M., Ebanks, C. M., Chaput, F., & Weissman, M. M. (1998). General medical problems among the offspring of depressed parents: A 10-year follow-up. *Journal of the American Academy of Child and Adolescent Psychiatry, 37*, 602–611.

Kumpfer, K. L., & Alvarado, R. (2003). Family-strengthening approaches for the prevention of youth problem behaviors. *American Psychologist, 58*, 457–465.

Langrock, A. M., Compas, B. E., Keller, G., Merchant, M. J., & Copeland, M. E. (2002). Coping with the stress of parental depression: Parents' reports of children's coping, emotional, and behavioral problems. *Journal of Clinical Child and Adolescent Psychology, 31*, 312–324.

Lewinsohn, P. M., Clarke, G. N., Hops, H., & Andrews, J. A. (1990). Cognitive-behavioral treatment for depressed adolescents. *Behavior Therapy, 21*, 385–401.

Lovejoy, M. C., Graczyk, P. A., O'Hare, E., & Neuman, G. (2000). Maternal Depression and parenting behavior: A meta-analytic Review. *Clinical Psychology Review, 20*, 561–592.

Malphurs, J. E., Field, T. M., Larraine, C., Pickens, J., Pelaez-Nogueras, M., et al. (1996). Altering withdrawn and intrusive interaction behaviors of depressed mothers. *Infant Mental Health Journal 17*, 152–160.

Matthews, G., & Wells, A. (1996). Attentional processes, dysfunctional coping, and clinical intervention. In M. Zeidner & N. S. Endler (Eds.), *Handbook of coping: Theory, research, and applications* (pp. 573–601). New York: Wiley.

McKee, L., Forehand, R., Rakow, A., Reeslund, K., Roland, E., Hardcastle, E., & Compas, B. E. (2008). Parenting specificity: An examination of the relation between three parenting behaviors and child problem behaviors in the context of a history of caregiver depression. *Behavior Modification, 32*, 638–658.

McMahon, R. J., & Forehand, R. (2003). *Helping the noncompliant child: Family based treatment for oppositional behavior* (2nd ed.). New York: Guilford Press.

Mrazek, P. J., & Haggerty, R. J. (Eds.). (1994). *Reducing risks for mental disorders: Frontiers for preventive intervention research.* Washington, DC: National Academy Press.

Nelson, D. R., Hammen, C., Brennen, P. A., & Ullman, J. B. (2003). The impact of maternal depression on adolescent adjustment: The role of expressed emotion. *Journal of Consulting and Clinical Psychology, 71*, 935–944.

Pineda, A. Q., Cole, D. A., & Bruce, A. E. (2007). Mother–adolescent interactions and adolescent depressive symptoms: A sequential analysis. *Journal of Social and Personal Relationships, 24*, 5–19.

Radke-Yarrow, M. (1998). *Children of depressed mothers: From early childhood to maturity.* New York: Cambridge University Press.

Radke-Yarrow, M., & Brown, E. (1993). Resilience and vulnerability in children of multiple-risk families. *Development and Psychopathology, 5,* 581–592.

Rakow, A., Forehand, R., McKee, L., Champion, J., Fear, J., & Compas, B. E. (2009). The relation of parental guilt induction to child internalizing problems when a caregiver has a history of depression. *Journal of Child and Family Studies, 18,* 367–377.

Rakow, A., Forehand, R., McKee, L., Roberts, L., Haker, K., Champion, J., et al. (in press). Parent guilt induction and child internalizing problems when a caregiver has a history of depression. *Journal of Family Psychology.*

Seifer, R., Dickstein, S., Sameroff, A. J., Magee, K. D., & Hayden, L. C. (2001). Infant mental health and variability of parental depression symptoms. *Journal of the American Academy of Child and Adolescent Psychiatry, 40,* 1375–1382.

Wadsworth, M. E., & Compas, B. E. (2002). Coping with family conflict and economic strain: The adolescent perspective. *Journal of Research on Adolescence, 12,* 243–274.

Warner, V., Weissman, M. M., Fendrich, M., Wickramaratne, P., et al. (1992). The course of major depression in the offspring of depressed parents: Incidence, recurrence, and recovery. *Archives of General Psychiatry 49,* 795–801.

Weissman, M. M., Warner, V., Wickramaratne, P., Moreau, D., & Olfson, M. (1997). Offspring of depressed parents: 10 years later. *Archives of General Psychiatry, 54,* 932–940.

Weisz, J. R., Jensen-Doss, A., & Hawley, K. M. (2006). Evidence-based youth psychotherapies versus usual clinical care. *American Psychologist, 61,* 671–689.

Wolchik, S. A., West, S. G., Sandler, I. N., Tein, J. -Y., Coatsworth, D., Lengua, L., et al. (2000). An experimental evaluation of theory-based mother and mother–child programs for children of divorce. *Journal of Consulting and Clinical Psychology, 68,* 843–856.

Index